1986

# Pediatric Esophageal Surgery

# The Principles and Practice of the Pediatric Surgical Specialties

*Series Editor*

*Stephen L. Gans, M.D.*
*Clinical Professor of Surgery*
*School of Medicine*
*University of California, Los Angeles*
*Attending in Surgery*
*Children's Hospital of Los Angeles*
*and Cedars-Sinai Medical Center*
*Los Angeles, California*

*This is the third book in the series*

# Pediatric Esophageal Surgery

*Edited by*

## Keith W. Ashcraft, M.D.
Clinical Professor of Surgery
University of Missouri at Kansas City
Chief of Urology
The Children's Mercy Hospital
Kansas City, Missouri

## Thomas M. Holder, M.D.
Clinical Professor of Surgery
University of Missouri at Kansas City
Chief of Cardio-Thoracic Surgery
The Children's Mercy Hospital
Kansas City, Missouri


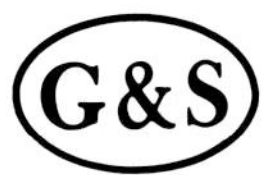

Grune & Stratton, Inc.
Harcourt Brace Jovanovich, Publishers
Orlando   New York   San Diego   Boston   London
San Francisco   Tokyo   Sydney   Toronto

**Library of Congress Cataloging-in-Publication Data**
Main entry under title:

Pediatric esophageal surgery.

(The Principles and practice of the pediatric
surgical specialties)
Includes bibliographies and index.
1. Esophagus—Surgery.  2. Children—Surgery.
I. Ashcraft, Keith W., 1935-      . II. Holder,
Thomas M., 1926-      . III. Series. [DNLM: Esophageal
Diseases—in infancy & childhood.  2. Esophagus—
surgery. WI 250 P371]
RD539.5.P43  1986    617'.548    85-27333
ISBN 0-8089-1776-5



**Grune & Stratton, Inc.**
**Orlando, FL 32887**

Distributed in the United Kingdom by
Grune & Stratton, Ltd.
24/28 Oval Road, London NW 1

Library of Congress Catalog Number 85-27333
International Standard Book Number 0-8089-1776-5

Printed in the United States of America
86 87 88 89 10 9 8 7 6 5 4 3 2 1

# Contents

# Contributors

**Raymond A. Amoury, M.D.,** *Katharine Berry Richardson Professor of Pediatric Surgery; Surgeon-in-Chief, The Children's Mercy Hospital, Kansas City Missouri*

**Keith W. Ashcraft, M.D.,** *Clinical Professor of Surgery, University of Missouri at Kansas City; Chief of Urology, The Children's Mercy Hospital, Kansas City, Missouri*

**Alfred A. deLorimier, M.D.,** *Professor, Department of Surgery, Division of Pediatric Surgery, University of California School of Medicine, San Francisco, California*

**Eric W. Fonkalsrud, M.D.,** *Professor and Chief of Pediatric Surgery, Department of Surgery, UCLA School of Medicine, Los Angeles, California*

**Jay L. Grosfeld, M. D.,** *Lafayette F. Page Professor; Chairman, Department of Surgery, Indiana University School of Medicine; Section of Pediatric Surgery, Department of Surgery, James Whitcomb Riley Hospital for Children, Indianapolis, Indiana*

**Michael R. Harrison, M.D.,** *Associate Professor, Department of Surgery, Division of Pediatric Surgery, University of California School of Medicine, San Francisco, California*

**John J. Herbst, M.D.,** *Professor and Chairman, Department of Pediatrics, Louisiana State University School of Medicine, Shreveport, Louisiana*

**Thomas M. Holder, M.D.,** *Clinical Professor of Surgery, University of Missouri at Kansas City; Chief of Cardio-Thoracic Surgery, The Children's Mercy Hospital, Kansas City, Missouri*

**Dale G. Johnson, M.D.,** *Chief of Surgery, Primary Children's Hospital, Salt Lake City, Utah*

**Lucian L. Leape, M.D.,** *Professor of Surgery, Tufts University School of Medicine; Chief of Pediatric Surgery, New England Medical Center, Boston, Massachusetts*

**Max L. Ramenofsky, M.D.,** *Professor of Surgery and Pediatrics, University of South Alabama Medical Center, Mobile, Alabama*

**L.R. Scherer, M.D.,** *Senior Resident, Department of Surgery, Indiana University Medical Center, Indianapolis, Indiana*

**Ronald J. Sharp, M.D.,** *Assistant Professor of Surgery, University of Missouri at Kansas City; Director of Burn Unit and Attending Surgeon, The Children's Mercy Hospital, Kansas City, Missouri*

# Preface

Probably no other lesion epitomizes the raison d'etre of pediatric surgery as does esophageal atresia and tracheo-esophageal fistula malformations. The solution to this difficult problem was born out of general and thoracic surgery almost coincidental with the birth of pediatric surgery as a specialty. Among the milestones in the treatment of this disease were the near simultaneous successful repair of esophageal atresia and distal tracheo-esophageal fistula in 1939 by Drs. Ladd in Boston, and Leven in Minneapolis, and the pioneering effort of Cameron Haight, a thoracic surgeon in Ann Arbor, who performed the first successful primary repair in 1941. In the intervening forty-four years practitioners of the specialty of pediatric surgery have been primarily responsible for the care and treatment of children born with these unfortunate malformations. The mortality has dropped from 100 percent for esophageal atresia to near zero if the esophageal lesion is unassociated with other major congenital defects.

Similar dramatic histories are not to be found for the other lesions described in this volume but then none were associated with universal mortality before successful treatment was devised. Nonetheless, most disorders of the esophagus interfere with the ingestion of food and drink and thus their correction is dramatic to the patient and his family. We bring together in this volume the surgical treatment of lesions of the esophagus in children. We hope that the reader will find a concise, up to date, readable work which will help improve the quality of life for these young patients.

*Keith W. Ashcraft*

# Pediatric Esophageal Surgery

Raymond A. Amoury

# 1

# Structure and Function of the Esophagus in Infancy and Early Childhood

The esophagus is a dynamic muscular tube designed primarily as a conduit of orally ingested material from the mouth to the stomach. Aboral organized peristalsis and regurgitation are complex processes which begin in utero and continue throughout life. The importance of the esophagus to nutrition is critical and its evolution in support of this function is most marked from early gestation throughout early childhood. This chapter will outline the development, basic structure, anatomical relationships, and function of the esophagus. Some aspects are highlighted as they are peculiar to the pediatric esophagus.

## DEVELOPMENTAL ANATOMY

The esophagus is derived from the foregut, as are the trachea, lungs, and stomach.[6] The esophagus and the developing trachea and bronchi separate from their common foregut anlage within the splanchnic mesoderm. This results in the partitioning of the common, single foregut tube into two separate tubes (Fig. 1-1). The trachea goes on to develop its cartilaginous supporting rings and lung buds. The esophagus becomes identifiable as a short tube between the pharynx and the stomach by the fourth week of gestation (Fig. 1-2). By the fifth week, the lung buds are present and distinct, as is the future stomach (Fig. 1-2). The esophagus continues to elongate with the linear growth of the embryo; its most rapid lengthening occurs in connection with the descent of the stomach.[2]

The esophageal mucous membrane is derived from the endoderm of the foregut. It consists of a stratified squamous epithelium beneath which is the lamina propria. Outside of the lamina propria is the muscularis mucosae. Primary longitudinal mucosal folds appear in the third month of gestation. Superficial esophageal glands appear at the 78-mm stage of the embryo (fourth month) and deep glands at the 240-mm stage.

Pediatric Esophageal Surgery
ISBN 0-8089-1776-5

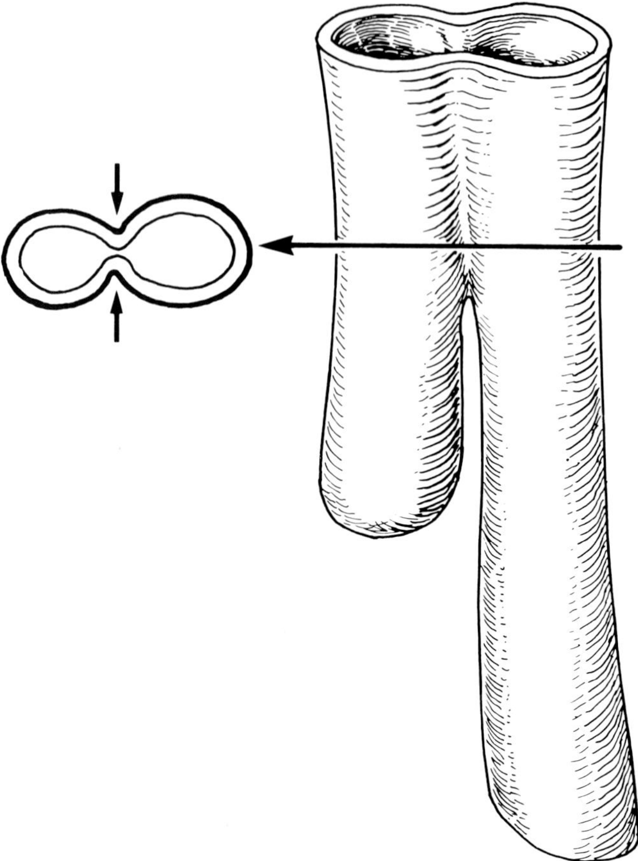

**Figure 1-1.** Division of the primitive foregut. The longer, tubular structure represents the future esophagus. Arrows show the local morphogenic movements which will result in partitioning of the foregut into the tracheobronchial tree and esophagus. Modified from: Gray SW, Skandalakis JE: Embryology for Surgeons. Philadelphia: W.B. Saunders Company, p. 64, 1972. With permission.

The endodermal tube first becomes invested with an inner layer of circular smooth muscle at about the 10-mm stage, followed by an outer, longitudinal layer in embryos of 17-mm length[2]. There is no serosal investment, but, rather, an outermost adventitial coat made of up fibrous tissue.

The esophagus is relatively longer in the newborn infant than in the adult.[2] Esophageal lengths have been determined for different age groups (Table 1-1).

## STRUCTURE

The layered structure of the esophagus is well defined and its components can be appreciated histologically. (Fig. 1-3).[1,2]

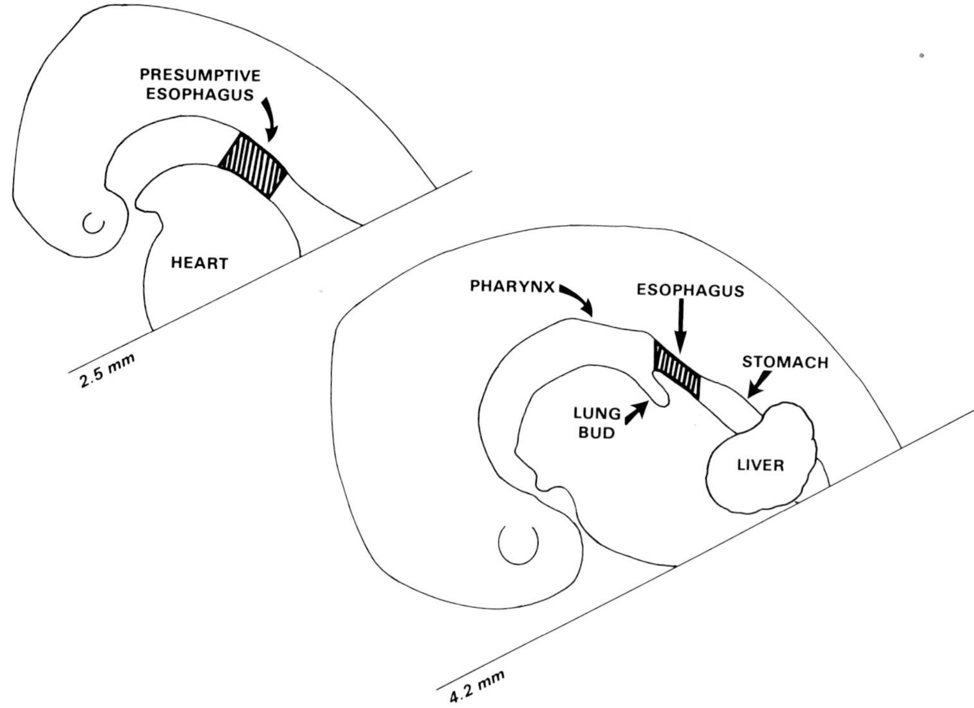


**Figure 1-2.** The esophagus elongates by cranial growth of the body of the embryo. At 2.5 mm (fourth week) the presumptive zone of the esophagus is shown. At 4.2 mm (fifth week) the lung bud has formed with partitioning of the foregut into its respiratory and esophageal components. Modified from: Gray SW, Skandalakis JE: Embryology for Surgeons. Philadelphia: W.B. Saunders Company, p. 64, 1972. With permission.

**Table 1-1**

*Length of Esophagus[10]*

| | Age | | | | | | |
|---|---|---|---|---|---|---|---|
| | 9 days | 14 months | 21 months | 3 years | 5 years | 9 years | 14 years |
| Centimeters from level of incisor teeth to: | | | | | | | |
| Lower border of cricoid | 7 | 10 | 10 | 10 | 10 | 11 | 11 |
| Bifurcation | 12 | 14 | 15 | 15 | 17 | 19 | 19 |
| Cardia | 17 | 22 | 23 | 23 | 26 | 28 | 31 |
| Total Length of Esophagus | 10 | 12 | 13 | 14 | 16 | 16 | 20 |

[10] Modified from: Lerche W: Surgery of the esophagus. Surg Gynecol Obstet 11:345–361, 1910

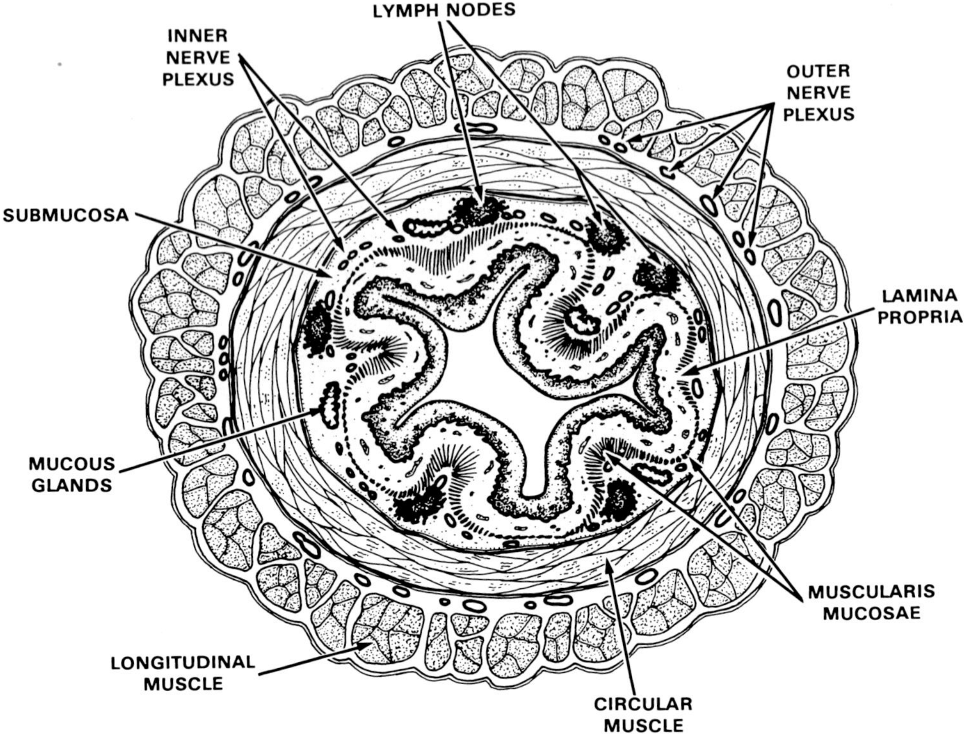


**Figure 1-3.** A cross-section of the esophagus is shown as a histologic study showing layers and mural components. Lymphoid nodules are prominent in the pediatric esophagus.

## Mucosa (Epithelium, Lamina Propria, Muscularis Mucosae)

The mucosa is thick and grayish in color. Its stratified squamous epithelium is arranged in the deep longitudinal folds noted before, which allow for distention and which give the lumen a stellate appearance in cross-section when empty. Beneath the mucosa is the lamina propria, which has many papillary projections and is limited externally by the muscularis mucosae. This is a comparatively thick layer composed of smooth muscle fibers arranged longitudinally. It contains the superficial or esophageal cardiac glands that resemble the fundic glands of the stomach.

## Submucosa

The submucosa is a wide, loose fibrous layer connecting the mucosa with its muscularis. It contains many vessels and nerves and mucous glands. The submucosal mucous glands are tubulo-alveolar in type. In addition to these structures, there are scattered lymphatic nodules which are often around the ducts of the mucous glands.

## Muscularis

The muscularis is a wide tunic with two distinct layers of approximately equal thickness. The fibers of the inner layer are arranged in circular fashion and are continuous with the inferior constrictor of the pharnyx cranially, and with the oblique fibers of the stomach caudally. The fibers of the outer layers are longitudinal and form a continuous layer that passes caudally into the muscular coat of the stomach.

The cranial one-third of the esophagus is distinct in that it is invested exclusively with striated muscle, as is the musculature of the pharynx. Caudal to this, there is a zone of intermingled smooth and striated muscle fibers. The caudal one-third of the esophagus has only smooth muscle fibers.

## Adventitia

The adventitia (tunica adventitia, fibrosa) is a relatively thin, loose layer of fibrous tissue external to the muscularis. It has no external covering layer of mesothelial cells like the serosa of the intestine, and it does not repair rapidly when breached, as occurs in perforation of the esophagus. This relative inability to seal off the esophagus—with its secretions, contents, and bacteria—makes this an especially dangerous viscus in which to sustain a perforating injury.

## ANATOMICAL RELATIONSHIPS

The esophagus consists of three parts: cervical, thoracic, and abdominal. It is narrowest at its commencement opposite the cricoid cartilage. This is the highest of its three levels of constriction and is at the apex of its cervical portion.[14,15]

## Cervical Portion

The cervical portion of the esophagus begins at its cranial attachments (Fig. 1-4). Here, its longitudinal muscle fibers arise as a short tendon from the dorsal aspect of the cricoid cartilage. This tendon, or ligament, then gives rise to two muscle bands which diverge and pass caudally around the sides of the esophagus to meet in the dorsal midline. The diverging bands leave a V-shaped area of the dorsal wall of the esophagus in which the circular muscle layer is exposed. The circular fibers of the esophagus are overlapped by, and intermingled with, the caudal fibers of the inferior constrictor of the pharynx (Fig. 1-4).

The cervical esophagus lies within the visceral fascia of the prevertebral fascia, which covers the prevertebral muscles (Fig. 1-5). Ventral to the esophagus, and separated from it only by areolar tissue, lies the trachea. The esophagus has a curvature to the left in the inferior part of the neck and protrudes here beyond the left margin of the trachea. This allows for an easier surgical approach from the left than from the right when an operation on the esophagus is required at this level. The recurrent laryngeal nerves pass cranially in the groove between the trachea and esophagus. They are in fairly intimate contact with the esophagus. Lateral to the esophagus lie the lateral lobes of the thyroid gland. These may actually cause dysphagia when sufficiently

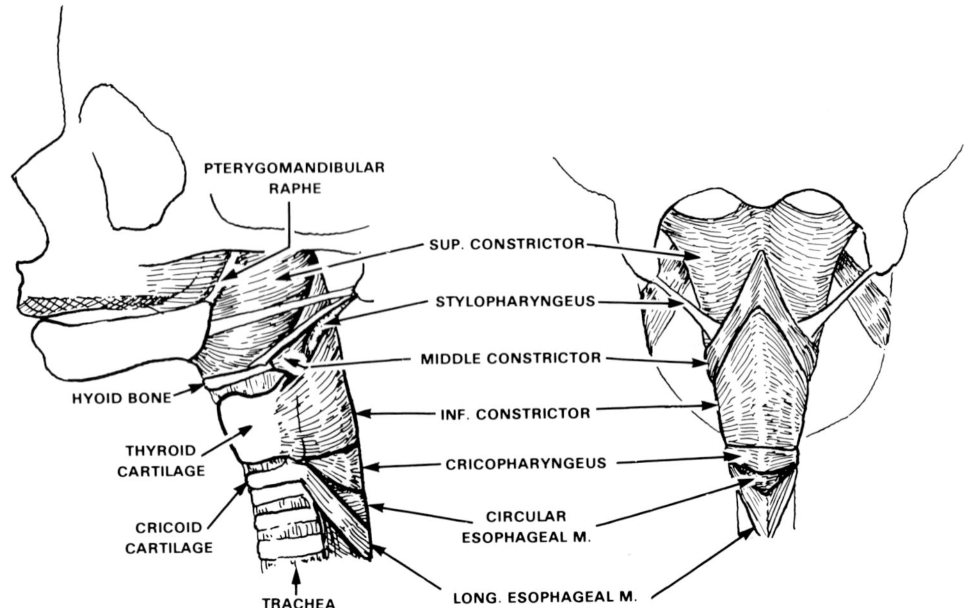



**Figure 1-4.** The pharyngeal constrictors, cricopharyngeus, and the musculature of the proximal esophagus are shown in lateral and posterior views. Note that the fibers of the cricopharyngeus blend with the lower fibers of the inferior constrictor above, while its lower fibers blend with the circular fibers of the esophagus. Modified from: Payne WS, Olsen AM, (Eds): The Esophagus. Philadelphia: Lea & Febiger, p. 8, 1974. With permission.

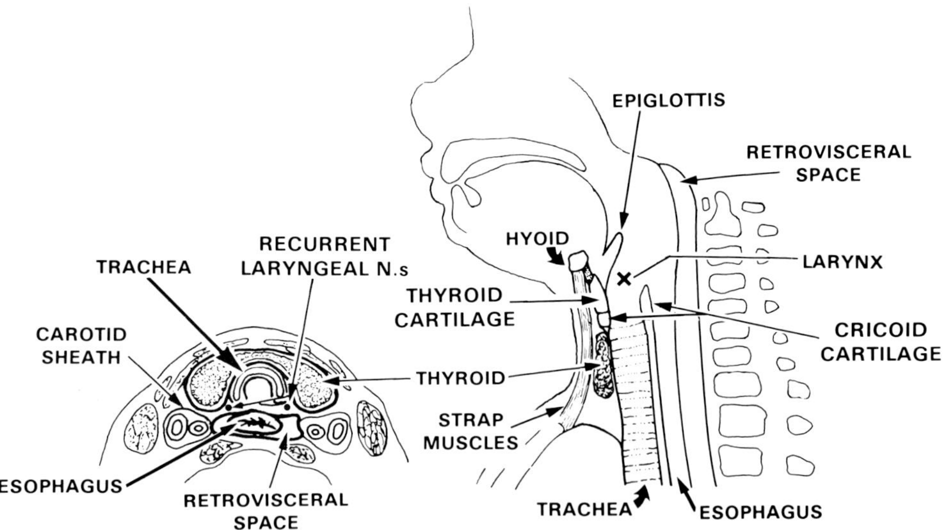



**Figure 1-5.** A sagittal section shows the relationships of the pharynx, larynx, and cervical esophagus. Note that the retrovisceral and the pretracheal spaces extend from the neck into the mediastinum. The insert shows a cross-section of the neck indicating major fascial planes and spaces. The retrovisceral space is usually involved in infections resulting from perforations of the cervical esophagus. The pretracheal space is affected by perforation injury of the pyriform fossa and anterior esophagus. Infection in either space in the neck may remain localized or may readily spread downwards into the mediastinum. Modified from: Payne WS, Olsen AM (Eds.): The Esophagus. Philadelphia: Lea & Febiger, p. 7, 1974. With permission.

6

enlarged, by encroaching on, or displacing, the esophagus. The carotid sheaths with their common carotid arteries, internal jugular veins, and vagus nerves are still more lateral to the cervical esophagus than are the lateral lobes of the thyroid (Fig. 1-5).

## Thoracic Portion

During its course through the thorax, the esophagus lies in the posterior medias-tinum and enters into important relations with the pleura and lungs, aorta, azygos vein, thoracic duct, trachea and bronchi, pericardium and heart, and vagus nerves (Figs. 1-6, 1-7, and 1-8). Continuity with the cervical esophagus is again noted (Fig. 1-7). The left pleura is closely related to the esophagus in the superior mediastinum. (Fig. 1-7). Although it basically lies against the vertebral column in its thoracic course, the esophagus is commonly separated from the vertebrae by pleural extensions into which the medial portions of the lungs glide during inspiration (Fig. 1-7). The mediastinal pleural membranes of the two sides often approach each other dorsal to the esophagus, so that only a thin layer of connective tissue remains between them. This arrangement approaches that of a mesentery of the esophagus (Fig. 1-7). The right pleura is in

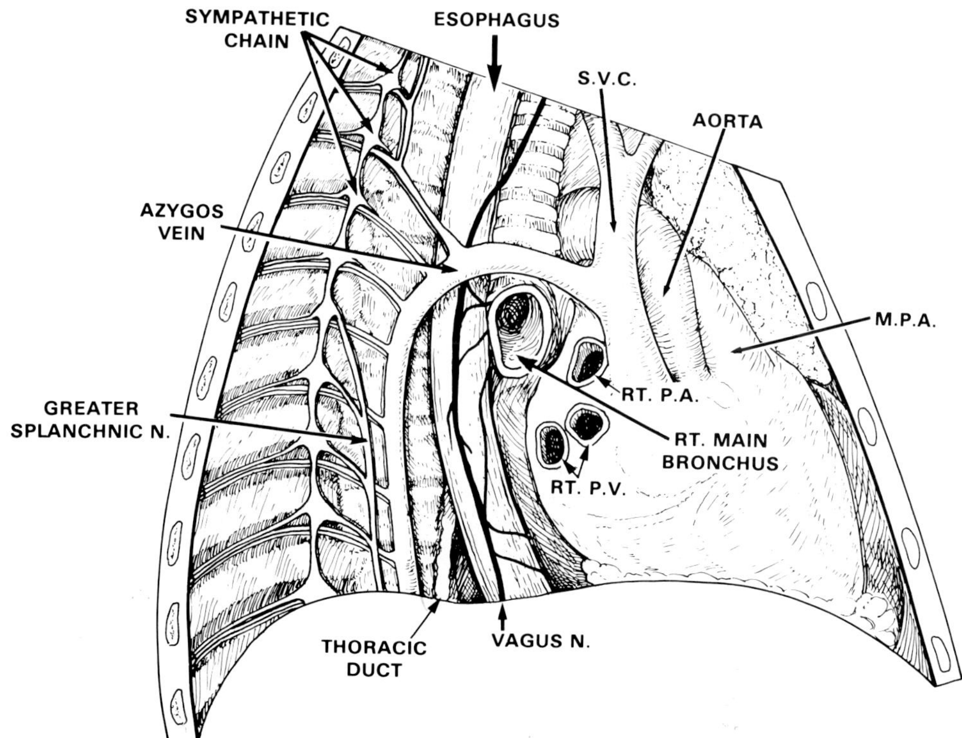


**Figure 1-6.**   Relationships of the thoracic esophagus and mediastinal structures (as viewed from the right side) are shown. The right lung is not shown in order to better demonstrate the azygos system, aorta, thoracic duct, heart, and pulmonary hilar structures. RT.P.A. = right pulmonary artery; RT.P.V. = right pulmonary veins; S.V.C. = superior vena cava. Modified from: Payne WS, Olsen AM, (Eds.): The Esophagus. Philadelphia: Lea & Febiger, p. 5, 1974. With permission.

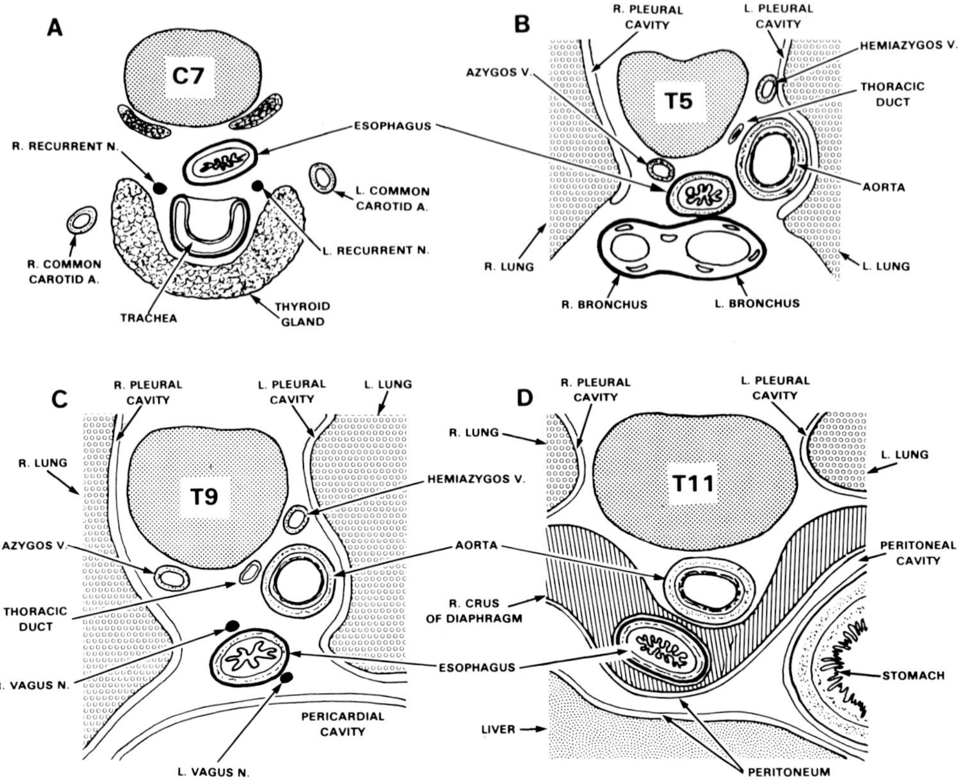



**Figure 1-7.** Cross-sections of the neck and thorax show relationships of the esophagus to adjacent structures at different levels. The cervical level is shown again for orientation. Modified from: Schaeffer JP (Ed.): Morris' Human Anatomy. (11th ed.) New York: The Blakiston Company, p. 1339, 1953. With permission.

particularly intimate contact with the esophagus, covering its right as well as its dorsal aspects as far distally as the level of the tenth thoracic vertebral body (Fig. 1-7).

As the arch of the aorta passes dorsally and to the left, it approaches the vertebral column and indents the esophagus from the left, producing the second of the three physiologic narrowings of the viscus (Fig. 1-8). In its further course, the descending aorta lies dorsally and to the left of the esophagus. Finally, as the esophagus turns toward the left to pass through its diaphragmatic hiatus to the stomach, the descending aorta comes to lie dorsally and to its right (Fig. 1-9). The trachea continues its ventral course from the inferior neck, remaining somewhat to the right of the esophagus as it passes through the superior mediastinum to its bifurcation. The left main bronchus then crosses over the ventral surface of the esophagus to reach the left lung. It may produce an additional impression on the lumen of the esophagus at this level (Figs. 1-8 and 1-9).

Three additional and clinically signficant causes of esophageal displacement at this level are: foregut-derived cysts, e.g., bronchogenic cysts and esophageal duplication cysts, and enlarged mediastinal lymph nodes. Any of these lesions can cause esophageal compression, and/or respiratory obstruction. Another rare anatomical

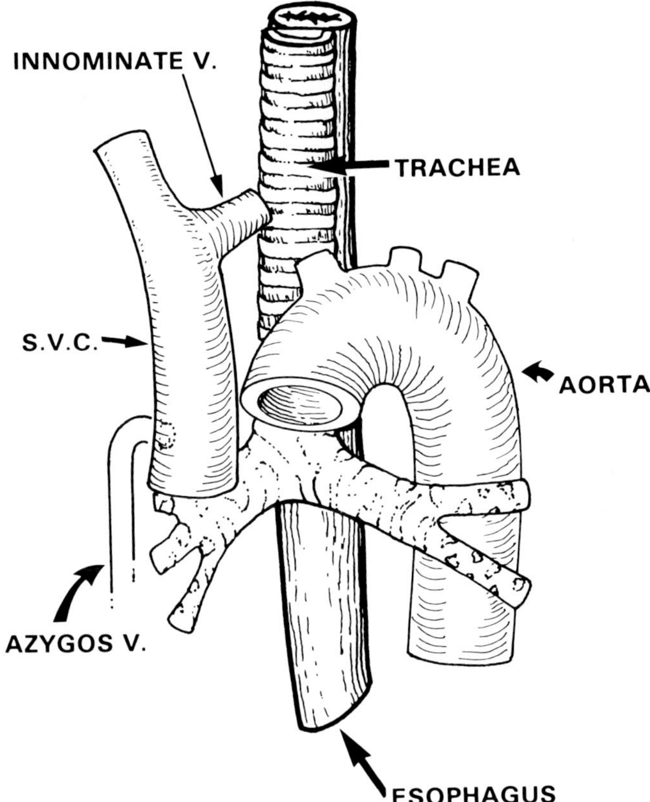



**Figure 1-8.** Regional anatomy of the esophagus at its middle third is shown. Note the relationships of esophagus to the aorta, tracheal bifurcation, left main stem bronchus, innominate vein, superior vena cava, and azygos vein. Modified from: Payne WS, Olsen AM (Eds.): The Esophagus. Philadelphia: Lea & Febiger, p. 4, 1974. With permission.

cause of esophageal and bronchial compression at the level of the carina is the pulmonary vascular sling. In this anomaly, the left pulmonary artery originates from the right pulmonary artery at its junction with the main pulmonary artery and passes to the left hilum between the trachea and esophagus.

Caudal to the carina, the pericardium lies ventral to the esophagus. The left atrium is in contact with the wall of the esophagus, separated from it only by the pericardium. Left atrial enlargement as in mitral stenosis and/or insufficiency may indent or displace the esophagus. In some cases, the displacement is severe enough to cause difficulty swallowing or dysphagia.

In its further course through the posterior mediastinum, the esophagus is surrounded by the esophageal plexus formed largely by the vagus nerves. As they emerge from the caudal part of the plexus as distinct nerves, the left vagus lies ventral and the right vagus lies dorsal to the esophagus. Further detailed description of esophageal innervation is given below.

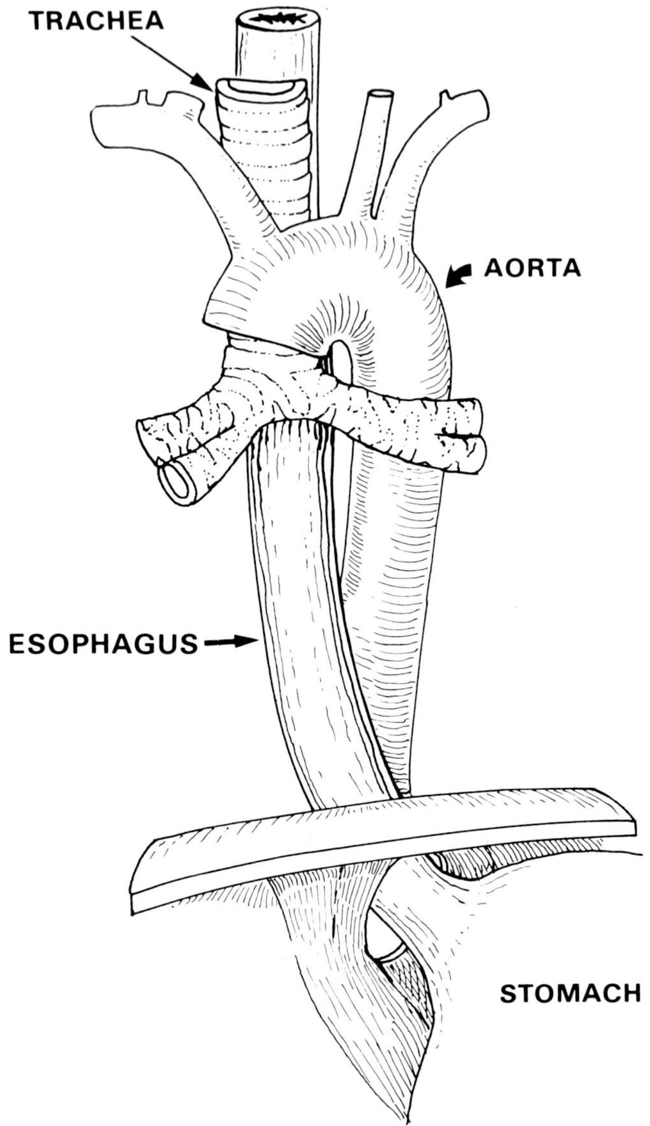



**Figure 1-9.** The relationship of the thoracic and abdominal esophagus is shown with adjacent structures. The arch of the aorta is a site of physiologic narrowing of the esophagus, as is the diaphragmatic hiatus. The hiatus is shown with the esophagus passing through it to its junction with the stomach. Modified from: Ellis FH Jr: In Sabiston DC Jr (Ed.): Davis-Christopher Textbook of Surgery (11th ed.). Philadelphia: W.B. Saunders Company, p. 792, 1977. With permission.

All of these relations are of great clinical interest, since esophageal ulcerations and/or strictures due to caustic ingestion, as well as acid-peptic or alkaline injuries due to gastroesophageal reflux, may occur with involvement of structures adjacent to the esophagus. Iatrogenic perforations from dilatation of esophageal strictures may occur at the three sites of physiologic narrowing, although perforation is more common in the two sites in the thorax than it is in the neck.

## Abdominal Portion

The terminal or abdominal portion of the esophagus lies below the diaphragm at about the level of the xyphoid process, just to the left of the midline. As it passes through the esophageal hiatus of the diaphragm, the esophagus is bounded dorsally by the decussating fibers of the crura of the diaphragm. Ventrally, it is bounded by the liver, which indents the esophagus. Medially, it is bounded by the caudate lobe of the liver (Fig. 1-7).

The diaphragmatic hiatus is a somewhat complex arrangement of slings or loops of crural musculature through which pass the esophagus and aorta (Fig. 1-10). The

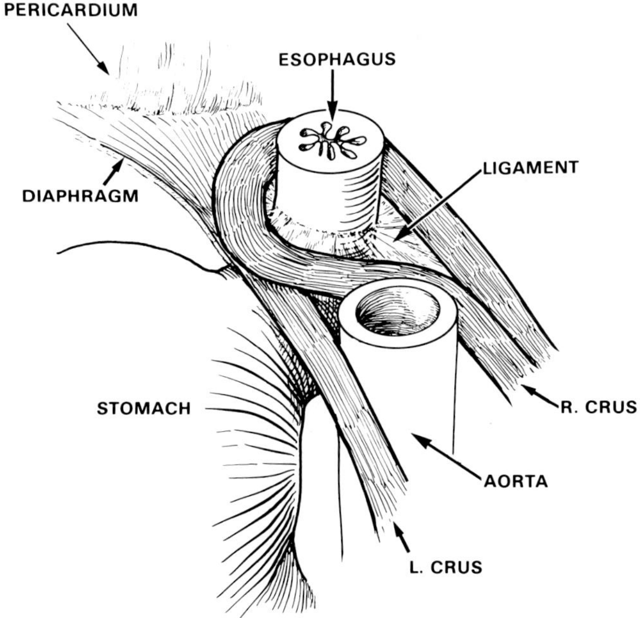


**Figure 1-10.**   The crura of the diaphragm are shown with the most common anatomic variation having both components arising from the right crus. The next most common variation has components from each bundle of crural musculature. The phrenoesophageal ligament is a continuation of the transversalis fascia. It is a supporting structure which inserts in a fan-like arrangement around the circumference of the esophagus at the hiatus. Modified from: Payne WS, Ellis FH Jr: In Schwartz SI (Ed.): Principles of Surgery. New York: McGraw-Hill Book Company, Inc., p. 870, 1969. With permission.

anatomy of the crura is variable. They originate from the second, third, and fourth lumbar vertebral bodies and extend past the aorta to form the margins of the esophageal hiatus. They insert (along with the other muscular components of the diaphragm) into the central tendon. In most cases, the right crus contributes all the fibers that form the esophageal hiatus, being reinforced by muscle from the left side. In the next most common case, the arrangement is similar, but a slip of muscle from the left crus passes behind the esophagus to form part of the right margin of the hiatus.

There are important supporting attachments within the hiatus that help to anchor the esophagus to the diaphragm. These include loose mediastinal connective tissue and reflections of parietal pleura above the diaphragm and peritoneum below. The phrenoesophageal ligament or membrane is the most important of these supporting structures (Figs. 1-10 and 1-11). This ligament is composed of collagen fibers and is a continuation of the transversalis fascia of the abdominal wall. It spreads over the undersurface of the diaphragm between the musculature and peritoneum (Fig. 1-11). At the hiatus, it inserts onto the circumference of the esophagus in a fan-like arrangement (Fig. 1-10). The ligament is not an easily identifiable, discrete structure seen during operations in the hiatal region. It is disrupted during mobilization of the distal esophagus, e.g., to achieve greater esophageal length during antireflux procedures.

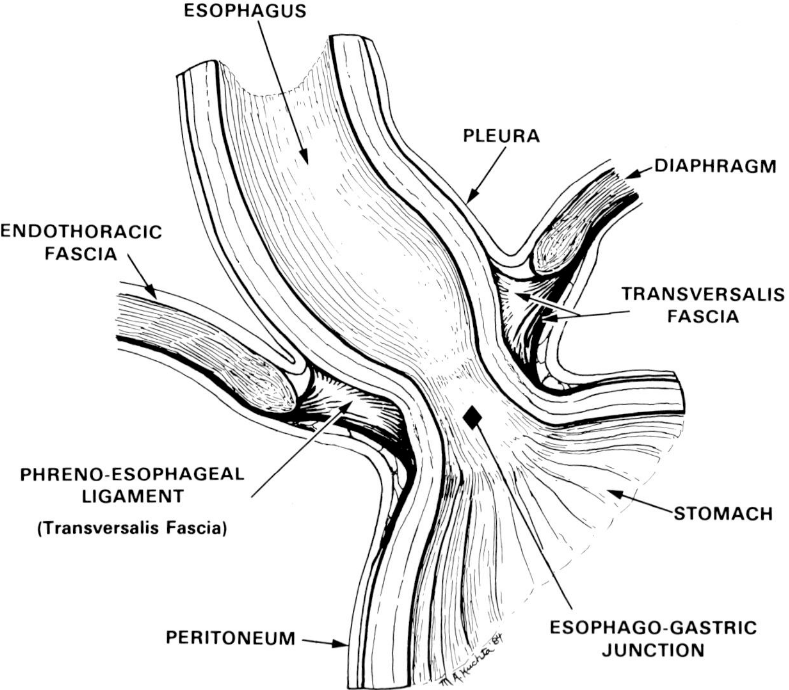


**Figure 1-11.** The anatomy of the esophagogastric junction is shown. The phrenoesophageal ligament is shown in continuity with the transversalis fascia (heavy line) as the latter reflects off the undersurface of the diaphragm. Here, it is in contiguity with the peritoneal lining. The ligament then fans out at the level of the crural musculature to insert into the circumference of the esophagus at the hiatal level shown here. Modified from: Payne WS, Ellis FH Jr: In Schwartz, SI (Ed.): Principles of Surgery (4th ed.). New York: McGraw-Hill Book Company, p. 1065, 1984. With permission.

The abdominal portion of the esophagus is short, usually one to two centimeters in length, and it behaves anatomically and functionally as part of the stomach. The esophageal smooth muscle blends imperceptibly with that of the stomach (Fig. 1-11). The cardiac sphincter of the stomach is formed by the circular muscle layer of the esophagus together with the adjacent fibers of the diaphragm. Although this distal esophageal musculature functions physiologically as a sphincter, it lacks any anatomic definition. It is indistinguishable both grossly and microscopically from the more proximal layers of muscle.

## BLOOD SUPPLY AND LYMPHATIC DRAINAGE OF THE ESOPHAGUS

### Arterial Supply

The esophagus can be considered in four segments when describing its arteries: (1) the cervical part; (2) that portion at the level of the aortic arch and tracheal bifurcation; (3) the lower thoracic part; and, (4) the abdominal part (Fig. 1-12).

#### Cervical Portion

The inferior thyroid artery, a branch of the thyrocervical trunk, supplies the cervical portion. In addition to its thyrocervical trunk branch, the subclavian artery may give off direct branches, as may the other major vessels in the neck. In the majority of cases, a tracheoesophageal branch arises from the inferior thyroid artery, courses downward with the recurrent laryngeal nerve, and supplies the esophagus and also the trachea and superior mediastinal lymph nodes. At times, this establishes an anastomotic connection with the superior bronchial arteries.

#### Aortic Arch and Tracheal Bifurcation

That portion of the esophagus at the level of the aortic arch and tracheal bifurcation receives its blood supply from the bronchial arteries, with occasional branches directly from the aorta. There are many anastomotic connections with adjacent vessels that supply the cervical and thoracic esophagus.

#### Thoracic Portion

The thoracic esophagus below the tracheal bifurcation is supplied usually by three unpaired esophageal branches arising directly from the aorta. These may anastomose with branches of the adjacent intercostal and bronchial arteries.

#### Abdominal Portion

The distal esophagus derives an additional blood supply from esophageal branches of the inferior phrenic and left gastric arteries.

The relatively small number and caliber of the arteries in the midthoracic esophagus is of practical importance, especially in newborns with esophageal atresia and tracheoesophageal fistula malformations. These vessels must be preserved during mobilization of the esophagus in order to avoid devascularizing the midportion of the esophagus just below the fistula. Devascularization may lead to anastomotic disruption and leakage. The proximal pouch may be safely mobilized well up into the neck

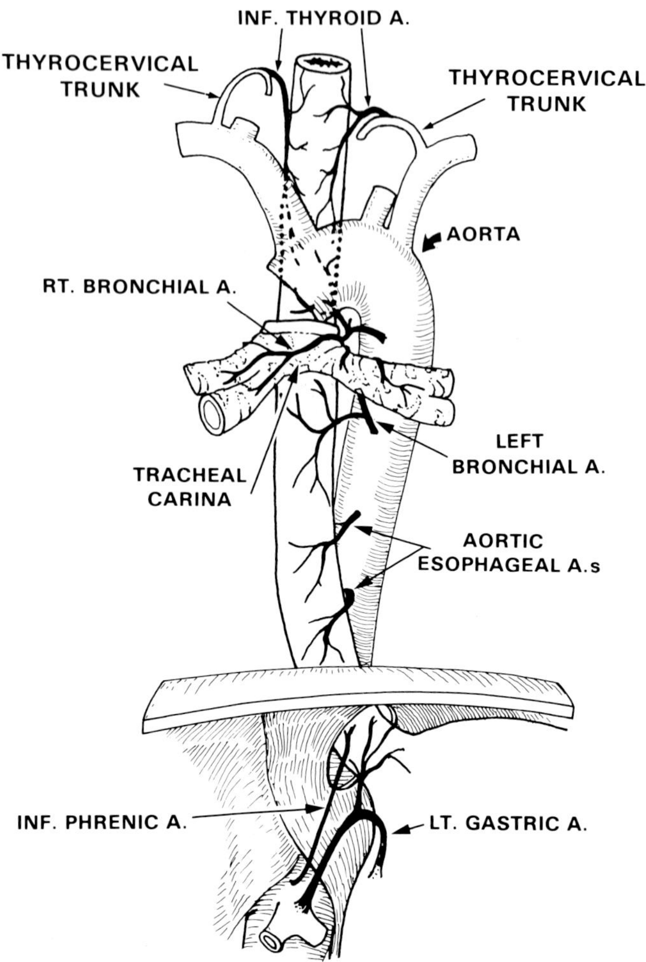


**Figure 1-12.** Arterial blood supply of the esophagus is shown. The cervical esophagus is well endowed with an arterial blood supply derived largely from the inferior thyroid artery. This is a branch of the thyrocervical trunk which originates from the subclavian artery. In most cases, each inferior thyroid artery sends a tracheoesophageal branch downward with the recurrent laryngeal nerves to supply the esophagus, trachea, and superior mediastinal nodes. Anastomotic connections with the bronchial arteries are shown (dotted lines). The esophagus at the level of the aortic arch and tracheal bifurcation receives its blood supply from the right and left bronchial arteries, which anastomose with adjacent vessels. Two of the usually three esophageal branches from the aorta are shown supplying the thoracic esophagus. The distal esophagus derives its blood supply from esophageal branches of the inferior phrenic and left gastric arteries. These are shown around the hiatus passing superiorly to anastomose with the direct branches from the aorta. Modified from: Ellis FH JR: In Sabiston DC Jr (Ed.): Davis-Christopher Textbook of Surgery (11th ed.). Philadelphia: W.B. Saunders Company, p. 792, 1977. With permission.

because of its abundant blood supply. The cervical esophagus is so well vascularized that it can also tolerate one or more myotomies for elongation without risk of critical ischemia.

## Venous Drainage

In general, the venous drainage parallels the arterial supply (Fig. 1-13). In addition, there are extensive submucosal intercommunications affording an excellent collateral venous circulation. A rich venous plexus is present throughout the entire

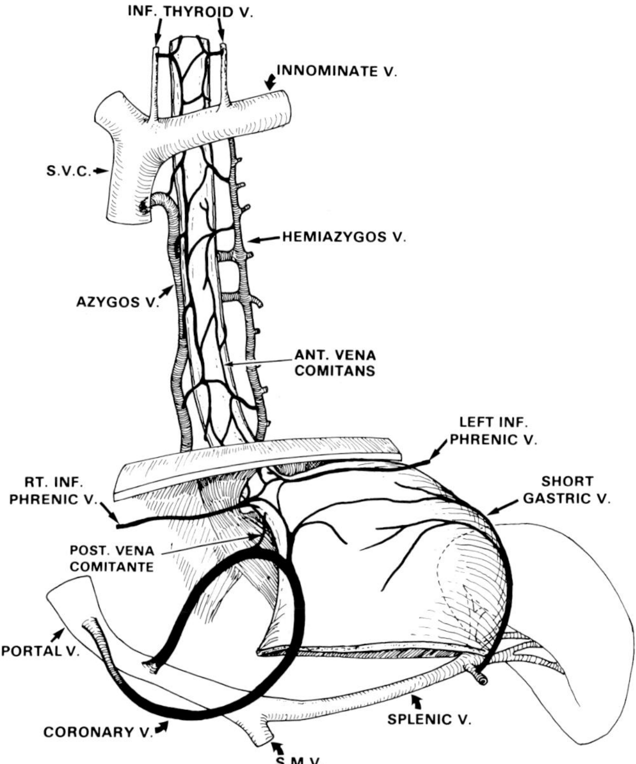


**Figure 1-13.** Venous drainage of the esophagus is shown. The cervical esophagus drains largely into the inferior thyroid veins and thereafter into the innominate vein. The venous drainage of the thoracic esophagus is into the azygos and hemiazygos systems, which communicate freely via the venal comitans. These major veins ultimately empty into the superior vena cava. Venous return from the abdominal portion of the esophagus is into the thoracic system via the inferior phrenic veins and into the portal system. The short gastric, splenic, and coronary veins drain a large part of the stomach into the portal vein. In cases of portal hypertension, these veins serve as collaterals, and, in the esophagus, can enlarge to form varices. Modified from: Postlethwait RW, Sealy WC: Surgery of the Esophagus. Springfield, IL: Charles C. Thomas, p. 454, 1961. With permission.

submucosa, which freely communicates with the abundant submucosal venous plexus in the stomach. This fine plexus of veins drains into larger submucosal venous channels that are evenly placed around the circumference of the esophagus and run longitudinally for the length of the esophagus.

Superiorly, these vertical veins intercommunicate with systemic veins that drain the cervical esophagus. In addition, these large vertical veins drain the thoracic esophagus via perforating and external esophageal veins into the hemiazygos and azygos systems, which in turn drain into the superior vena cava.

Inferiorly, at the esophagogastric junction, these large vertical veins have direct connections with the portal venous system via the left gastric (cardinal) veins, thereby providing major connections between the portal and systemic venous circulations. Clinically, this is commonly seen in patients with portal venous hypertension where these veins form tortuous esophageal varices. The latter circumstance may be due to increased resistance to flow in the liver parenchyma, as for example in neonatal cirrhosis or as a result of extraheptic portal vein blockage following umbilical vein-portal vein phlebitis. The latter may occur as a consequence of omphalitis or following venous cannulation of the umbilical vein for exchange transfusion. These submucosal varices generally do not ascend the esophagus any higher than the perforating connections with the azygos system. They are, therefore, within the lower two-thirds of the esophagus.

### Lymphatic Drainage

Lymphatic channels (Fig. 1-14) run longitudinally in the wall of the esophagus. They penetrate the muscular layers of the esophagus to reach the regional lymph nodes which are scattered throughout the length of the esophagus in the periesophageal connective tissue[14,15] At times, enlarged periesophageal nodes may cause esophageal symptoms. There is free intercommunication between the esophageal lymphatics and nodes and neighboring lymphatic systems such as the tracheal, tracheobronchial, subcarinal, posterior mediastinal, and diaphragmatic nodes. The thoracic duct is another major drainage system of the esophagus.

## INNERVATION OF THE ESOPHAGUS

The innervation of the esophagus is largely via the autonomic nervous system, with essentially the same elements as in the rest of the gastrointestinal tract.[5,8] Classically, the autonomic nervous system is considered to consist of its two major subdivisions: the sympathetic and parasympathetic systems. In both systems, innervation involves a two-neuron chain consisting of a preganglionic neuron located in the central nervous system which projects onto a postganglionic neuron located in the periphery.

In the sympathetic nervous system, the preganglionic neurons are situated in the thoracic and upper lumbar spinal cord forming the thoracolumbar division. Postganglion neurons are situated in either the paravertebral (sympathetic) chains that parallel the vertebral column or in prevertebral ganglia, such as in the celiac plexus which serves the esophagus (Figs. 1-15 and 1-16).

The parasympathetic neurons innervating the esophagus are located chiefly in the vagal nuclei, with preganglionic fibers passing in the vagus nerves to the esophagus

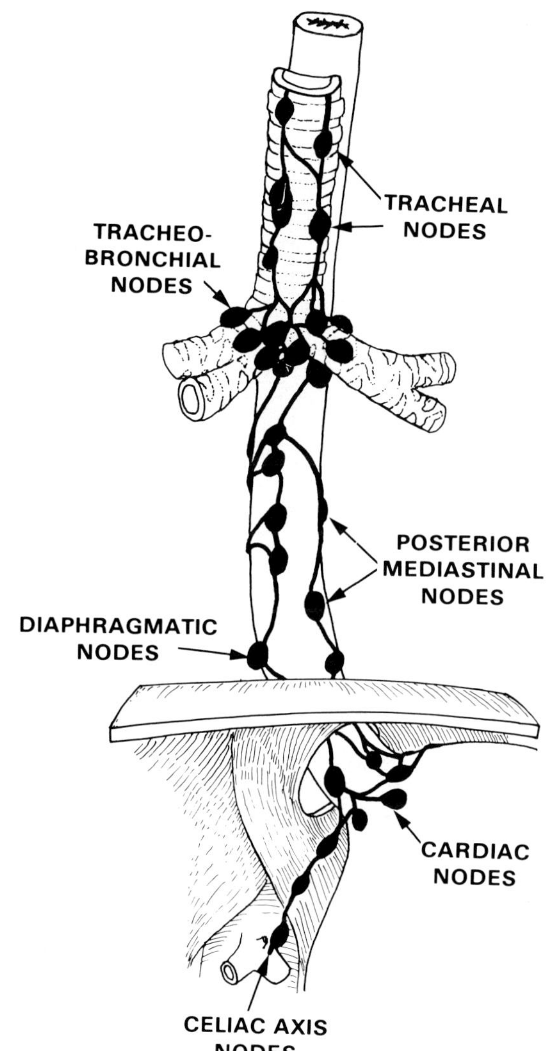


**Figure 1-14.**    Lymphatics of the mediastinum are shown. Enlargement of any of these nodes can occur and produce esophageal and/or respiratory symptoms. In pediatric patients, such involvement is most often secondary to lymphomas or infectious processes. Modified from: Ellis FH Jr: In Sabiston DC Jr (Ed.): Davis-Christopher Textbook of Surgery (11th ed.). Philadelphia: W. B. Saunders Company, p. 792, 1977. With permission.

(Fig. 1-17). Typically, postganglionic neurons of the parasympathetic system are located in close proximity to their target organs. In the esophagus, preganglionic fibers pass from the vagal plexus into the esophageal wall to synapse with postganglionic neurons in the intramural myenteric and submucosal plexuses. These ganglionic cells then function as postganglionic, parasympathetic neurons that innervate the smooth muscle and secretory cells of the gastrointestinal tract. Parasympathetic input usually

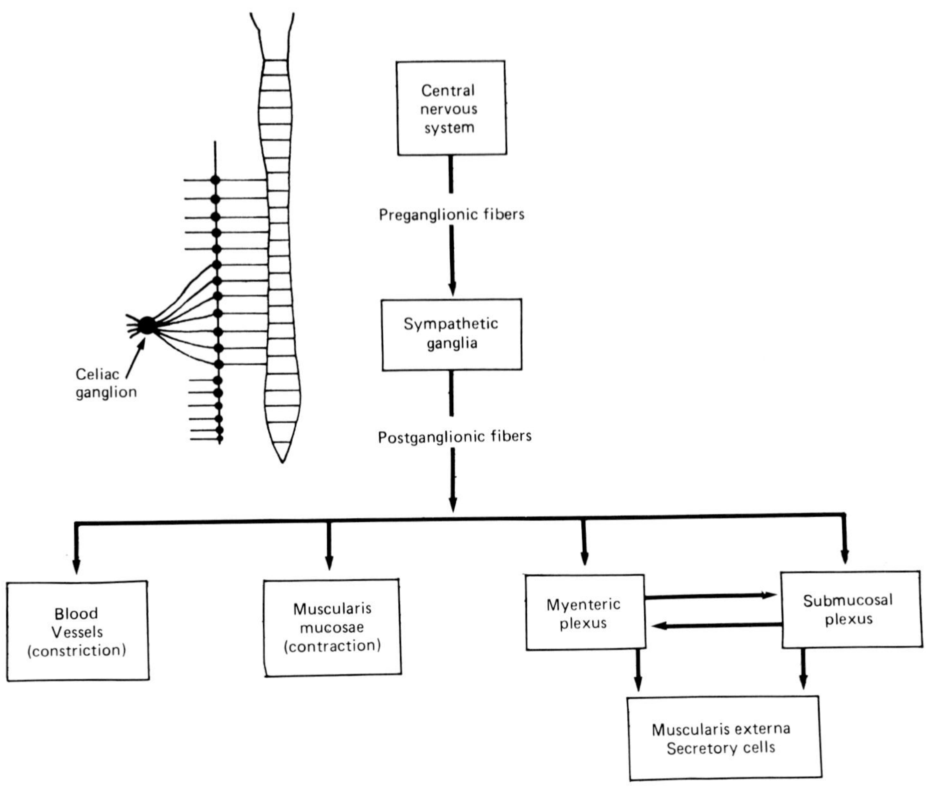



Major aspects of the sympathetic innervation of the gastrointestinal tract.

**Figure 1-15.** Sympathetic efferent pathways include preganglionic fibers from the spinal cord, which synapse in the sympathetic ganglia or in the celiac ganglion. Postganglionic fibers then terminate in the various mural elements shown. The integrated relationships of the myenteric and submucosal plexuses, the muscularis externa, and secretory cells are indicated. Also shown are the effects on the muscularis mucosae and blood vessels. Many autonomic effects are mediated by known neurotransmitters, while, in some, the transmitter remains unrecognized. In the sympathetic system, preganglionic neurons all use acetylcholine as a neurotransmitter, while postganglionic neurons most commonly use norepinephrine. Norepinephrine has an excitatory action on blood vessels and muscularis mucosae, while it has an inhibitory effect on the smooth muscle of the muscularis externa. This led to the classification of receptors as alpha-adrenergic or beta-adrenergic, depending on the response of a given receptor to norepinephrine. In the gastrointestinal tract, adrenergic impulses acting on alpha and beta receptors cause a decrease in motility and tone, while stimulation of alpha receptors causes contraction of sphincters and inhibition of secretions. The effect of the sympathetic nerves on the muscularis externa is not a direct action on the smooth muscle cells, since there are few sympathetic nerve endings in the muscularis externa. Rather, the sympathetic nerves act to influence neurons in the intrinsic myenteric and submucosal plexuses that provide input to the smooth muscle cells. This effect may be reinforced by the action of the sympathetic nerves in cuasing constriction of vessels and so reducing blood flow to the muscularis externa.[5,8] Modified from: Kutchai HC: In Berne RM, Levy MN (Eds.): Physiology. St. Louis: The C.V. Mosby Company, p. 744, 1983. With permission.

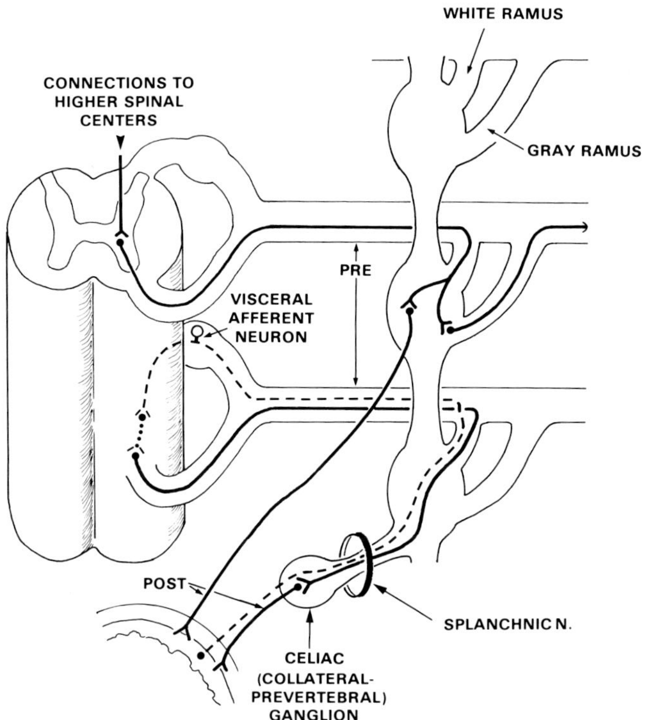



**Figure 1-16.** Afferent and efferent sympathetic pathways are shown in detail. Preganglionic neurons lie in the intermediolateral cell column of the spinal cord. They project their axons through a white ramus (so named because the sympathetic preganglionic fibers are myelinated) to the sympathetic ganglia and celiac ganglion. Postganglionic neurons are situated in either the paravertebral (sympathetic) chains that parallel the vertebral column or in the collateral prevertebral (celiac) ganglion. As can be seen, the celiac ganglion receives preganglionic fibers via the splanchnic nerves, which have bypassed the sympathetic chains without synapsing. After reaching this ganglion, synapse with postganglionic neurons occurs and, like the postganglionic neuron in the sympathetic chains, postganglionic unmyelinated fibers continue onward to penetrate the wall of the esophagus and upper stomach. The path of afferent fibers to the visceral afferent neuron in the dorsal root ganglion is shown (dotted line) from the wall of the esophagus via the splanchnic nerves. Afferent impulses continue centrally from these neurons into the spinal cord, where they make connections with efferent neurons. Shown is a synapse with an internuncial neuron and then with the sympathetic preganglionic, efferent neuron. Modified from: Ganong WF: Review of Medical Physiology (11th ed.). Los Altos, CA: Lange Medical Publishers, p. 174, 1983. With permission.

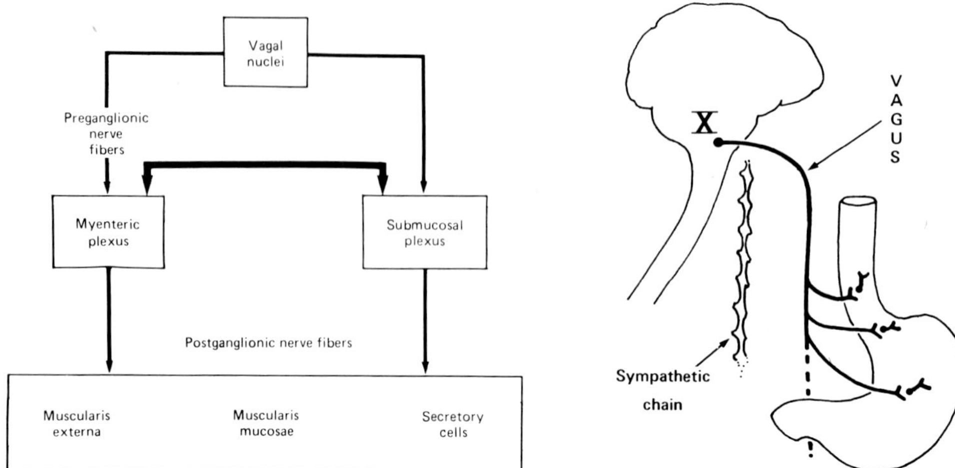



Parasympathetic innervation of the esophagus and upper gastrointestinal tract.

**Figure 1-17.** Organization of parasympathetic innervation of the esophagus and upper gastro-intestinal tract is shown. Within the vagal nuclei are located the preganglionic nerve cells which give rise to preganglionic (VAGUS) fibers. These axons synapse to the postganglionic neurons in the wall of the target organs. Postganglionic neurons are in the myenteric and submucosal plexuses and send postganglionic nerve fibers to specific mural components which include those indicated—the muscularis externa, the muscularis mucosae, and secretory cells. As in the sympathetic system, the parasympathetic preganglionic fibers release acetylcholine as their neurotransmitter. In contrast to the sympathetic innervation, however, the parasympathetic postganglionic fibers are also cholinergic. In general, they cause increased motility and tone, relaxation of sphincters, and stimulation of secretions. Their synapses are blocked by atropine.[5,8] Modified from: Kutchai HC: In Berne RM, Levy MN (Eds.): Physiology. St. Louis: The C.V. Mosby Company, p. 745, 1983. With permission.

stimulates the muscularis externa and secretory activity of the gut (Fig. 1-17). The two divisions produce a cooperative, reciprocally integrated action on the esophagus as well as on the rest of the gastrointestinal tract (Fig. 1-18).

## Function

Early, organized esophageal function begins in utero with fetal ingestion of amni-otic fluid. This is an established process by the fourth month of gestation. Swallowing activity may be integrated with the development of a sense of taste in the fetus. Taste buds are present in the human fetal tongue epithelium by 14 weeks of gestation, about the time swallowing begins. Using fetal lambs, attempts have been made to determine whether or not fetal taste buds respond to stimuli by making recordings of neural activity in the fetal chorda tympani nerve while applying chemicals to the tongue.[4] These studies demonstrated that the peripheral taste system of the fetal lamb is func-tional over the last third of gestation. Responsiveness or perceptiveness to taste stimuli have also been tested in utero by using fetal swallowing as an index of taste percep-tion.[4] Swallowing activity was measured with an electromagnetic flow transducer

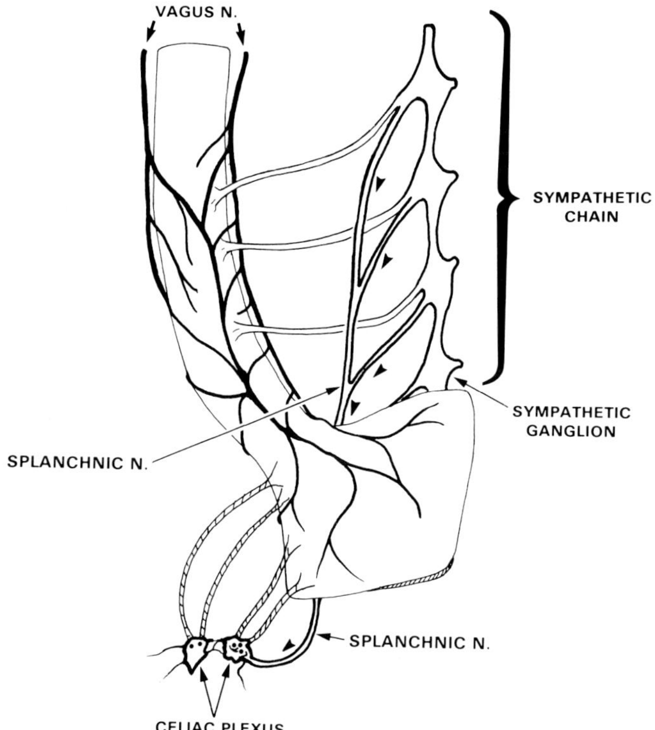



**Figure 1-18.** The relationships of the sympathetic and para-sympathetic systems to the esophagus and upper stomach are shown. Sympathetic innervation is from the sympathetic chains and from the splanchnic nerves via the celiac plexus (Figs. 1-15 and 1-16). Parasympathetic innervation of the esophagus is largely via the vagus nerves. The recurrent laryngeal nerves supply the upper portion of the esophagus, while the vagi below the recurrent nerves supply the remainder of the esophagus. The vagus nerves lie on both sides of the esophagus, forming the plexus shown. The nerves usually emerge at the hiatus as two major trunks. Following gasric rotation (during early gestation), the left trunk is oriented anteriorly and the right posteriorly as they pass onto the stomach.[15]

implanted in the fetal esophagus. The results were inconclusive regarding the stimulation of swallowing by altering taste; however, the experiments clarified some of the physiology of in-utero swallowing. Results showed that the fetus swallows large volumes of amniotic fluid in two–seven "bouts" each day. A bout consisted of a period of swallowing of from 20 ml to 200 ml of amniotic fluid. In between these episodes, the fetus frequently swallowed small volumes. No obvious pattern of swallowing was established.

Following birth, sucking with reflex swallowing is established. This is a well-developed function in the term infant, but may be less well-developed in the premature, in whom there may be a delay in the opening of the cricoid sphincter and in whom esophageal contractions may not have organized peristalsis.

The neonate is a nosebreather capable of closing off the oral passageway by elevation of the tongue to the palate during sleep. This capability of physical partitioning of the nasal and oral passages is functionally complemented by inhibition of respiration during sucking movements.[14] In essence, the primary function of the esophagus is to transmit nutrients from the mouth to the stomach. This requires an integrated effort between the voluntary striated muscles of the pharynx, the constrictors, and the smooth musculature of the esophagus. This effort, in turn, is dependent upon the complex neural circuits involved in the control of esophageal motility (Fig. 1-19).

Classically, swallowing has been divided into three stages: the oral, the pharyngeal, and the esophageal. The process is continuous, however, and its uninterrupted sequence is outlined and illustrated in Figure 1-20.

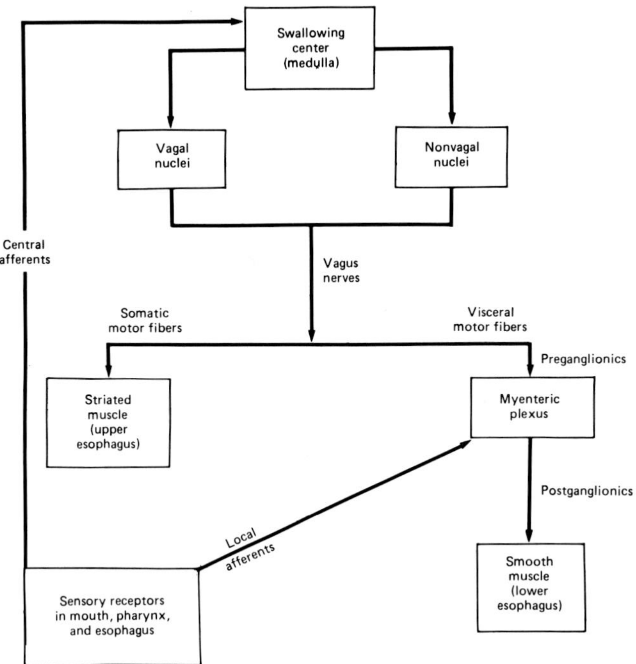


Local and central neutral circuits involved in the control of esophageal motility.

**Figure 1-19.** Coordinated esophageal motility is dependent on both the local and central neural circuits shown. Vagal components are emphasized. Sensory receptors feed stimuli to the smooth muscle of the lower esophagus via local afferents to the intramural (myenteric) plexuses and via central afferents to the swallowing center in the medulla oblongata. The swallowing center initiates impulses through vagal and nonvagal nuclei, largely through the vagus nerves, to both the striated muscles of the upper esophagus and to its lower visceral smooth musculature. Modified from: Kutchai HC: In Berne RM, Levy MH (Eds.): Physiology. St. Louis: The C.V. Mosby Company, p. 756, 1983. With permission.

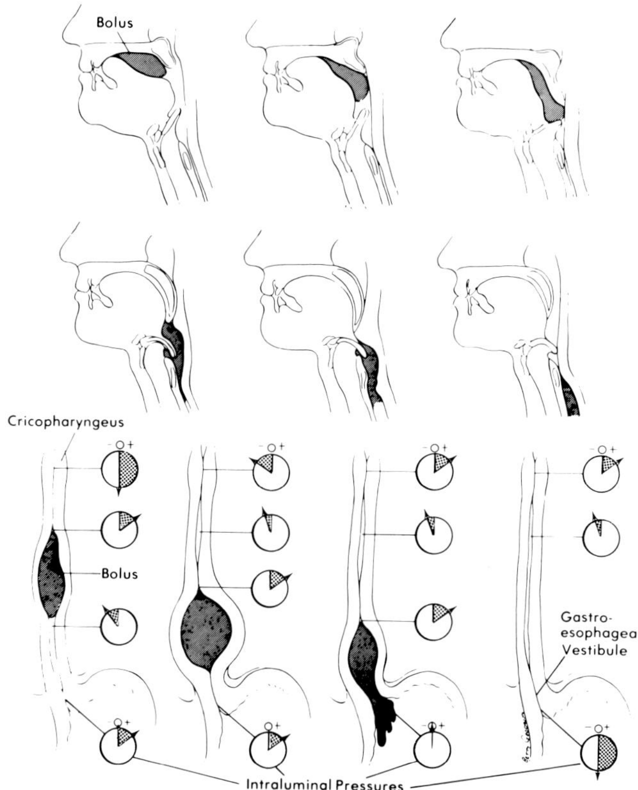



**Figure 1-20.** Coordinated acts of deglutition are illustrated. Included are pressure changes indicated by position of the arrows in positive and negative zones of adjacent circles. These pressure deflections occur with swallowing and propulsive peristalsis of an ingested bolus from the mouth into the stomach. The mechanisms of deglutition are shown with pressure relationships of oral, pharyngeal, and esophageal waves indicated. The function of the cricopharyngeal and cardiac sphincters is noted. Modified from: Othersen HB Jr: In Holder TM, Ashcraft KW (Eds.): Pediatric Surgery. Philadelphia: W.B. Saunders Company, p. 255, 1980. With permission.

The sequence can be seen in the diagrams as follows:

1. Tongue pushes bolus into oropharynx.
2. Tongue rises to close oral cavity.
3. Palate closes nasopharynx.
4. Larynx elevates and moves forward to close supraglottic area and open hypopharynx.
5. Pharynx contracts to propel bolus to esophagus.
6. Cricopharyngeal sphincter relaxes to receive bolus.
7. Esophageal motility propels bolus toward stomach.
8. Gastroesophageal sphincter relaxes as bolus passes to stomach.

The cricopharyngeal and gastroesophageal sphincters are true sphincters with resting tone. They relax to receive the bolus, contract to propel it, and then return to resting tone. Modified from: Payne WS, Olsen HM, (Eds): The Esophagus. Philadelphia: Lea & Febiger, p. 13, 1974. With permission.

Initial phases of swallowing are voluntary, beginning with the intake of food and, when necessary, chewing.[14] It is noteworthy that normal infants are born with a vigorous suck and tend to develop negative pressures up to 250 cm of water.[13] Thereafter, the propulsion of formula or solids from the mouth to the throat is involuntary. The tongue rises to the hard palate and the soft palate partitions the nasopharynx. As the bolus progresses, the larynx and epiglottis are pulled upward by the thyroglossal and mylohyoid muscles and the airway is temporarily obstructed. The bolus is further propelled by the pharyngeal constrictor muscles. The cricoid sphincter relaxes simultaneously, thereby permitting the bolus to enter the esophagus, after which the cricoid contracts forcefully. The high resting tone of this sphincter normally prevents regurgitation of esophageal contents. It is pertinent that newborn infants swallow in a manner different than that of older children. In the latter, the teeth are opposed and the jaw muscles contract, while in infants, the gums are held apart with the tongue against them and the circumoral muscles contract. The activity of the masseter and the temporalis muscles is minimal. After the initiation of the swallow, further passage of material to the stomach depends upon organized esophageal peristalsis.

Peristaltic activity has been classically divided into three types: (1) Primary—a contraction wave in continuity with oral and pharyngeal swallowing; (2) secondary—a wave originating in the esophagus below the cricopharyngeal sphincter and independent of pharyngeal swallowing; and, (3) tertiary—a wave occuring only in the smooth

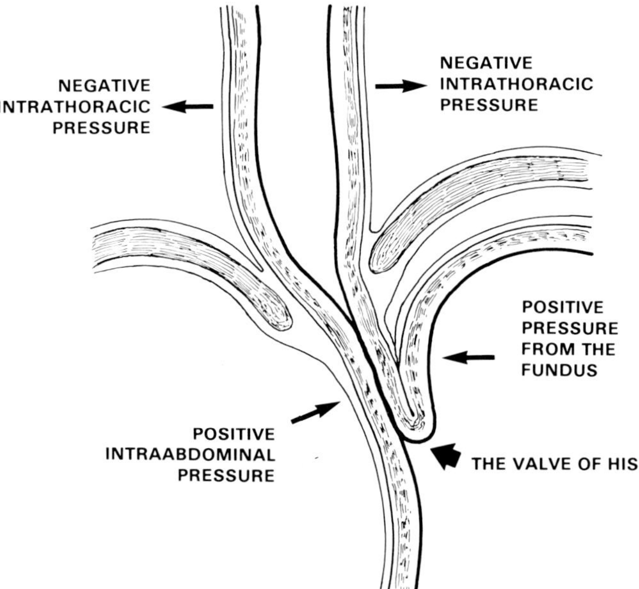


**Figure 1-21.**   Diagram of the region of the lower esophageal sphincter. Negative intrathoracic pressure and postive intraabdominal pressure act to close the gastroesophageal junction, as does intragastric fundic pressure. Part of the fundus forms the valve of His, where the terminal esophagus joins in continuity with the stomach. This mechanism also acts to prevent gastroesophageal reflux. Modified from: Flavell G: The Oesophagus. London: Butterworth and Company, 1963. With permission.

muscle of the innervated esophagus. It is important that the gastroesophageal sphincter relax as the oncoming wave of peristalsis approaches it. This sphincter, or high-pressure zone, is in the region of the gastroesophageal junction; it is not a clearly defined anatomic entity. Its location is identified physiologically by manometric studies. Its importance in preventing gastroesophageal reflux has been emphasized. This is a complex function involving multiple factors. One of these involves the pressure of relationships of the region and the acute angle of the esophagogastric junction which forms the valve of His (Fig. 1-21). This valve is formed by the esophagus making an acute angle of entry into the stomach in relation to the longitudinal axis of the fundus. It lies between the intra-abdominal esophagus and fundus of the stomach as the fundus lies cephalad on the left under the dome of the diaphragm. On the right, however, the lower esophagus continues on an almost straight line with the lesser curvature of the stomach.

## THE ESOPHAGOGASTRIC JUNCTION

Over the past two decades, a great deal of information on the function of the distal esophagus has accumulated. Most of this has been derived from studies of adults; however, information on pediatric subjects has become available.

The lower end of the human esophagus is separated from the stomach by a zone of increased pressure that acts as a barrier to reflux of stomach contents into the esophagus but also allows material to pass in both directions. In theory, this zone could be recongized in two different ways: It could possess distinguishing anatomic features or it could have characteristic patterns of behavior.[11] There is no anatomic or histologic definition of the gastroesophageal sphincter in the human. The "sphincter" may be a physiologic function of the *tone* of the intrinsic muscle of the region, or it may be a function of the structures surrounding the distal end of the esophagus, or it may be a function of the shape of the junctional zone which creates a mechanical valve at the cardia.

When the musculature of the esophagogastric junction is excised or seriously damaged, reflux esophagitis commonly occurs, even if the hiatus is carefully repaired. Satisfactory sphincteric function is maintained even if diaphragmatic factors have been eliminated by paralysis, surgical resection, or transposition of the esophagogastric junction away from the hiatus. When the esophagogastric junction is displaced into the thorax, the development of reflux esophagitis appears to be related to a diminution or absence of the intrinsic pressure barrier at the esophagogastric junction rather to the loss of any direct contribution by the diaphragm to the competency at the junction.[11]

A valve-like action of the abdominal segment of esophagus has been proposed as a barrier to gastroesophageal reflux, although some investigators deny the existence of a portion of esophagus lying within the abdomen. Most of the conflicting views could be resolved by the acceptance of the existence of a so-called crural tunnel.[11] The fact that the esophagus passes from a low-pressure zone above to a higher pressure zone below the hiatus has functional signficance whether or not such a tunnel exists. Deep inspiration increases the holdup of material at the hiatus and this has been shown to be due to increased differences between the intrathoracic and intra-abdominal pressures. Positive intra-abdominal pressure probably plays little part in the closing mechanism of the gastroesophageal junction.

The importance of the sling fibers of the stomach and the oblique angle of entrance of the esophagus into the stomach in the prevention of reflux have been questioned. The mechanism of action of the latter feature, the so-called angle of His, (Fig. 1-21) is based on the theory that when intragastric pressure rises, the terminal portion of the esophagus is compressed by the enlarging fundus and reflux is thus prevented. In contradiction to this theory, many species of mammals with competent esophagogastric sphincters do not have an oblique angle of entry of the esophagus into the stomach. In man, the angle is variable and is sometimes so obtuse as to be almost nonexistent.

Evidence *against* external influences on an antireflux mechanism is accumulating, while data to support the concept of an intrinsic muscular tone as the most important antireflux mechanism increase.[11] The distal portion of the esophagus is found to behave differently from the rest of the esophagus, despite the absence of an anatomic or histologic distinction. Manometric studies have shown that active relaxation and contraction occur in this region in response to appropriate stimuli. In some conditions, such as scleroderma and polymyositis, where the function of the muscle of the gastroesophageal junction is destroyed but normal anatomy otherwise persists, reflux often develops. This indicates that competency of the sphincter depends largely upon a factor present in the muscle of the esophagus itself.[11] There is a high-pressure zone distinct from the esophagus above or the stomach below. This so-called "pressure barrier" is presumed to be maintained by an increase in tone of the circular muscle of the junctional zone. In adults, this segment of increased pressure is between three and five cm in length and is located above and below the hiatus. In response to a swallow, this high-presure zone normally relaxes preceding the arrival of a contraction wave traveling down the esophagus. After passage of the bolus, there is an elevation of pressure above resting values, following which pressure in the sphincteric zone returns to a resting level.

Antegrade and/or retrograde determinations of pH and manometric changes across the distal esophageal sphincter measured in 159 patients demonstrated variability in sphincter data obtained by these techniques.[17] Contrary to popular opinion, the majority of patients who reflux have distal esophageal sphincter pressures greater than 10 torr. It is to be emphasized that, while distal esophageal pressure is a useful guide to the presence of reflux when it is grossly abnormal, the presence of a normal distal esophageal resting pressure does not exclude the possibility of gastroesophageal reflux. From these data, it was concluded that esophageal manometry is useful only in locating the position of the sphincter prior to doing a standard acid reflux test and in evaluating motility disturbances.

The value of manometry in the evaluation of motility disorders should not be underestimated. Sphincteric behavior is altered by some diseases so consistently that manometrics are pathognomonic of each disorder.[11] For example, in achalasia, the sphincter does not relax and there is disordered motility between the body of the esophagus and the cardia. In sliding hiatal hernias, the barrier zone is longer than normal and pressures may be reduced; additionally, the sphincter often relaxes poorly and contracts prematurely. In scleroderma, the sphincter may be destroyed so that in extreme cases there is no pressure barrier and no relaxation or contraction is recognizable. The so-called "hypertensive sphincter" is a cause of pain and dysphagia and is characterized by great elevation of resting pressure and failure of the sphincter to respond properly to deglutition.

The innervation of the sphincter appears to be important. In the foregoing section on innervation, the intimate relationship of the vagus nerves to the esophagus and the gastroesophageal junction, as well as the sympathetic nerve supply, have been examined. Regarding the sphincter, the effect of the vagus nerves is controversial. Some investigators believe that stimulation of the nerves can cause either contraction or relaxation of the sphincter, depending upon the rate and intensity of the stimulus and the tone of the sphincter at the time of impulse propagation. There is evidence to suggest that although the vagus nerves are accepted as part of the normal relaxation mechanism of the sphincter, some relaxation can occur in their absence. Alternatively, the sympathetic nerves should cause contraction; however, most researchers indicate that the sympathetic nerves play little or no part in regulating the tone of the esophagogastric sphincter.

The response of the sphincter to the neurotransmitter acetylcholine and the effect of adrenergic drugs have not been uniform. In some experimental animals, acetylcholine causes contraction of both the circular and longitudinal muscles of the sphincter, while epinephrine relaxes the circular muscle. The role of parasympathomimetic drugs and gastrin on the pathogenesis of lower esophageal sphincter incompetence has been studied.[9] Two groups of adults were examined: the first had symptomatic gastroesophageal reflux, and the second, which had no symptoms, served as a control. In both the symptomatic and control groups the lower esophageal sphincter response to direct muscle stimulation by the parasympathomimetic drug benthanechol chloride was identified. The effect of the cholinesterase inhibitor edrophonium chloride was identical. Dose-response curves of lower esophageal sphincter pressure to exogenous intravenous pentagastrin were also similar in both groups. The response to endogenous gastrin release was diminished in those patients having reflux. This suggested that diminished release of endogenous gastrin might be responsible for sphincteric hypotension in patients with gastroesophageal reflux.

Finally, it is pertinent to note that a significant number of infants and children with severe brain damage have gastroesophageal reflux. Experiments producing chronic brain injury in cats by elevating intracranial pressure using balloon catheters have demonstrated reduced lower esophageal sphincter (LES) pressures when intracranial pressure was elevated. The mechanism to explain this observation has not been established.

In summary, although an anatomic sphincter is not identifiable at the gastroesophageal junction, a physiologic sphincter is present and is a function of the intrinsic musculature of the junction. This intrinsic high-pressure zone is the main barrier to reflux of gastric contents. Its ability to maintain tone and to respond normally to swallowing appears to be dependent on the vagus nerves as well as on a mechanism in the wall of the esophagus itself. The sympathetic nerves appear to play little part in this mechanism. Although the diaphragm is not part of this sphincter in the human and does not have a direct role in the prevention of reflux, it does affect esophageal emptying by altering the pressures in the pleural and peritoneal cavities. The angle of His and the oblique gastric sling fibers do not appear to be important in the prevention of gastroesophageal reflux. Esophageal manometric studies performed in infants and children largely confirm the data derived from adult patients and controls[3,7,12,16] Two of these studies[3,16] have shown that the normal neonate has a low distal esophageal pressure which matures to an adult level by six weeks of age.

## REFERENCES


1.  Bloom W, Fawcett DW: In: A Textbook of Histology (10th ed.). Philadelphia: W. B. Saunders Company, pp. 639–643, 1975.
2.  Blount RF, Lachman E: In Schaeffer JP (Ed.): Morris' Human Anatomy (11th ed.). New York: The Blakiston Company, pp. 1327–1342, 1953.
3.  Boix-Ochoa J, Canals J: Maturation of the lower esophagus. J Pediatr Surg 11:749–756, 1976.
4.  Bradley RM, Mistretta CM: The sense of taste and swallowing activity in foetal sheep. In Emline KS, Cross KW, Dawes GS, et al. (Eds.): Foetal and Neonatal Physiology. London: Sir Joseph Barcroft Centenary Symposium, Cambridge University Press, pp. 77–81, 1973.
5.  Cohen DH, Sherman SM: In Berne RM, Levy MN (Eds.): Physiology. St Louis: The C.V. Mosby Company, pp. 314–335, 1983.
6.  Gray SW, Skandalakis JE: In: Embryology for Surgeons. Philadelphia: W.B. Saunders Company, pp. 63–100, 1972.
7.  Gryboski JD: The swallowing mechanism of the neonate. 1: Esophageal & gastric motility. Pediatrics 35:445–452, 1965.
8.  Kutchai HC: In Berne RM, Levy MN (Eds.): Physiology. St. Louis: The C.V. Mosby Company, pp. 743–761, 1983.
9.  Lipshutz, WH, Gaskins RD, Lukash WM, et al: Pathogenesis of lower-esophageal-sphincter incompetence. N Engl J Med 289:182–184, 1973.
10. Lerche W: Surgery of the oesophagus. Surg Gynecol Obstet 11:345–361, 1910.
11. Mann CV, Greenwood RK, Ellis FH Jr: The esophagogastric junction. Surg Gynecol Obstet 118:853–862, 1964.
12. Moroz SP, Espinoza J, Cumming WA, et al: Lower esophageal sphincter function in children with and without gastroesophageal reflux. Gastroenterology 71:263–241, 1976.
13. Othersen HB Jr: In Holder TM, Ashcraft KW (Eds.): Pediatric Surgery. Philadelphia: W.B. Saunders Company, pp. 253–265, 1980.
14. Payne WS, Olsen AM: In Payne WS, Olsen AM (Eds.): The Esophagus. Philadelphia: Lea and Febiger, pp. 1–54, 1974.
15. Postlethwait RW, Sealy WC: In: Surgery of the Esophagus. Springfield, IL: Charles C. Thomas, pp. 445–478, 1961.
16. Strawcynski H, Beck IT, McKenna RD, et al: The behavior of the lower esophageal sphincter in infants and its relationship to gastroesophageal regurgitation. J Pediatr 64:17–23, 1964.
17. Thurer RL, DeMeester TR, Johnson LF: The distal esophageal sphincter and its relationship to gastroesophageal reflux. J Surg Res 16:418–423, 1974.

Thomas M. Holder

# 2

# Esophageal Atresia and Tracheoesophageal Fistula

The most common and most serious of congenital anomalies of the esophagus is esophageal atresia (EA). While tracheoesophageal fistula (TEF) may occur independently, it is usually associated with EA. By far the most frequent combination is EA with a fistula from the trachea to the distal esophagus.

This anomaly was first described by Thomas Gibson in 1697. The first two survivors occurred in November, 1939, reported independently by Ladd[30] and by Levin.[33] Both infants were treated with multiple operations—gastrostomy, cervical esophagostomy, and subsequent esophageal reconstruction. In 1941, Cameron Haight accomplished the first successful primary repair with division and suture of the tracheoesophageal fistula and direct esophageal anastomosis.[18]

Primary repair rapidly became the standard approach to treatment of EA. A steady reduction of mortality has come about because of refinements in technique, improvement in pediatric anesthesia, and the recognition and care of special groups of patients at high risk. The latter include those with pneumonia, prematurity, and major associated anomalies.[47] Currently, about 95 percent of patients who come for repair leave the hospital alive.

The incidence of esophageal atresia and/or tracheoesophageal fistula is about 1 in 3000–4500 births,[35,46] which makes it one of the most common of major congenital anomalies. Twins are affected slightly more frequently than are singletons.[14]

The etiology of EA and TEF is not known. As with most common birth defects, the pathogenesis is probably related to both genetic and environmental factors. Chromosomal abnormalities have not been implicated, although the anomaly has been seen in patients with chromosomal defects. While more than one affected child in a family has occasionally been observed, no evidence of a Mendelian inheritance pattern has been established.[40]

Associated congenital anomalies occur in about half of the infants with EA and/ or TEF, suggesting a diffuse process which occurs during organogenesis in many of the affected babies.

Pediatric Esophageal Surgery
ISBN 0-8089-1776-5

## EMBRYOLOGY

The trachea and lungs form as an out-pouching of the primitive foregut. As the embryo grows, the trachea elongates in a caudal direction, while the esophagus and pharynx proceed cranially. Lateral mesodermal ridges proceed in a cranial direction, joining in the midline to separate the trachea and esophagus.

The embryogenesis of esophageal atresia and tracheoesophageal fistula is not completely understood. Misdirection of the lateral ridges can obliterate a portion of the developing esophagus. Incomplete septation of the trachea and esophagus may result in a tracheoesophageal fistula to the proximal or distal esophagus.[45]

Another possibility is that cell proliferation of the foregut fails to keep up with the elongation of the primitive trachea and esophagus. The attenuation results in a single tube—the trachea—with atresia of the esophagus.[17]

## ANATOMY

The anomaly of esophageal atresia and/or tracheoesophageal fistula occurs in five general forms. Esophageal atresia with distal TEF is by far the most common type (85 percent). Esophageal atresia with proximal TEF, esophageal atresia with both proximal and distal TEF, esophageal atresia without TEF, and TEF without esophageal atresia are much less common. Figure 2-1 shows the relative frequency of the different types of lesions. There are innumerable variations on the above general categories of anomalies.[29]

In the case of esophageal atresia, the proximal segment ends blindly, usually at the level of the second to fourth thoracic vertebra. The proximal pouch is dilated with a thickened muscular wall because of the bougienage effect of continuous swallowing of amniotic fluid by the fetus. The blood supply is generous and arises from the thyrocervical trunk. If a proximal TEF is present, it arises not from the tip, but, rather, usually a centimeter or two proximal to the tip of the proximal esophageal pouch and runs obliquely from the esophagus upward to enter the membranous trachea.

If there is no distal TEF, the distal esophageal segment is a small pouch extending one–two cm above the diaphragm. A long gap exists between the two ends of the esophagus and presents a major technical problem in esophageal reconstruction. The distal segment is narrow and has a thinner musculature than does the proximal segment. The distal atretic esophagus has an adequate blood supply which does not limit mobilization.

A distal TEF anchors the distal esophagus at its upper end and prevents retraction and shortening of the distal esophageal segment. The distal esophagus is smaller in diameter and has a thinner musculature than does the proximal segment. Usually, the TEF enters the membranous trachea just above the carina. Occasionally, the fistula communicates with the trachea inferiorly between the two major bronchi. On rare occasion, the fistula arises from a bronchus. There is commonly a gap of a centimeter or more between the upper and lower esophageal segments, which may cause major problems at reconstruction. This is especially true when the fistula is at the carina or below. The upper end of the distal esophagus has a segmental blood supply arising directly from the aorta and intercostal vessels and should not be freed extensively to approximate the ends because of the possibility of serious ischemia. Rarely, the atretic ends of the esophagus overlap and may even have a continuous musculature.

RELATIVE FREQUENCY OF EA AND/OR TEF ANOMALIES

| | | SURVEY (23) 1058 PTS (1964) | PRESENT SERIES 100 PTS (1984) |
|---|---|---|---|
|  | EA WITH DISTAL TEF | 86.5 | 82 |
| 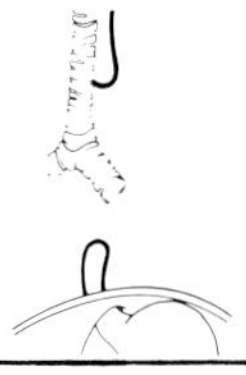 | EA WITHOUT TEF | 7.7 | 2 |
| 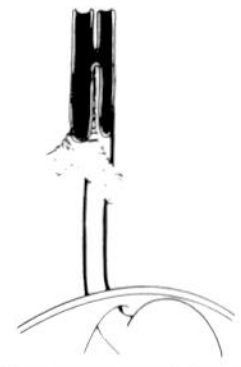 | TEF WITHOUT EA | 4.4 | 7 |
| 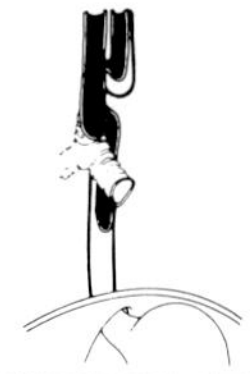 | EA WITH PROXIMAL AND DISTAL TEF* | 0.7 | 6 |
| 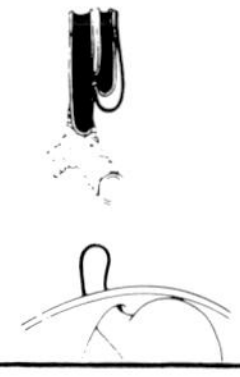 | EA WITH PROXIMAL TEF* | 0.8 | 3 |

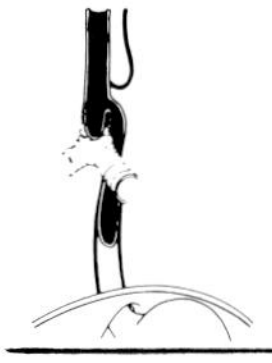

**Figure 2-1.** The incidence of the different types of tracheoesophageal anomalies is presented from both a large collective series and the current personal series. While the present series is considerably smaller, the much higher incidence of TEF to the proximal pouch (9% vs 1.5% for the survey) is probably more accurate and is the result of current better diagnostic methods.

TEF without esophageal atresia, the isolated, or "H", type TEF, occurs at any level from the cricoid cartilage to the carina, but most often occurs at or above the second thoracic vertebra. The tracheal end of an isolated fistula is always proximal as compared with the esophageal end. Double fistulas have rarely been reported, as is also true of fistulas from the intact esophagus to both the stem bronchi and segmental bronchi.[6]

## PHYSIOLOGY

Anatomic anomalies lead to altered function. With esophageal atresia, the infant cannot swallow its saliva and hence drools from birth. If fed, the infant cannot swallow and is apt to aspirate what it is offered.

The most severe symptoms occur in patients with esophageal atresia and TEF to the distal esophagus. When these infants cry, cough, or strain, the intratracheal pressure is elevated and air is forced through the fistula into the stomach, which becomes distended. The small intestine likewise becomes dilated, the diaphragm elevated, and ventilation decreased. Periodically, the stomach decompresses through the fistula into the tracheobronchial tree. The acid gastric secretions are irritating to the respiratory mucosa, leading to atelectasis and pneumonitis.

The same sequence of events occurs in isolated tracheoesophageal fistula with intact esophagus, but to a lesser degree. Decompression of the gastric contents results in regurgitation into the pharynx rather than directly into the trachea.

Esophageal motility in the patient with isolated tracheoesophageal fistula is abnormal in that there is discoordinated peristalsis from the level of the fistula down to the stomach. Manometric studies done via a gastrostomy in patients prior to repair of EA and distal TEF have also demonstrated abnormal motility in the distal esophagus.[44] Altered esophageal motility is therefore associated with the anomaly and is not secondary to operative manipulation. This contention is supported by the observation in experimental animals that transection and anastomosis of the esophagus is not associated with similar disturbance in motility.[19]

## DIAGNOSIS

Infants with esophageal atresia and tracheoesophageal fistula are, as a group, small. One-third weigh less than 2250 gm. Those who have EA without TEF often have had associated polyhydramnios, since the fetus is unable to swallow and absorb fluid from the gut. The infant with EA with or without TEF presents with drooling because the saliva cannot be swallowed. When fed, the infant regurgitates what has been taken, chokes, coughs, and may become cyanotic. The respiratory symptoms usually worsen with the passage of hours. Delay in diagnosis allows atelectasis and pneumonitis to develop. These symptoms develop more rapidly in infants with distal TEF than in those without. If not recognized and treated, esophageal atresia is uniformly fatal.

Symptoms in the infant with an isolated TEF start from birth, but are more subtle and tend to be recognized somewhat later. Some patients go for months before diagnosis. Feeding is associated with coughing. Liquids cause more symptoms than do solids.

Pneumonia is common and will recur after treatment. Abdominal distention is often present and is associated with excessive burping and flatus.

If the diagnosis of esophageal atresia is suspected, it is imperative that this diagnosis be promptly confirmed or excluded. Time is important, since significant pulmonary involvement can develop rather rapidly.

The simplest and safest way to settle the question is to pass a stiff radio-opaque, plastic 10F catheter down the mouth and into the stomach and confirm its position by chest roentgenogram. If the tube has reached the stomach, there is no esophageal atresia. The tube will pass only to about nine cm in the patient with EA. A soft, small plastic or rubber catheter may curl in the upper atretic esophagus. Infants have been encountered whose diagnosis was significantly delayed because it was assumed that the tube had reached the stomach when, in fact, it had coiled in the upper esophagus. Roentgenograms are simple and diagnostic. These roentgenograms also reveal the status of the lungs, heart size and configuration, the intestinal gas pattern, and the presence of vertebral anomalies. Absence of abdominal gas indicates esophageal atresia without a distal TEF (Fig. 2-2). In the presence of esophageal atresia, gas in the stomach confirms a distal TEF (Fig. 2-3). Associated intestinal obstruction will usually be recognizable on this one study.

Strongly suspected esophageal atresia may be confirmed by the injection of one ml of dilute barium. The upper esophagus ends blindly in the upper mediastinum, usually at the first through the fourth thoracic vertebra (Fig. 2-3). The one condition which may produce a radiographic picture which can be confused with that produced by EA is a traumatic pseudodiverticulum of the pharynx (Fig. 2-4). This is a rare occurrence, with symptoms similar to those of EA. Barium-contrast roentgenograms may show a pouch extending below the carina. The pouch may not be as smooth as is the usual proximal esophageal pouch. The barium may stain the mediastinum and will not be removed by suction. Finally, the esophagus is in continuity with the stomach.[15]

If the contrast enters the trachea, it may have done so through a proximal TEF, through a laryngeal cleft, or simply by aspiration (Fig. 2-5). In any case, bronchoscopy done at the time of the first anesthetic can detect a cleft or proximal TEF. If not specifically looked for, a proximal pouch fistula may be overlooked. Such a fistula missed both preoperatively and at operation has occasionally been fatal.[9,16,27]

Demonstration of an isolated TEF (or of a postoperative recurrent TEF) may be very difficult indeed. Roentgenographic demonstration utilizing videotape or cinefluoroscopy may demonstrate a fistula which is not seen with an ordinary barium swallow. This should be the first alternate approach, since it does not require an anesthetic (Fig. 2-6). If a fistula is demonstrated, its level should be accurately determined, since this factor will dictate a cervical or thoracic operative approach.

If a suspected isolated fistula is not demonstrated by the above procedure, bronchoscopy should be undertaken under general anesthetic using a ventilating bronchoscope with a fiberoptic light source and a telescopic lens system. Careful inspection of the membranous trachea will usually demonstrate the fistula if one is present (Fig. 2-7). Suspicious areas should be probed with a 3F or 4F ureteral catheter. If a fistula is present, the catheter should be passed through it and the esophageal end retrieved endoscopically and brought out through the mouth. Manipulation and palpation of the catheter help to localize the fistula at operation. A roentgenogram documents the level of the fistula (Fig. 2-8).

Esophagoscopy may be utilized to locate the difficult isolated TEF if bronchos-

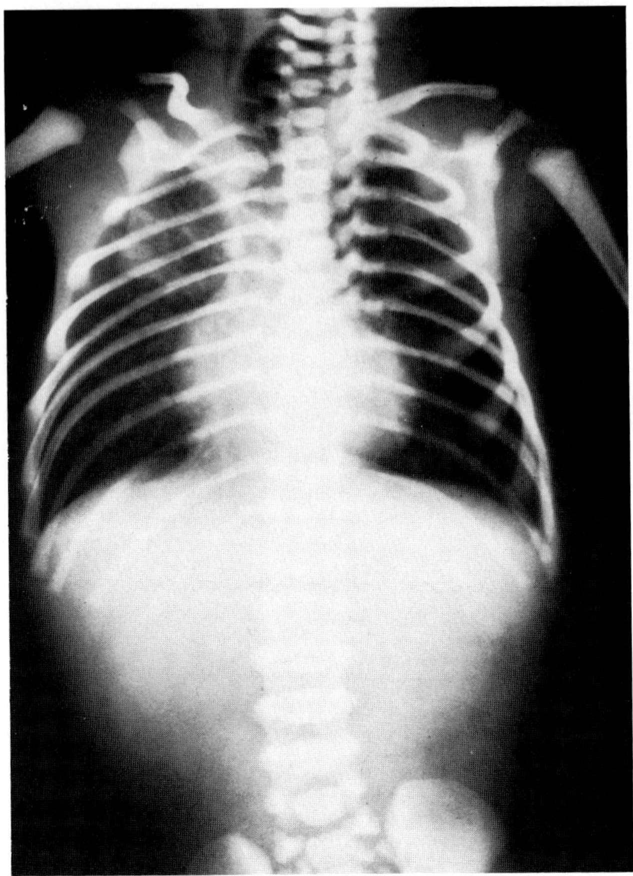

**Figure 2-2.** Esophageal atresia without tracheoesophageal fistula. There is a dilated, air-filled proximal esophagus. Lack of gas in the abdomen implies a lack of fistula to the trachea. (A rare patient who is not vigorous or who has a small distal tracheoesophageal fistula will not show abdominal air on early films.)

copy has not been successful. Methylene blue placed through the endotracheal tube may be observed coming through the esophageal end of the fistula during positive pressure ventilation.

## OTHER CONSIDERATIONS

The infant's pulmonary status is of particular concern. Pneumonia and atelectasis are common and are detected by auscultation and chest roentgenogram. Small, premature infants should be evaluated for Idiopathic Respiratory Distress Syndrome (IRDS).

Associated anomalies are present in half the patients (Table 1-1). They are the major cause of death in patients with esophageal atresia and TEF. The lesions which

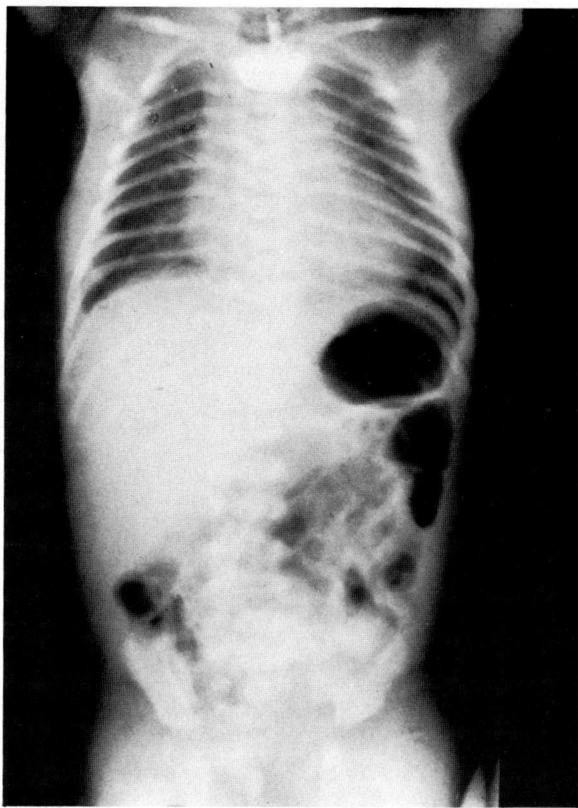

**Figure 2-3.** Esophageal atresia and distal tracheoesophageal fistula. The barium-filled proximal esophageal pouch ends blindly at the level of T4. Gas in the stomach and intestine confirms the presence of a fistula from the trachea to the distal esophagus.

**Table 2-1**
*Incidence of Associated Anomalies*

|  | Survey[23] (1058 patients) | Present Series (100 patients) |
|---|---|---|
| CHD | 113 (10%) | 17 |
| GI | 241 (23%) | 15 |
| MS | 161 (15%) | 15 |
| Pulmonary | 19 (1.5%) | 7 |
| CNS | 35 (3%) | 5 |
| GU | 109 (10%) | 5 |
| Chromosomal | 28 (2.5%) | 3 |
| Other | 43 (4%) | 33 |

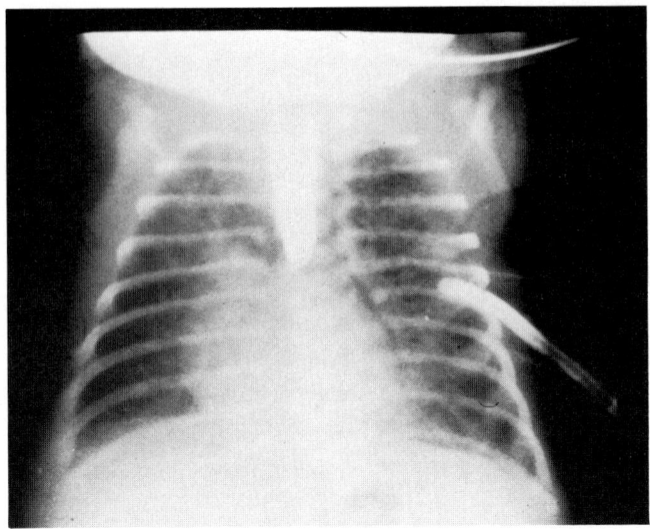

**Figure 2-4.** Pharyngeal pseudodiverticulum. Symptoms and roentgenogram may be confused with those of esophageal atresia. The diverticulum tends to be irregular and may extend to a lower level than is true in esophageal atresia. This X-ray was taken 18 hours after the barium was injected. In the case of esophageal atresia, the barium is easily removed.

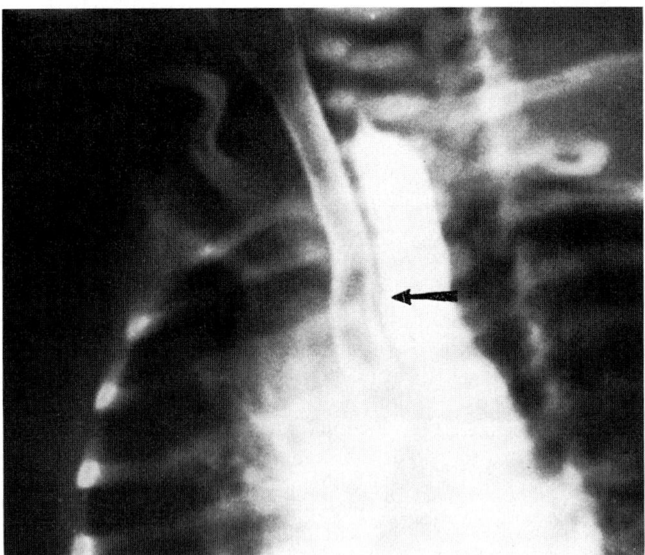

**Figure 2-5.** Esophageal atresia and proximal tracheoesophageal fistula. Barium injected into the proximal pouch reached the trachea through a proximal tracheoesophageal fistula which can be seen (arrow) in this patient. Aspirated barium or a laryngeal cleft can cause similar findings. Bronchoscopy is usually necessary to make the distinction.

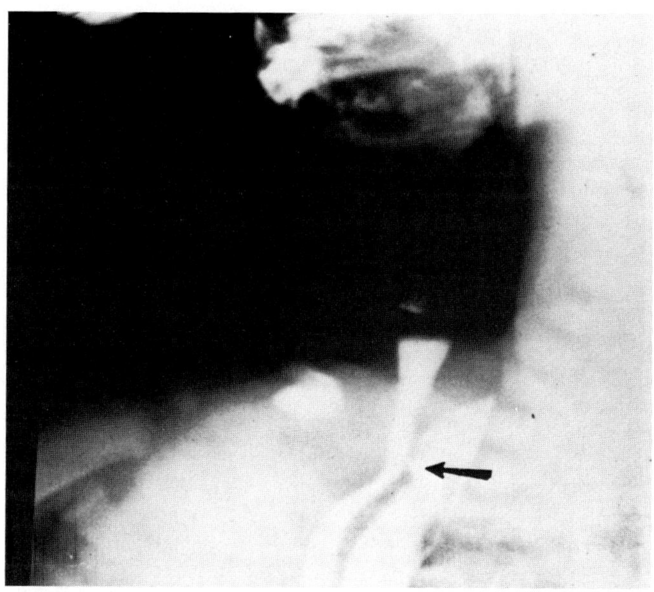

**Figure 2-6.** Isolated tracheoesophageal fistula without esophageal atresia. While demonstrated nicely here (arrow) by barium swallow, it is often not seen radiographically.

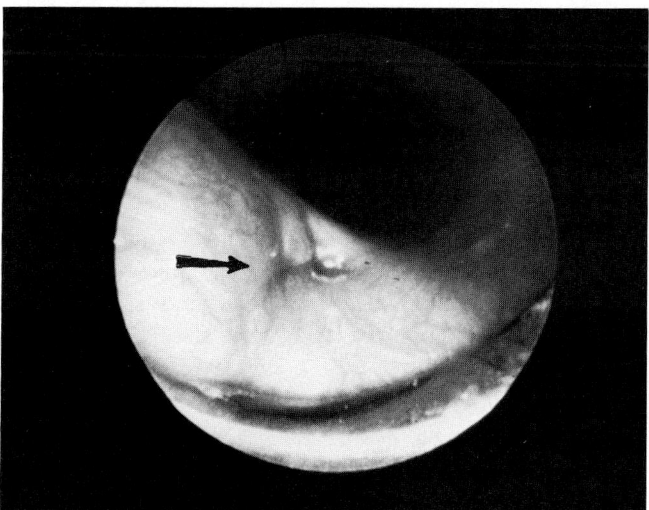

**Figure 2-7.** Isolated tracheoesophageal fistula (arrow) without esophageal atresia is seen endoscopically in the membranous
portion of the trachea at any level from the cricoid to the carina.

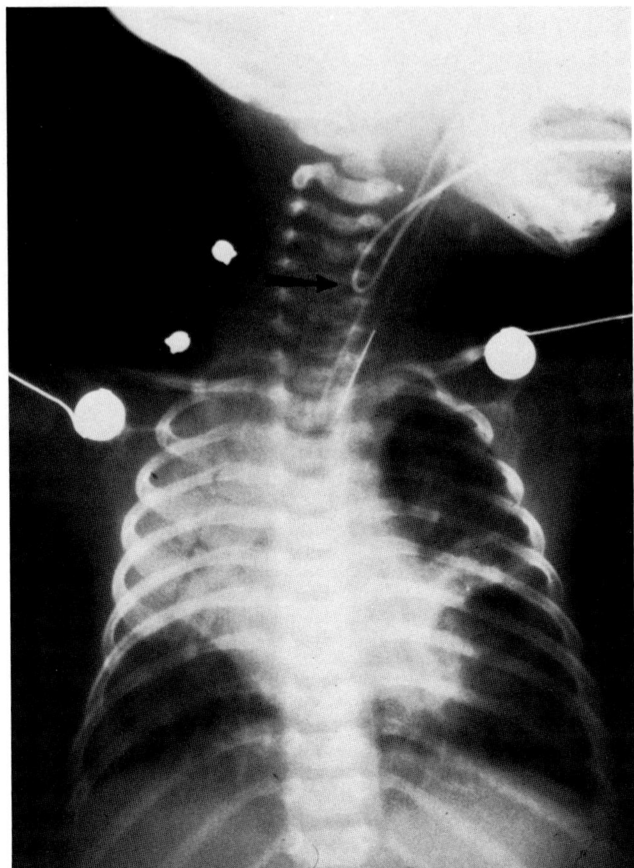

**Figure 2-8.** Esophageal atresia with proximal and distal tracheoesophageal fistula. The proximal tracheoesophageal fistula
is located in the midcervical level and is demonstrated by the
loop of the ureteral catheter passed through the fistula (arrow).
There are extensive right upper-lobe and left mid-lung field
infiltrates.

pose the greatest immediate threat to life are congenital heart disease and intestinal or
anal atresia. Each patient should be specifically evaluated for heart disease. Cardiac
investigation should be done if there is a murmur, cyanosis, or heart failure, or if the
chest roentgenogram reveals an abnormality of heart size or configuration. The patient
with cyanotic congenital heart disease or congestive heart failure should undergo
cardiac catheterization prior to esophageal repair.

One specific associated anomaly, the only effect of which is to present technical
problems at the time of repair, is a right aortic arch, which occurs in about five percent
of infants with esophageal atresia.[5,20,40] A right-sided aortic arch is present in one-
fourth of patients with Fallot's tetralogy. Often, on plain films of the chest the side of
the arch is obvious. If not, a CAT scan or sonogram may be used in localizing the side
of the arch. The location of an umbilical artery catheter to the right of the thoracic
spine indicates a right arch.

Duodenal atresia is the most commonly associated intestinal atresia. This is readily detected on the original roentgenogram, which should include the entire abdomen. Jejunal or ileal atresia should also be obvious. An imperforate anus is easily detected by physical examination. Many other associated anomalies are important, but not likely to be an immediate threat to life or to interfere with the surgical treatment of the esophageal atresia. Associated congenital anomalies occur with greater frequency and severity in the premature than in the full-term infant.[13]

A pattern of associated anomalies has been described which is referred to as the VATER association.[39] This includes vertebral defects, anal atresia, tracheoesophageal fistula with esophageal atresia, and radial and renal dysplasia.[28] Often, only two or three of the defects are present in a given patient. This association does not represent a distinct, simple, etiologic syndrome, but does suggest that when one of these anomalies is present a search should be made for the others.[3] Perhaps the CRAVET association would be a more accurate acronymn, since it includes cardiac anomalies, which are not only common but are the most lethal of the associated anomalies.

## THERAPY

In order to minimize further respiratory deterioration, all infants with esophageal atresia should have the proximal pouch immediately decompressed with a sump suction catheter. Both the sitting position at 45 degress or the prone position minimize regurgitation through the TEF into the trachea. The infant should be started on antibiotics as soon as the diagnosis is made. The patient is then evaluated for size and maturity, pulmonary status, and the presence and severity of associated anomalies. The complicating factors will determine the therapeutic approach.

Healthy babies of over 1300 grams who have no pneumonia or major associated anomalies are candidates for prompt primary repair. The author performs gastrostomy at the time of repair. While it is not essential in all patients, it is helpful in most.

Those who have pneumonia-atelectasis as their only complicating factor are treated by correction of the pulmonary complication, followed by primary repair. This is best accomplished by proximal pouch sump suction and by decompression gastrostomy to prevent further gastric reflux into the trachea. Antibiotics, pulmonary physiotherapy, high humidity, and occasional tracheal aspiration are added. Clearing the pneumonitis may require two or three days, but sometimes extends to a week or more. During this time, the patient is maintained on intravenous feedings. When the lungs have cleared as determined by physical examination and chest roentgenogram, the primary repair is undertaken.

Recognition of the importance of improving the pulmonary status prior to repair has been a major factor in improving survival rates.

The small premature baby (less than 1300 grams) who is not vigorous may require more time than is usual for evaluation and to establish a positive nitrogen balance. Proximal pouch suction should be combined with gastrostomy for decompression to prevent gastroesophageal reflux into the trachea. Parenteral nutrition, either central or peripheral, will allow the infant to establish a positive metabolic state. If there are no major associated anomalies, usually one to two weeks is sufficient to allow stabilization and satisfactory weight gain. This delayed primary repair has been most helpful in treatment.

An occasional premature infant will develop Idiopathic Respiratory Distress Syndrome and will require ventilatory support. This may be difficult or impossible in the presence of a distal TEF. Positive-pressure ventilation will force air through the fistula into the stomach or the proximal pouch rather than expanding the lungs. Satisfactory ventilation may not be possible without division of the TEF. After the lungs have cleared, esophageal repair is undertaken. (Fig. 2-9)

The most challenging group of patients to manage are those with major associated anomalies. The plan of management for each of these infants must be individualized. Many of the anomalies, such as skeletal, facial, hand, and genitourinary anomalies, pose no initial threat to life and will not interfere with primary repair of the esophageal atresia and TEF. Every patient should undergo a radiographic evaluation of the urinary tract following repair of EA/TEF because many abnormalities are occult yet very serious.[2]

The more serious anomalies require an early estimation as to which is the more immediate risk to life: the esophageal atresia or the associated anomaly. The most threatening condition should be corrected first. Delayed primary approach with proximal pouch decompression and prompt gastrostomy can be undertaken while the associated anomaly is treated. Associated anomalies requiring a neonatal operation in a series of 100 patients are listed in Table 2-2.

The patient with a low imperforate anus may have a perineal fistula of sufficient size to require merely dilatation until after the EA/TEF is corrected. Colostomy for a high rectal atresia may be performed concomitantly with gastrostomy as the initial procedure. Delayed primary repair of the esophageal anomaly should then follow in a day or two.

Intestinal atresia presents a somewhat more complicated problem. If the intestinal atresia is at the duodenal level, gastrostomy for gastric decompression to prevent reflux is the first order of business. Either the duodenal atresia or the esophageal atresia may be repaired at the time of gastrostomy if the baby is in good general condition (Fig. 2-10). It is probably wise not to proceed with repair of both the esophageal and duodenal

**Table 2-2**
*Associated Anomalies Requiring
Neonatal Operation
(100 patients)*

| | |
|---|---|
| Cardiac | |
|     tetralogy complex | 3 |
|     PDA | 2 |
| GI | |
|     imperforate anus (colostomy) | 5 |
|     duodenal atresia | 3 |
|     gastroschisis | 1 |
|     gastric web | 1 |
|     pyloric stenosis | 1 |
| Pulmonary | |
|     laryngeal cleft | 1 |
|     tracheal stenosis (tracheostomy) | 1 |
|     tracheomalacia (tracheostomy) | 1 |

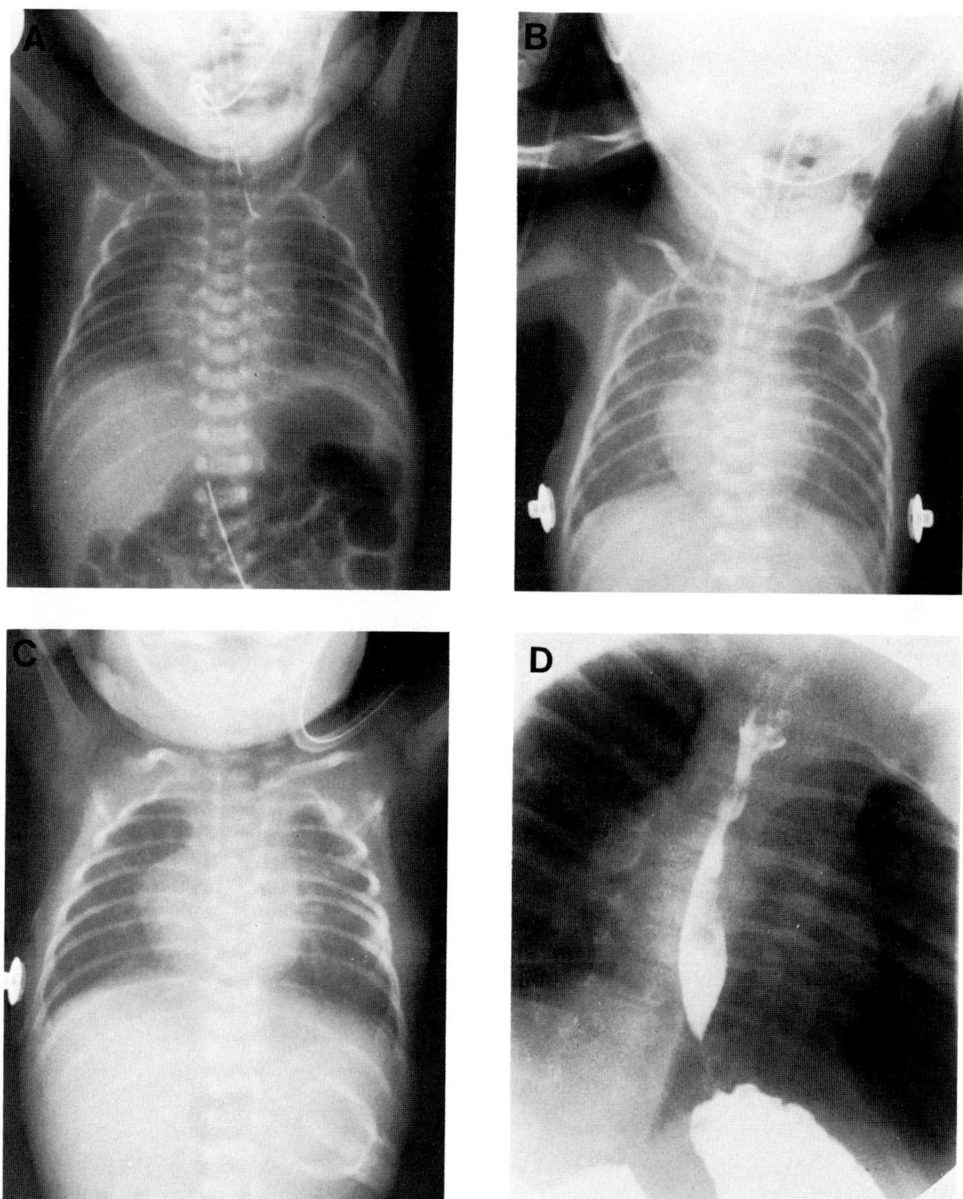

**Figure 2-9.** (A) A one-day-old, 1320-gm male with esophageal atresia with distal tracheoesophageal fistula and Idiopathic Respiratory Distress Syndrome. (B) Shortly after admission, a gastrostomy was performed for decompression and a central venous line positioned for nutrition. (C) His IRDS worsened, requiring ventilatory support. He also developed congestive heart failure secondary to a patent ductus arteriosus. Through the left chest, the tracheoesophageal fistula was divided and sutured (to facilitate ventilatory support) and the patent ductus was ligated (day 4). (D) Ten days later, the esophagus was repaired through the right chest.

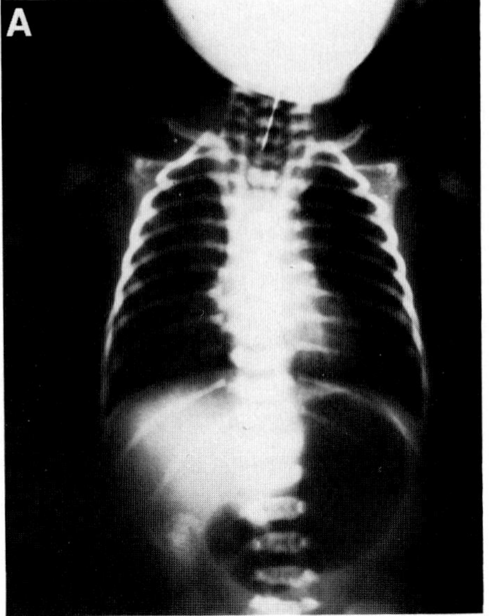

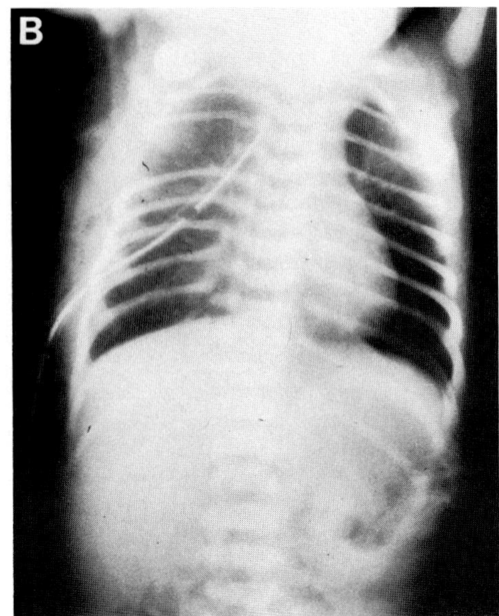

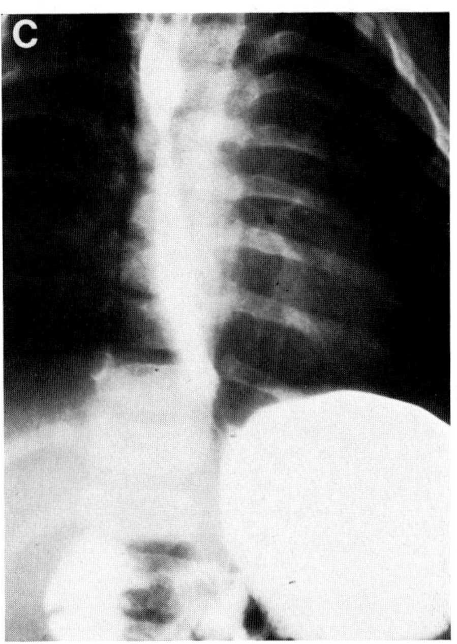

**Figure 2-10.** (A) A six-hour-old, 1800-gm female with dilated, air-filled, proximal esophagus (esophageal atresia), air in the dilated stomach (distal tracheoesophageal fistula), and air in the duodenum but not in the small bowel (duodenal atresia). There is also a hemivertebra at L5. Shortly after admission, a gastrostomy and repair of the duodenal atresia and insertion of a ventral venous line were performed. (B) One week later, the esophageal atresia and tracheoesophageal fistula were repaired. (C) She did well, with good function of the esophagus and duodenum.

atresia at the same time. A central venous line should be placed for parenteral nutrition at the time of gastrostomy. Jejunal or ileal atresia prevents a gastrostomy from providing adequate intestinal decompression. The intestinal atresia should be corrected at the time of gastrostomy, followed a few days later by esophageal repair.

Associated cardiac anomalies present the most difficult problem. Cyanotic congenital heart disease is apt to require operative intervention in the neonatal period. Cardiac catheterization will probably be required for accurate diagnosis and estimate of the seriousness of the lesion. For patients with transposition of the great vessels, a balloon septostomy at the time of catheterization often provides adequate palliation. For many patients with a tetralogy complex (including pulmonary and tricuspic atre-sia), a systemic pulmonary artery shunt may be required (Fig. 2-11); this is often more urgent than the esophageal repair. A Blalock subclavian-pulmonary artery shunt is the preferred shunt procedure and, like the esophageal repair, is best performed through the side of the chest opposite the aortic arch. This usually means that the esophageal repair follows a few days after the shunt through the same incision.

An isolated ventricular septal defect rarely produces neonatal congestive heart failure. A patent ductus arteriosus, on the other hand, may cause congestive heart failure in the neonatal period or may complicate the care of a premature infant with IRDS. Symptoms produced by a patent ductus arteriosus may necessitate its ligation. Division and suture of the TEF may be done through the left chest at the same time. Subsequent esophageal repair will be by means of a right thoracotomy.

## OPERATIVE TECHNIQUE

Operative repair of esophageal atresia with distal TEF may be a technically difficult procedure because of the disparity in size between the upper and lower esophageal segments and because the anastomosis must often be performed under some tension. The approach is through the chest opposite the aortic arch. A retropleural repair is safer than is a transpleural repair. An esophageal anastomotic leak produces the least morbidity when the intact pleura confines the leak and allows it to seal. A leak following transpleural repair results in empyema and is more often associated with continued leakage and sepsis than is retropleural repair. The retropleural approach is best accomplished by resecting the fourth rib subperiosteally, incising the deep layer of periostium to reach the plane between the endothoracic fascia and the pleura. The parietal pleura is reflected from the inner surface of the ribcage. Dissection is carried posteriorly from the apex of the chest to well below the incision. As the mediastinum is approached, the first two or three intercostal veins are divided and the azygos vein reflected anteriorly with the pleura. This is done to reduce the chance of entering the pleura. If a small opening is made in the pleura, it should be closed and the advantages of the retropleural approach preserved. The vagus nerve is a good landmark, since it courses down the mediastinum and runs along the distal esophageal segment. The latter should be freed to its junction with the trachea. The fistula is then transected at the trachea so that no residual pouch is left on the back of the trachea and the trachea is not narrowed. The tracheal end is then closed with fine, interrupted nonabsorbable sutures. The distal pouch should not be extensively dissected because of its segmental blood supply.

The proximal pouch is then identified in the upper mediastinum. Identification and dissection of the upper pouch can be facilitated by intermittent pressure on a large tube placed in the upper pouch by the anesthesiologist. Traction sutures are placed in the tip of the proximal pouch, which should be dissected well up into the neck. A known proximal fistula is dissected free, divided, and the ends sutured. Adjacent pleural or mediastinal tissue is pulled between the divided ends of the fistula. Even without prior knowledge of a proximal fistula, it is important to dissect the plane between the proximal pouch and the trachea as far as possible into the neck in order to expose a previously unrecognized fistula if one is present.

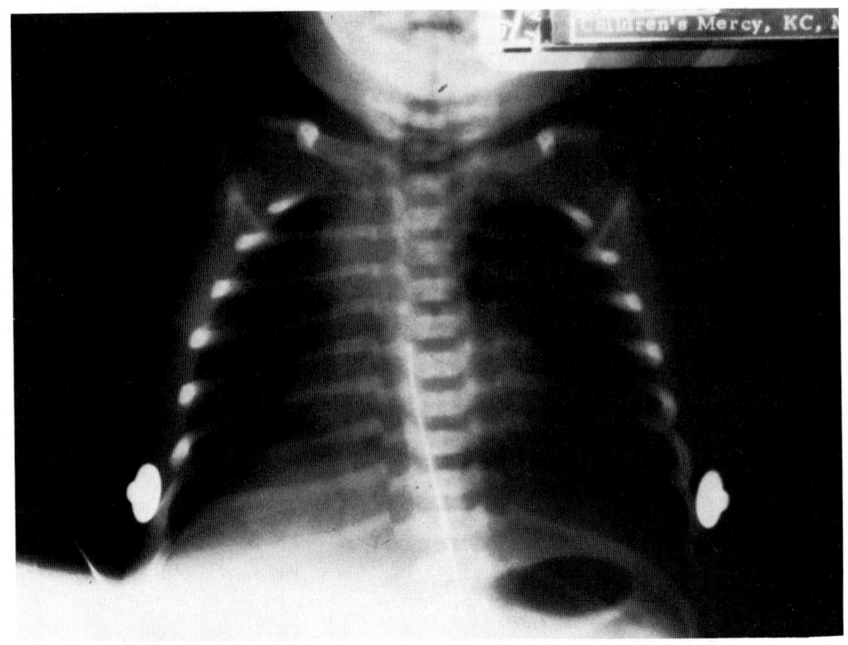

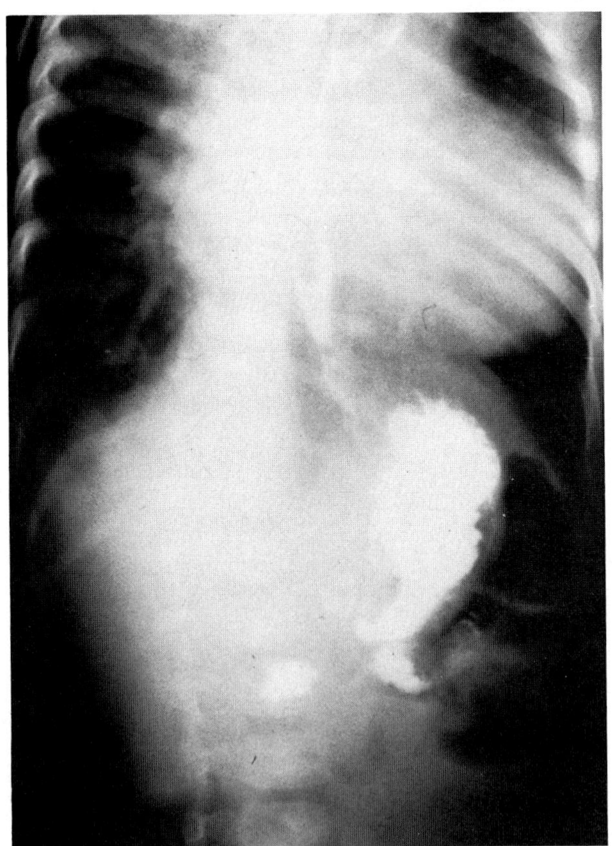

Figure 2-11

After freeing the proximal pouch as far as is feasible, the ends of the esophagus are approximated. The gap may be so long that there is too much tension for a safe anastomosis. A circular myotomy down to the submucosa allows elongation of the upper pouch.[34] Two or three myotomies may be safely performed with about a centimeter of length obtained from each.[8]

The tip of the proximal pouch is then excised. There is always a considerable disparity in size and thickness of the esophageal wall between the proximal and distal segments. Two types of anastomosis are popular. The simplest is a full-thickness single layer using fine, nonabsorbable, interrupted sutures. The other is the telescoping anastomosis described by Haight. The proximal pouch muscularis is freed from the mucosa for a centimeter. The mucosa of the proximal pouch is then sutured full thickness to the distal esophagus. A second layer of sutures is then placed to pull the upper pouch muscularis down over the first suture line. Fine, nonabsorbable sutures are used throughout. The single layer anastomosis carries the slightly higher risk of leak, while the Haight anastomosis is a little more likely to form a stricture. The differences are not great. A drainage tube is left in the retropleural, periesophageal space for ten days, because leaks have occurred as late as nine days after repair.

The greatest technical problem is encountered in the management of the patient with a long gap between the two ends of the esophagus. This is most pronounced in those patients with esophageal atresia without a distal TEF (either with or without a proximal pouch fistula). A long gap also results if the proximal pouch is short and/or the distal fistula connects with the airway at the carina or lower. Stretching of the proximal pouch probably is worthwhile if a proximal fistula is not present.[24] This is accomplished by passing a Bakes dilator into the proximal pouch, stretching it downward into the mediastinum for a few seconds two or three times a day. Three or four weeks may be required to obtain maximum length. The distal pouch can also be stretched upward by passing the dilator through the gastrostomy and into the distal segment.[31] This manual technique has been modified to include the placement of metal cylinders in the proximal and distal sections of the pouch, placing the patient in an intermittent magnetic field which causes magnetic attraction of the metallic dilators to each other. This allows the esophagus segments to be stretched hundreds of times during a day.[21]

The patients in whom a long gap is recognized or suspected preoperatively should have the neck as well as the chest prepared at operation. This allows a second cervical incision, permitting a much easier dissection of the proximal pouch to a significantly higher level than is possible through the thoracic incision alone. It also greatly facilitates the exposure of the proximal pouch for one, two, or even three circular myotomies (Fig. 2-12). A short distal segment (without TEF) may be extensively mobilized and a circular myotomy may be performed without impairing the blood supply.

---

**Figure 2-11.** A one-day-old, 2920-gm male with esophageal atresia and distal tracheoesophageal fistula was cyanotic on admission with a PaO2 of 25. He had a dilated proximal pouch, air in the stomach, a boot-shaped heart, and oligemic lung fields. The umbilical artery catheter along the right side of the vertebral column indicated a right aortic arch. Cardiac catheterization revealed a severe Fallot's tetralogy. A Waterston aorta to pulmonary artery shunt was performed through the right chest. (B) He improved and one week later the esophageal atresia and tracheoesophageal fistula were repaired through the left chest (opposite side from the aortic arch).

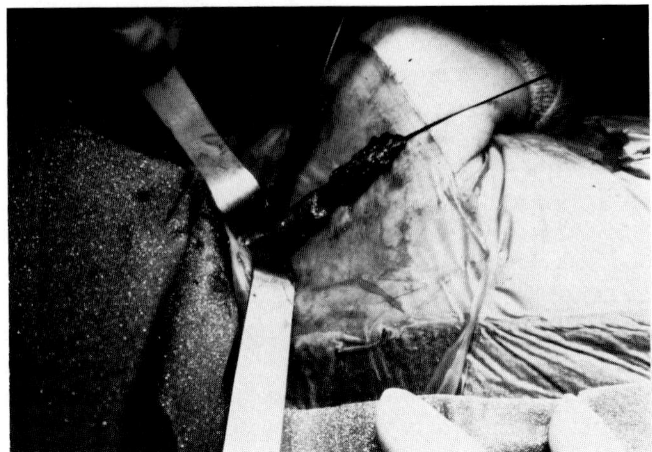

**Figure 2-12.** When a long gap between the esophageal ends is suspected, either because of esophageal atresia without distal fistula or because of a high pouch, prepping and draping of the neck permits a cervical incision which greatly facilitates high proximal pouch dissection and circular myotomy. Only one myotomy is shown here, but two or three can be made with much better exposure than is possible through a thoracotomy alone.

Through the use of some or all of these maneuvers, the esophageal ends can usually be approximated even though there may be considerable tension. The use of a retropleural approach with a chest drainage tube usually allows satisfactory management of an anastomotic leak with anticipated healing.

There are still a few patients in whom the ends cannot be approximated. In these patients, the proximal pouch is brought out as a cervical salivary fistula and the distal pouch sewn over. At about a year of age, the gap between the two ends is bridged using a colon interposition or a reverse gastric tube (See Chapter 5).

Patients with isolated TEF without associated atresia usually present a less challenging technical problem. Once the diagnosis and level have been confirmed, the approach can be selected. If the fistula is at T2 or higher, the approach should be cervical; if it is at T3 or T4, a thoracic retropleural approach gives better exposure. A ureteral catheter placed through the fistula endoscopically, with both ends brought out the mouth, facilitates location of the fistula at operation.

For the high TEF, a right cervical approach is usually employed. The plane between the trachea and esophagus is developed. The fistula is identified and divided. The ends are closed with fine, nonabsorbable, interrupted sutures. Adjacent tissue is interposed between the ends or the esophagus is rotated slightly and fixed in this position in order to prevent contact between suture lines. In the rare patient with a recurrence of high isolated TEF, the second operation is best done through the side of the neck opposite the original procedure. This approach affords the least scarring and least chance for damage to the recurrent nerve.

The thoracic approach to the isolated TEF is on the side opposite the aortic arch. Division and suture of the fistula is similar to that employed during the cervical approach.

**Table 2-3**
*Waterston Risk Classification—*
*EA and TEF**

|         | Birth Weight  | Associated Major Anomalies |
|---------|---------------|----------------------------|
| Group A | >2500 gm      | none                       |
| Group B | 1800–2500 gm  | none                       |
| Group C | <1800 gm      | present                    |

* The presence of significant pneumonia moves the patient into the next greater risk group.

## POSTOPERATIVE CARE

The patient is maintained on intravenous fluid replacement and antibiotics with particular attention to pulmonary toilet. The endotracheal tube is usually removed when the patient fully reacts from anesthesia. The pharynx is suctioned frequently with a catheter marked so that it is not long enough to reach and disturb the esophageal anastomosis. Occasionally, endotracheal suction is required. If thick secretions or atelectasis are a problem, a dilute solution of N-acetylcystine is injected into the trachea and suctioned.

Gastrostomy feedings are started on the first or second postoperative day (in the uncomplicated case) and clear liquids by mouth on the next day. Formula is offered the following day. Formula not taken by mouth is fed by gastrostomy. The gastrostomy tube is usually removed at about the tenth day.

The healthy infant who is treated by immediate primary repair usually enjoys a benign postoperative course. For those infants who have had significant pulmonary problems preoperatively, small, premature infants, or those who have major associated anomalies, the postoperative period tends to be a greater problem.

A variety of complications may arise which must be recognized and treated. Mortality is closely related to the Waterston high-risk group, i.e., those who have major associated anomalies (Table 2-3).[47] Prematurity and pulmonary problems are less serious. Table 2-4 depicts the overall mortality rate, both early and late, in 100

**Table 2-4**
*EA-TEF (100 patients) Deaths Related to Waterston*
*Risk Groups*

|                    | Group A (41 pts.) | Group B (31 pts.) | Group C (28 pts.) | Total |
|--------------------|-------------------|-------------------|-------------------|-------|
| Preoperative deaths | 0                | 0                 | 3                 | 3     |
| Post-repair deaths  | 0                | 2                 | 1                 | 3     |
| Late deaths         | 1                | 3                 | 6                 | 10    |
| Total               | 1                | 5                 | 10                | 16    |

consecutive patients with EA and/or TEF. Three patients died in the neonatal period prior to repair of associated anomalies. Three patients died in the postoperative period related to the operative repair—two from esophageal anastomotic leak and sepsis and one from a ruptured stomach and peritonitis. Two other patients died of associated anomalies a month or more after repair of associated anomalies. (One had patent ductus arteriosus and persistent fetal circulation; the other had associated duodenal atresia, imperforate anus, and laryngotracheoesophageal cleft.) All other patients left the hospital alive. There was one late death from esophageal atresia at the time of gastric tube repair for long gap atresia. The other late deaths were related to associated anomalies, particularly congenital heart disease.

An esophageal anastomotic leak is the most frequent early major postoperative complication of the treatment described. It occurs in about one-sixth of patients. If the anastomosis has been performed extrapleurally and if the mediastinum is well drained, contamination does not usually result in uncontrollable infection. The leak usually heals spontaneously. Antibiotics are administered, oral intake is stopped, and nutrition is maintained by vein, gastrostomy, or duodenal tube feeding. In the last 100 patients of the author's group, there have been 16 anastomotic leaks, nine of which responded to the above therapy and healed spontaneously. Five patients developed a recurrent tracheoesophageal fistula, presumably resulting from a leak. Two patients died with sepsis as the major cause of death.

Symptoms of a recurrent TEF are the same as those of an isolated tracheoesopha-geal fistula. The diagnosis is difficult and is approached in the same manner as was previously described for isolated TEF. A recurrent fistula occurs at the site of the previous fistula. It is important to consider the possibility of a previously unrecognized upper pouch fistula.[16] A recurrent fistula will not close spontaneously, so it requires operative division and suture. Recurrent fistulas are usually approached through the previous operative incision. The exception to this is the recurrent high, isolated TEF, which is best approached through the side of the neck opposite the original approach.

Anastomotic esophageal strictures are the most common late postoperative com-plication and are frequently associated with gastroesophageal reflux.[38] Control of gastroesophageal reflux (GER) is important in control of the stricture. Aggressive treatment for GER has been associated with a significant reduction in anastomotic strictures. Strictures should be treated by means of dilatation in order to prevent aspiration and weight loss; most will respond. An occasional patient who does not respond will be improved by an injection of triamcinolone into the stricture site.[22] Rarely, a tenacious stricture will require resection. Of the last 100 patients in the author's series, 24 required at least one esophageal dilatation and two required resec-tion of a persistent stricture. Most strictures develop and become symptomatic in the first year or two of life. An occasional older child who has had no esophageal symp-toms for years will present with an esophageal foreign body, usually lodged at the anastomotic site.

Gastroesophageal reflux is common in patients with esophageal atresia. Symptoms are the same as in patients without EA: cough, apnea, recurrent pneumonia, failure to thrive, and stricture (either anastomotic or distal esophageal). In this group of patients, there are often other explanations for these symptoms, so a thorough evaluation is necessary. Barium esophagram or barium through the gastrostomy is usually diagnos-tic. The magnitude of the gastroesophageal reflux is assessed by esophageal pH moni-toring.

The mechanism of reflux is probably related to altered anatomy as well as disturbed function. There is almost always sufficient gap between the two ends of the esophagus to necessitate some freeing of the distal esophagus in order to create an anastomosis with only modest tension. This may result in some decrease in the length of the intra-abdominal esophagus and may straighten the angle of His. Esophageal peristalsis is always disturbed as a part of the lesion which interferes with prompt clearing of the esophagus after a reflux episode. Prolonged esophageal contact with refluxed gastric contents promotes stricutre formation. In some patients, delayed gastric emptying is a contributing factor.[26] Whatever the mechanism, gastroesophageal reflux is frequently a problem for patients following repair of esophageal atresia.[1,37,43] A study of Haight's early patients as adults showed that 60 percent still had moderate to severe gastroesophageal reflux.[36] Twenty-four of the last 100 patients in the author's series had significant symptomatic reflux. Nine of these responded to medical therapy, while 15 required fundoplication.

## POSTOPERATIVE RESPIRATORY DISTRESS

Stridor, persistent barking cough, respiratory distress, and even apnea will occur in some patients. Causes of these symptoms include tracheomalacia,[4,7] a distended proximal pouch pressing on the back of the trachea as well as anterior compression,[12] gastroesophageal reflux with aspiration,[1] and recurrent tracheoesophageal fistula. Barium esophagram to demonstrate the size of the proximal esophagus and to detect gastroesophageal reflux is necessary. Bronchoscopic assessment of tracheomalacia and a possible recurrent tracheoesophageal fistula are also indicated. Recurrent TEF requires division. Gastroesophageal reflux may be treated medically or surgically. Proximal pouch dilatation requires a search for the obstruction, which is treated if present. Aortopexy to relieve anterior vascular compression as well as to pull the trachea forward away from the dilated pouch may be helpful. Aortopexy is also useful in some patients with tracheomalacia.[41]

Associated anomalies are not only the major cause of death in the neonatal period, they also pose the greatest risk for the next several years of life. Congenital heart disease remains the leading cause of mortality.

Altered esophageal motility with poorly coordinated peristalsis involves the distal esophagus and, to some extent, the proximal esophageal segment.[11] Esophageal dysfunction of this sort lasts forever. It can be documented with both manometric studies and cine-esophagrams.[42] As children grow, they learn to compensate for their altered peristalsis. The upright position uses gravity to help esophageal emptying. Frequent swallowing of liquids helps wash down ingested food. A long-term study of esophageal function in 42 patients with esophageal atresia and TEF found that 26 percent were asymptomatic, 64 percent had occasional dysphagia, and 10 percent had frequent dysphagia.[32]

Patients who have required a circular myotomy of the proximal pouch will demonstrate ballooning at the myotomy site on a postoperative barium study. (Fig. 2-13) Swallowing function, however, is similar to that in other patients following repair of esophageal atresia.[25]

Postoperatively, a hacking cough is present in most patients, which decreases with time and has usually disappeared by one year of age. The etiology of this cough is

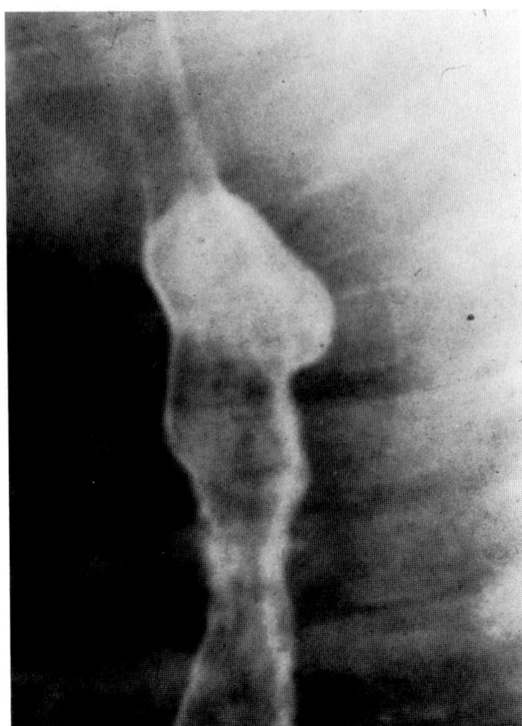

**Figure 2-13.** Barium swallow following circular myotomy
shows a ballooning at the myotomy site which does not appear
to hamper function.

not known, but it may be secondary to chronic aspiration. Pulmonary symptoms such
as cough, bronchitis, and pneumonia occur more frequently in children suffering from
EA or TEF than in normal children. Fifty-eight of 100 patients followed for more than
a year post-repair had been hospitalized for a respiratory infection.[10] Those patients
followed over eight years post-repair had an average of three bouts of bronchitis/year.

While some patients continue to have esophageal and respiratory symptoms even
after years, most of these symptoms are minor. The large majority of patients do well
over the years.

## REFERENCES


1.  Ashcraft KW, Goodwin CD, Amoury RA, et al: Early recognition and aggressive treat-
    ment of gastroesophageal reflux following repair of esophageal atresia. J Ped Surg 12:317–
    321, 1977.
2.  Atwell JD, Beard RC: Congenital anomalies of the upper urinary tract associated with
    esophageal atreasia and tracheoesophageal fistula. J Ped Surg 9:825–831, 1974.
3.  Barry JE, Auldist AW: The VATER association—One end of a spectrum of anomalies.
    Am J Dis Child 128:769–771, 1974.
4.  Benjamin B, Cohen D, Glasson M: Tracheomalacia in association with congenital tra-
    cheoesophageal fistula. Surgery 79:504–508, 1976.

5. Berdon WE, Baker DH, Schullinger JN, et al: Plain film detection of right aortic arch in infants with esophageal atresia and tracheoesophageal fistula. J Ped Surg 14:436–437, 1979.
6. Blackburn WR, Amoury RA: Congenital esophago-pulmonary fistulas without esophageal atresia: An analysis of 260 fistulas in infants, children and adults. Rev Surg 23:153–175, 1965.
7. Davies MRQ, Cywes S: The flaccid trachea and tracheoesophageal anomalies. J Ped Surg 13:363–367, 1978.
8. deLorimier AL, Harrison MR: Long gap esophageal atresia. J Thorac Cardiovasc Surg 79:138–144, 1980.
9. Dudgeon DL, Morrison CW, Woolley MM: Congenital proximal tracheoesophageal fistula. J Ped Surg 7:614–619, 1972.
10. Dudley NE, Phelan PD: Respiratory complications in long-term survival of esophageal atresia. Arch Dis Child 51:279, 1976.
11. Duranceau A, Fisher SR, Flye MW, et al: Motor function of the esophagus after repair of esophageal atresia and tracheoesophageal fistula. Surgery 82:116–123, 1977.
12. Filler RM, Rossello PA, Lebowitz RL: Life-threatening anoxic spells caused by tracheal compression after repair of esophageal atresia: Correction by surgery. J Ped Surg 11:739–748, 1976.
13. German JC, Mahour GH, Woolley MM: Esophageal atresia and associated anomalies. J Ped Surg 11:299–306, 1976.
14. German JC, Mahour GH, Woolley MM: The twin with esophageal atresia. J Ped Surg 14:432–435, 1979.
15. Girdany BR, Sieber WK, Osman MF: Traumatic pseudodiverticulum of the pharynx in newborn infants. New Engl J Med 2:237–240, 1969.
16. Goodwin CD, Ashcraft KW, Holder TM, et al: Esophageal atresia with double tracheoesophageal fistula. J Ped Surg 13:269–273, 1978.
17. Gray SW, Skandalakis JE: Gray SW, Skandalakis JE (Eds.): Embryology for Surgeons. Philadelphia: WB Saunders Company, pp. 69–79, 1972.
18. Haight C, Towsley HA: Congenital atresia of the esophagus with tracheoesophageal fistula and end to end anastomosis of esophageal segments. Surg Gynecol Obstet 76:672–688, 1943.
19. Haller JA Jr, Brooker AF, Talbert JL, et al: Esophageal function following resection studies in newborn puppies. Ann Thorac Surg 2:180, 1966.
20. Harrison MR, Hanson BA, Mahour GH, et al: The significance of right aortic arch in the repair of esophageal atresia. J Ped Surg 12:861–870, 1977.
21. Hendren WH, Hale JR: Electromagnetic bougienage to tighten esophageal segments in congenital esophageal atresia. New Engl J Med 293:428–432, 1975.
22. Holder TM, Ashcraft KA, Leape LL: The treatment of patients with esophageal strictures by local steroid injections. J Ped Surg 4:646–653, 1969.
23. Holder TM, Cloud DT, Lewis JE, et al: A survey of its members by the Surgical Section of the American Academy of Pediatrics. Pediatrics 34:542–549, 1974.
24. Howard R, Meyers N: Esophageal atresia: A technique for elongating the upper pouch. Surgery 58:725, 1965.
25. Janik JS, Filler RM, Ein SH, et al: Long term follow-up of circular myotomy for esophageal atresia. J Ped Surg 15:835–841, 1980.
26. Jolley SG, Johnson DG, Roberts CC, et al: Patterns of gastroesophageal reflux in children following repair of esophageal atresia and distal tracheoesophageal fistula. J Ped Surg 15:857–862, 1980.
27. Kafrouni G, Baich CH, Woolley MM: Recurrent tracheoesophageal fistula: A diagnostic problem. Surgery 68:889–894, 1970.
28. Kirkpatrick JA, Wagner ML, Pilling CP: A complex of anomalies associated with tra-

cheoesophageal fistula and esophageal atresia. Am J Roentgenol Radium Ther Nucl Med 95:208–211, 1965.

29. Kluth D: Atlas of esophageal atresia. J Ped Surg 11:901–919, 1976.
30. Ladd WE: The surgical treatment of esophageal atresia and tracheoesophageal fistula. New Engl J Med 230:625, 1944.
31. Lafer DJ, Boley SJ: Primary repair in esophageal atresia with elongation of the lower segment. J Ped Surg 1:585–587, 1966.
32. Laks H, Wilkinson RH, Schuster SR: Results following correction of esophageal atresia with tracheoesophageal fistula: A clinical and cinefluorographic study. J Ped Surg 7:591–597, 1972.
33. Levin NL: Congenital atresia of the esophagus with tracheoesophageal fistula: Report of successful extrapleural ligation of fistulous communication and cervical esophagostomy. J Thoracic Surg 10:648, 1940–1941.
34. Livaditis A: Esophageal atresia: A method of overbridging large segmental gaps. Z Kinderchir 13:298, 1973.
35. Myers NA: Oesophageal atresia: The epitome of modern surgery. Ann R Coll Surg Engl 54:277, 1974.
36. Orringer MB: Discussion of Randolph JG, Altman RP and Anderson KD, Selective Status in Infants With Esophageal Atresia. J Thorac Cardiovasc Surg 74:335–342, 1977.
37. Parker AF, Christie DL, Cahill JL, et al: Incidence and significance of gastroesophageal reflux following repair of esophageal atresia and tracheoesophageal fistula and the need for anti-reflux procedures. J Ped Surg 14:5–8, 1979.
38. Pieretti R, Shandling B, Stephens CA: Resistant esophageal stenosis associated with reflux after repair of esophageal atresia: A therapeutic approach. J Ped Surg 9:355–357, 1974.
39. Quan L, Smith DW: The VATER Association. J Ped Surg 82:104, 1973.
40. Schimke RN, Leape LL, Holder TM: Familial occurrence of esophageal atresia: A preliminary report. Birth Defects: Original Article Series 8:22–23, 1972.
41. Schwartz MZ, Filler RM: Tracheal compression as a cause of apnea following repair of tracheoesophageal fistula: Treatment by aortopexy. J Ped Surg 15:842–848, 1980.
42. Shepard R, Fenn S, Sieber WK: Evaluation of esophageal function in postoperative esophageal atresia. Surgery 59:609–617, 1966.
43. Shermeta DW, Whitington PF, Seto DS, et al: Lower esophageal sphincter dysfunction in esophageal atresia: Nocturnal regurgitation and aspiration pneumonia. J Ped Surg 12:871–876, 1977.
44. Sieber WK, Sieber AM: Esophageal manometry in postoperative esophageal atresia with tracheoesophageal fistula. Kinderchir (supplement) 17:109, 1974.
45. Smith EI: The early development of the trachea and esophagus in relation to atresia of the esophagus and tracheo-esophageal fistula. Contr Embryol Carnegie Inst Wash #245, 36:41, 1957.
46. Sulamaa M, Gripenberg L, Ahvenainen EK: Prognosis and treatment of congenital atresia of the esophagus. Acta Chir Scandinav 102:141, 1952.
47. Waterston DJ, Bonham-Carter RE, Aberdeen E: Oesophageal atresia: Tracheo-oesophageal fistula: A study of survival in 218 infants. Lancet, April 21, 1962, pp. 819–822.

L. R. Scherer
Jay L. Grosfeld

# 3

# Congenital Esophageal Stenosis, Esophageal Duplication, Neurenteric Cyst and Esophageal Diverticulum

Congenital anomalies of the esophagus present a significant challenge to the clinician with respect to both diagosis and treatment. If one excludes the variants of esophageal atresia and tracheoesophageal fistula, many of the remaining anomalies are relatively rare. These unusual lesions may become clinically apparent in the newborn period and, in some instances, the anomaly may present in the adult. Since esophageal atresia with or without tracheoesophageal fistula is covered extensively elsewhere in this text, this chapter will concern itself with esophageal stenosis due to a congenital web or tracheobronchial remnant, esophageal cyst or duplication, neurenteric cyst, or congenital esophageal diverticulum.

## EMBRYOLOGY

In order to understand these unusual esophageal anomalies, a review of the embryologic development of the esophagus is helpful. Initially, the embryo forms as a flat disc consisting of an ectodermal and entodermal layer. During the third week of development, there is an invagination of ectodermal cells along the primitive streak.[32] Once these cells have invaginated, they migrate between the ectodermal and entodermal layers laterally, forming the mesodermal germ-cell layer. Specialized ectodermal cells extending cephalad from the primitive pit form a tube-like structure, known as the notochordal process, extending to the prochordal plate by the 17th day of development (Fig. 3-1). By the 18th day of development, the floor of the notochordal process fuses with the underlying entoderm and the lumen of the notochordal process disappears as notochordal cells proliferate to form the solid notochord. With the formation of the notochord, differentiation of intraembryonal mesoderm into segmented blocks of epithelial cells and somites occurs, which causes separation of the notochord and

Pediatric Esophageal Surgery  
ISBN 0-8089-1776-5

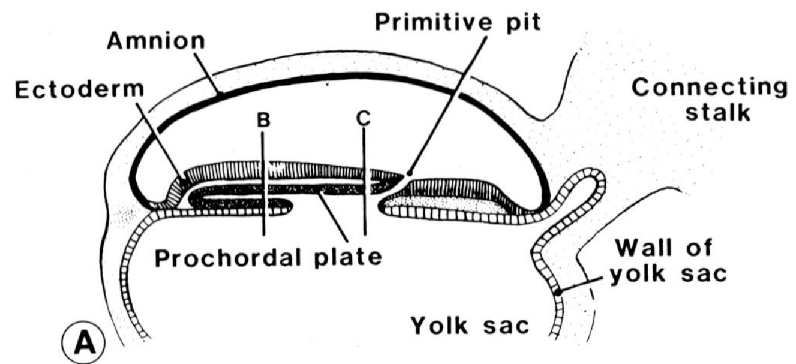


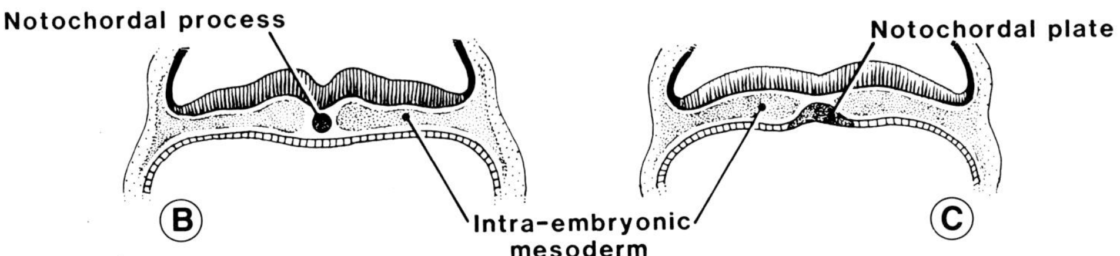


**Figure 3-1.** (A) Drawing of a cephalocaudal midline section through a 17-day-old embryo, depicting the formation of the notochord process extending from the primitive pit in a cephalic direction. By the 18th day, the process has fused, forming the notochord. (B) A transverse section through the trilaminar germ disc where the notochordal process persists. (C) Transverse section of disc where the entoderm and notochordal process are absent, while the entoderm and notochordal plate remain temporarily fused.

entoderm by the 20th day after fertilization. The embryo remains flat until the end of the third week, when cephalocaudal folding caused by rapid longitudinal growth of the central nervous system and lateral folding due to the shaping of rapidly forming somites creates flexion and lengthening of the embryo (Fig. 3-2). The formation of the gut occurs passively during this event with the inversion of the entodermal-lined yolk sac and incorporation of part of the yolk sac into the coelomic cavity (Fig. 3-2). The foregut differentiates into the esophagus and ventrally placed respiratory diverticulum (lung bud) at 22–23 days of development. The esophagus will develop from a small area between the diverticulum and the posteriorly located stomach dilatation (Fig. 3-2). As the esophagus and respiratory diverticulum lengthen, a groove in the floor of the esophagus forms. The lateral ridges that form along the posterior rim of the trachea begin to proliferate and join in the midline, dividing the foregut into the trachea and esophagus (tracheoesophageal septum). Due to the simultaneous elongation of the trachea and esophagus and the separation of the two foregut structures, the process is not completed before 34–36 days of gestation. At four weeks of development, the submucosal and muscular layers of the two foregut structures are present. The elongation process is actually an ascension of the pharynx from the diaphragm rather than a descent to the stomach, as the transverse septum of the diaphragm is stationary (Fig. 3-2). The final length of the fetal esophagus is achieved by the seventh week. At the completion of the separation phase and while the esophagus is lengthening, four primary folds develop by the tenth week. During the seventh and eighth weeks of development, there is rapid proliferation of epithelial cells, nearly filling the esophageal lumen, except for areas of vacuoles.[10] The vacuoles coalesce by the end of the tenth week to form a hollow tube. The primary epithelium of the fetal esophagus is ciliated epithelium, and, during the fourth month of development, stratified squamous epithelium begins to replace the ciliated cells intially in the midesophagus. Critical events in esophageal development include the separation of the notochord from the entoderm, the coalescence of the intraluminal vacuoles to form a lumen, and the partitioning of the foregut into the esophagus and trachea during the fourth intrauterine week.

## CONGENITAL ESOPHAGEAL STENOSIS AND ESOPHAGEAL DIAPHRAGM (WEB)

### Embryology and Histopathology

Esophageal stenosis in infancy can result from a congenital abnormality or from an acquired lesion related to esophageal mucosal injury. The most common cause of esophageal stenosis is related to reflux esophagitis. Other acquired causes include injury as a result of caustic chemical ingestion and trauma from foreign bodies.

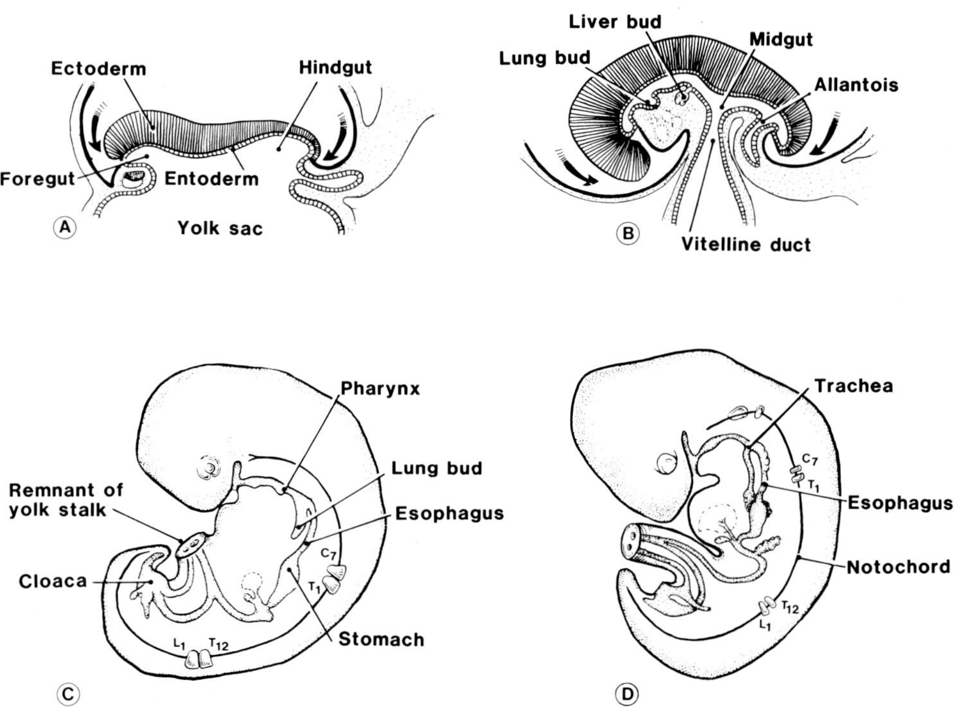


**Figure 3-2.** Drawings of various stages of embryologic development, using sagittal sections to demonstrate the cephalocaudal flexion and its effect on the development and position of organs in the entodermal-lined cavity. (A) 21-day-old embryo. (B) 28-day-old embryo. (C) 5-week-old embryo. (D) 6-week-old embryo. The lung bud develops between Stages A and B. As the drawings demonstrate, the lengthening of the esophagus occurs with cephalic lengthening and development of the pharyngeal pouches.

Three types of congenital esophageal stenosis have been described: (1) segmental hypertrophy of the muscularis and submucosal layers of the esophageal wall; (2) membranous web or diaphragm; and, (3) intramural rests of cartilagenous tracheobronchial tissue. The etiology of segmental hypertrophy is poorly understood, but may be related to a remnant of a perforated membranous web. The development of an esophageal web is similar to that of other mucosal diaphragms encountered elsewhere in the gastrointestinal tract. This developmental defect is associated with a failure to recanalize the lumen after the temporary solid cord stage at ten weeks' gestation. Using wax models, it has been theorized that the failure to recanalize the lumen of the esophagus is the probable cause of esophageal web as well as the etiology of the esophageal cyst.[10,30] Histologically, segmental hypertrophy and mucosal web contain only submucosal and mucosal components and not the wall of the esophagus.

The occurrence of tracheobronchial remnants in the esophagus was first reported in 1936 by Frey and Duschl[19] and, more recently, similar cases have been documented by other authors (Table 3-1). In the developing embryo, the respiratory diverticulum (lung bud) forms during the fourth week (Fig. 3-2). A tracheoesophageal septum forms from cellular proliferation from lateral ridges originating in the lateral walls of the foregut between the diverticulum and the esophagus. With the subsequent cranial elongation of the esophagus and respiratory tree, it is conceivable that mesenchymal cells of the respiratory diverticulum may become embedded in the wall of the developing esophagus. The remnant of tissue consists of respiratory seromucinous glands, respiratory epithelium, and crescent-shaped mature cartilage; a single case report exists of pancreatic remnant causing stenosis.[11] The resulting stenosis is due to the extrinsic compression of the heterotopic tissue and the inelasticity of the cartilage.

There have been several case reports of stenosis or web associated with tracheoesophageal fistula. A very unusual form of esophageal stenosis was reported, in which a short fistulous tract connected the lower and upper pouch of an infant with esophageal atresia and tracheoesophageal fistula.[29] One patient has been reported to have esophageal stenosis along with an H-type tracheoesophageal fistula.[46] Several cases have been described in which esophageal atresia without tracheoesophageal fistula have been associated with stenosis due to a failure in foregut epithelial cellular proliferation with continued foregut elongation.[42] An esophageal web with tracheoesophageal fistula has also been reported.[4]

## Clinical Presentation

The clinical presentation of a complete esophageal web is similar to that of esophageal atresia. Symptoms include excessive salivation, choking spells, and respiratory distress. Inability to pass a catheter into the stomach confirms the diagnosis. The infant with a web almost always presents in the newborn period, while those babies with a ruptured or incomplete web, segmental hypertrophy of the muscularis, or stenosis secondary to a tracheobronchial remnant tend to present later in infancy when solid food intake begins. Table 3-1 lists a collective review of published series concerning tracheobronchial remnants. Although the age at the time of clinical presentation varies from one day to 57 years, the age of onset of symptoms is usually less than one year. This condition affects both sexes equally. As a group, all causes of congenital stenosis of the esophagus have a similar presentation, which includes dysphagia, vomiting during meals, failure to thrive, and regurgitation of undigested food particles.

Recurrent respiratory infection secondary to aspiration is also a common occurrence. These infants and children may have an increased incidence of associated anomalies, as also occurs in babies with esophageal atresia. Congenital esophageal web and esophageal stenosis are known to coexist with esophageal atresia, although the frequency is not truly known. In 1981, a review of the English, German, and Japanese literature collected 81 cases of tracheobronchial remnants causing congenital esophageal stenosis.[35] These cases were surveyed for the presence of associated anomalies, with a reported incidence of 17.3 percent, which is significantly lower than the 30–75-percent incidence of associated anomalies reported with esophageal atresia. The most commonly occurring anomalies included esophageal atresia with or without tracheoesophageal fistula, imperforate anus, and Down's syndrome.

## Diagnosis and Differential Diagnosis

Both radiologic and endoscopic evaluation are useful in obtaining a diagnosis. The chest X-ray will document the location of the oral gastric tube and presence of air in gastrointestinal tract below the diaphragm, which is helpful in the evaluation of an esophageal web or associated anomalies. A barium esophagram using an image intensifier, fluoroscopy, and cineradiography will identify the exact anatomic location of the lesion, allow for the evaluation of esophageal motility, and determine the presence of gastroesophageal reflux (Fig. 3-3). Over 90 percent of cases of congenital stenosis due to tracheobronchial remnant occur in either the lower third or distal end of the esophagus, whereas a majority of instances of congenital esophageal mucosal diaphragm occur in the middle third. On barium esophagram, the congenital web presents as a sharp shelf at the point of obstruction, whereas the tracheobronchial remnant reveals an abrupt narrowing of the distal esophagus with proximal esophageal dilatation. Endoscopy is another important diagnostic tool and may be therpeutic as well. Endoscopy may demonstrate the presence of a lesser degree of stenosis. Evidence of mucosal injury or esophagitis due to gastroesophageal reflux may be seen. Biopsy or dilatation of the esophagus may be performed if necessary.

Gastroesophageal reflux may present as esophageal stenosis due to stricture, even in the young infant. Diagnostic evaluation should include pH testing, manometry, and scintillation scanning if necessary to rule out reflux esophagitis. An adequate history will reveal whether or not stenosis is due to caustic ingestion, which is more commonly observed in toddlers than in small infants. Radiologic study should precede endoscopy, since occasionally a form of blind pouch may lie just beyond the stricture and, if not previously identified, may lead to esophageal perforation during endoscopy.

## Treatment

The initial therapy for congenital esophageal stenosis is dilatation. If the dilator passes easily, this can be continued first on a weekly basis, followed by bimonthly dilatations and calibrations of the esophagus for several months, until the stenosis is no longer destructing. At this time, the patient should be asymptomatic. Relief of the stricture should be documented by a contrast swallow.

If the bougie is difficult to pass, however, a gastrostomy should then be performed, followed by antegrade passage of a string through the gastrostomy site from a

**Table 3-1**
*Clinical and Histologic Findings of Esophageal Stenosis Due to Cartilaginous Tracheobronchial Remnants*

| Author | Age | Sex | Age at onset of Stenosis | Site of Stenosis | Histologic Components | | | Operative Method |
|---|---|---|---|---|---|---|---|---|
| | | | | | Carti-lage | Glands | Respi-ratory Epithe-lium | |
| Frey[19] | 19 yrs. | F | ? | distal end | + | + | − | Diagnosed at postmortem exam |
| M.G.H.(1947) | 43 yrs. | M | 28 yrs. | ? | − | − | + | Extramucosal excision |
| M.G.H.(1956) | 52 yrs. | M | 3 yrs. | distal end | + | + | + | Resection |
| Bergmann[7] | 57 yrs. | F | childhood | lower third | − | + | + | Resection |
| Spath[44] | 49 yrs. | F | birth | lower third | − | + | + | Resection |
| Kumar[31] | 10 mos. | F | 4 mos. | distal end | + | + | − | Resection |
| Paulino[37] | 8 mos. | F | birth | lower third | + | − | + | Resection |
| | 14 mos. | F | 6 mos. | distal end | + | + | + | Extramucosal excision |
| Ishida[27] | 17 mos. | M | 7 mos. | distal end | + | + | + | Resection |
| | 4 mos. | M | 6 mos. | distal end | + | + | + | Resection |
| | 5 mos. | M | 1 yr. | distal end | + | + | − | Resection |
| Goldman[21] | 1 day | F | birth | upper third (atresia) | + | + | − | Cervical esophagostomy |
| Fonkalsrud[18] | 1 yr. | F | 6 mos. | lower third | − | + | + | Resection |
| Anderson[2] | 8 yrs. | F | 7 mos. | distal end | + | − | + | Resection |
| Deiraniya[14] | 2 yrs. | F | 6 mos. | lower third | − | + | − | Resection (with colon interposition) |
| | 10 mos. | M | 5 mos. | lower third | + | + | − | Diagnosed at postmortem exam |
| Ohkawa[36] | 4 yrs. | M | 18 mos. | lower third | + | + | − | Resection |
| | 20 mos. | M | 9 mos. | distal end | + | + | + | Resection |
| | 19 mos. | M | 4 mos. | distal end | + | + | + | Resection |

| | | | | | | | | |
|---|---|---|---|---|---|---|---|---|
| | 4 yrs. | M | 8 mos. | distal end | + | + | ? | Resection |
| | 13 mos. | F | 7 mos. | distal end | + | + | ? | Myomectomy |
| Rose[40] | 7 mos. | ? | 7 mos. | distal end | + | + | + | Resection |
| | 8 yrs. | F | birth | distal end | + | + | + | Resection |
| Sneed[43] | 20 mos. | F | 6 mos. | distal end | + | + | + | Resection |
| Ibrahim[26] | 13 mos. | M | 6 mos. | distal end | + | + | + | Resection |
| | 6 yrs. | F | 18 mos. | distal end | + | + | − | Resection |
| Bar Maur[5] | 8 mos. | M | birth | distal end | + | + | − | Resection |


[19] From: Frey EK, Duschel L: Der Kardiospasmus. Ergeb Chirur Orthop 29:637, 1936. With permission.

From: Case Records of Massachusetts General Hospital (MGH) 1947. Case 33182. Congenital tracheobronchial cysts of the esophageal wall. N Engl J Med 236:172–174, 1947

From: Massachusetts General Hospital (MGH) 1956. Case 42411. N Engl J Med 255:707–710, 1956.

[7] From: Bergmann M, Charna RM: Tracheobronchial rests in the esophagus, their relation to some benign strictures and certain types of cancer of the esophagus. J Thorac Surg 35:97, 1958. With permission.

[44] From: Spath F, Ratzenhofer M: Ueber die angkborene Oesophagusstenose. Wien Klin Wochenschr 71:723, 1959. With permission.

[31] From: Kumar R: A case of congenital oesophageal stricture due to a cartilaginous ring. Br J Surg 49:533, 1962. With permission.

[37] From: Paulino F, Roselli A, Aprigliano F: Congenital esophageal stricture due to tracheobronchial remnants. Surgery 53:547, 1963. With permission.

[27] From: Ishida M, Tsuchida Y, Saito S, et al: Congenital esophageal stenosis due to tracheobronchial remnants, J Pediatr Surg 4:339, 1969. With permission.

[21] From: Goldman RL, Ban JL: Chondroepithelial choristoma of the esophagus associated with esophageal atresia. J Thorac Cardiovasc Surg 63:318, 1972. With permission.

[18] From: Fonkalsrud EW: Esophageal stenosis due to tracheobronchial remnants. Am J Surg 124:101, 1972. With permission.

[2] From: Anderson LS, Shackelford GD, Mancilla-Jimenez R, et al: Cartilaginous esophageal ring: A cause of esophageal stenosis in infants and children. Radiology 108:665, 1973. With permission.

[14] From: Deiraniya AK: Congenital oesophageal stenosis due to tracheobronchial remnants. Thorax 29:720, 1974. With permission.

[36] From: Ohkawa H, Takahashi H, Hoshino Y, et al: Lower esophageal stenosis in association with tracheobronchial remnants. J Pediatr Surg 10:453, 1975. With permission.

[40] From: Rose JS, Kassner EG, Jurgens KH, et al: Congenital esophageal strictures due to cartilaginous rings. Br J Radiol 48:16, 1975. With permission.

[43] From: Sneed WF, LaGarde DC, Kogutt MS, et al: Esophageal stenosis due to cartilaginous tracheobronchial remnants. J Pediatr Surg 14:786, 1979. With permission.

[26] From: Ibrahim NB, Sandry GJ: Congenital oesophageal stenosis caused by tracheobronchial strictures in the oesophageal wall. Thorax 36:465, 1981. With permission.

[5] From: BarMaor JA, Posen JA, Hamilton DG, et al: Congenital oesophageal stenosis due to cartilaginous tracheobronchial remnants. South Afr J Surg 21(1):43, 1983. With permission.

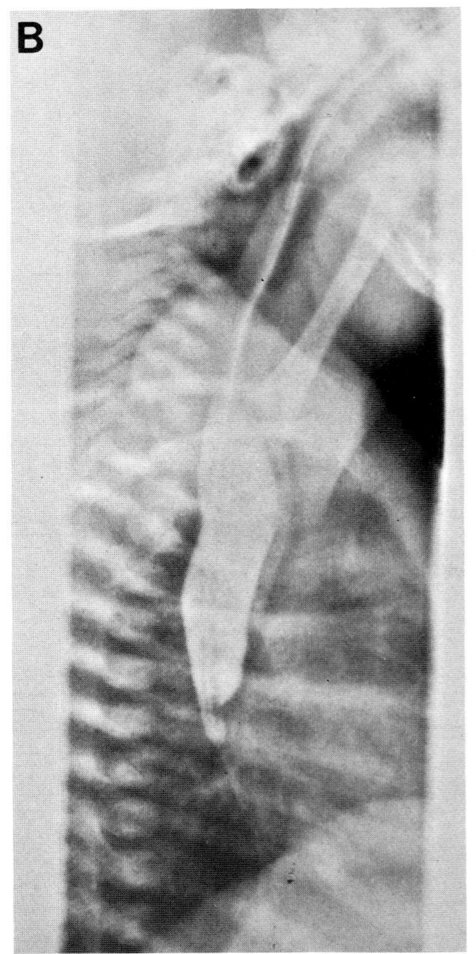

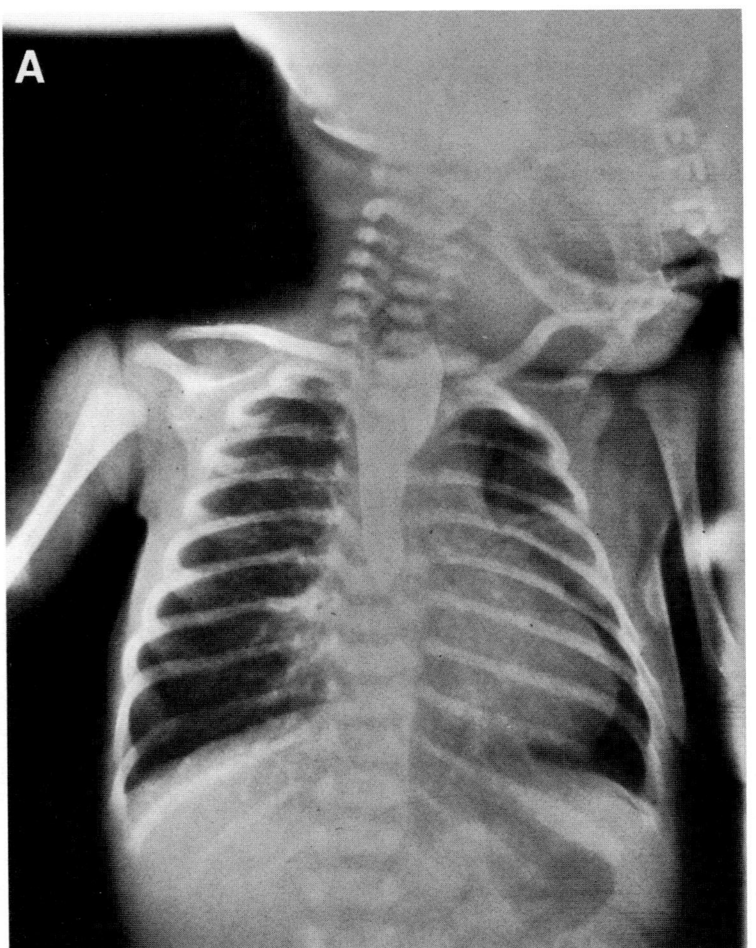

**Figure 3-3.** Posterantero and lateral projection of an esophagram revealing significant narrowing of the esophagus with proximal dilatation. This segmental hypertrophic congenital stenosis of the midesophagus responded well to repeated esophageal dilatation.

week to ten days later. Using the string as a guide, the stenosis is gently dilated with progressively larger tapered dilators of the Tucker type.

Esophageal dilatation has not been a successful method of treating tracheobronchial remnant stenosis and can actually be dangerous. One infant died following esophageal perforation secondary to dilatation of stenosis due to a tracheobronchial remnants[14] The remnant of tracheobronchial tissue includes a circumferential crescent of cartilage around the stenotic portion which prevents stretching and may lead to perforation. Surgical excision of the stenosis is required. Primary esophageal anastomosis is almost always possible. This resection may be accomplished either by a thoracic or abdominal approach, depending on the location of the lesion.

Endoscopic treatment of an esophageal web has been reported, with the web incised using electrocautery; an orogastric tube is passed and esophageal dilatation proceeds a week later.[25]

## FOREGUT DUPLICATION

### Embryology and Histopathology

The nomenclature of foregut duplication varies considerably according to whether the lesions are classified by anatomic site, embryology, or type of epithelial lining. A very practical classification of these congenital lesions is based on anatomic location and embryologic origin. According to this classification, three categories of intrathoracic foregut anomalies: bronchogenic cysts, intramucosal esophageal cysts, and enteric cysts (neurenteric cysts).[22] The term neurenteric cyst will be used in this discussion, as it most appropriately describes the origin of this anomaly. The current discussion will be limited to the latter two anomalies, leaving out bronchogenic cysts.

Intramural esophageal cysts or duplications share a common wall and may or may not communicate with the lumen of the normal esophagus. The cyst wall includes one or more layers of muscularis and includes a myenteric plexus. The epithelial lining may be ciliated columnar, squamous, or gastric. The embryologic origin of this lesion is considered to be a defect in the vacuolization process during the phase of epithelial proliferation in the seventh to tenth week of gestation. During the sixth week of embryologic life, there is a rapid proliferation of esophageal epithelial cells, which may occlude the esophageal lumen. Normally, the lumen is re-established by the formation and coalescence of vacuoles. It has been theorized that abnormalities in this process could lead to chains of fused vacuoles separate from the main lumen and thus result in the formation of esophageal duplications.[10] This appears, therefore, as an intramural lesion. The epithelial lining varies due to differences in the fetal mucosal origin.

Neurenteric cysts are anatomically closely related to esophageal duplication cysts, since they occur in the posterior mediastinum, adjacent or adherent to the esophagus and vertebral column (Fig. 3-4). The cyst wall is composed of the same histologic components; the difference is in their embryologic origin. Neurenteric cysts are derived from the foregut, prior to the development of the respiratory deverticulum. In the third week of gestation, the notochord forms from specialized cells of the ectoderm.[34,41] The notochord migrates dorsally with the proliferation of the mesodermal cells. If an adhesion forms between the notochord and the entoderm prior to this dorsal migration, two lesions may form: (1) the spinal column may not close ventrally in the

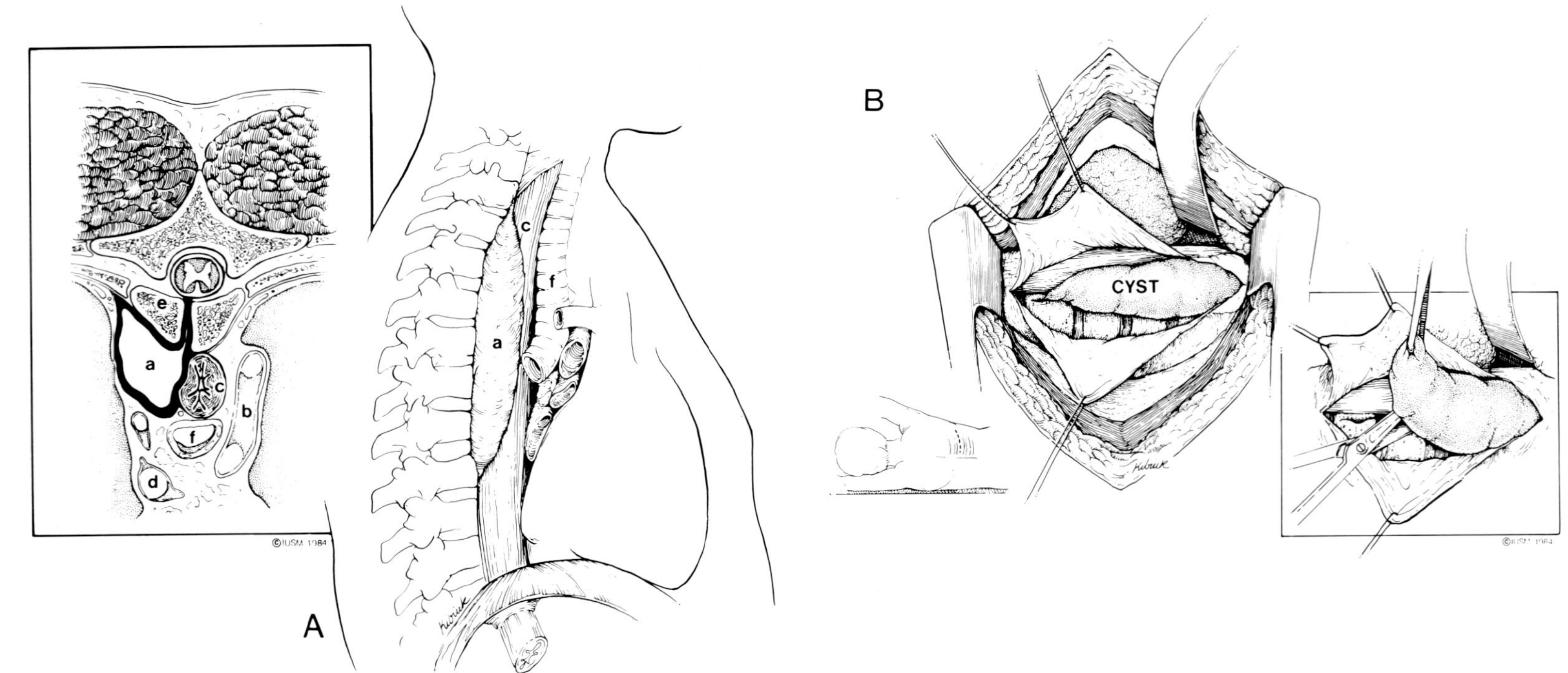



**Figure 3-4.** (A) Anatomic relationship of a neurenteric cyst: (a) neurenteric cyst; (b) aortic arch; (c) esophagus; (d) brachiocephalic artery; (e) bifid thoracic vertebrae; and, (f) trachea. The cyst in this drawing is attached to the dura of the spinal cord. The cyst may only have a fibrous attachment to the vertebrae or it may extend into the spinal cord. The cyst is only loosely attached to the esophagus whereas an esophageal duplication has a common wall with the esophagus. (B) Drawing depicting the surgical excision of a neurenteric cyst with the mediastinal pleura reflected as viewed from a right posterolateral thoracotomy. The cyst's vertebral attachment should be completely excised. During exploration, the surgeon should be aware of possible transdiaphragmatic extension.

area of that somite; and, (2) an entodermal tract or diverticulum associated with the notochord and foregut may persist, resulting in the formation of a neurenteric cyst. The cyst may remain in the thorax or it may have an intra-abdominal component as well, often attached to the duodenum or jejunum and possibly also communicating with their lumen. There may also be a communication with the spinal canal as a mass or a patent canal of Kovalevski. Intraspinal anomalies coexist with mediastinal masses in 25 percent of these patients (Fig. 3-4).[47]

## Associated Anomalies

The most frequent coexisting abnormality associated with the development of a neurenteric cyst are anomalies of the vertebral bodies of the lower cervical and upper thoracic regions. These include instances of spinabifida, hemivertebrae, fused verte-brae, or intraspinal mass. A majority of neurenteric cysts show only fibrous attachment to the vertebral column, but these are reported cases in which the cyst communicates within the dura.[39,47] The vertebral anomaly is associated only with neurenteric cysts. The overall incidence of vertebral anomalies in cases of neurenteric cyst is 80 percent (Table 3-2).

The second most common associated anomaly is an additional duplication of the small intestine. In a series of 65 patients with mediastinal cysts, eight instances of separate abdominal duplications were observed.[15] Similar observations in somewhat smaller series of duplications have been reported.[6,8,9,16]

## Clinical Presentation

Infants and children with esophageal duplication and neurenteric cyst present at any age and with a variety of symptoms (Table 3-2). Duplications should be consid-ered in the differential diagnosis of severe respiratory distress of the newborn.[24] In one review of the literature, 22 percent of esophageal duplications were found to occur in the upper third of the esophagus and were diagnosed in patients less than two years of age.[3] In older infants and children, symptoms include stridor, pneumonia, hemoptysis, chest pain, and cough. The older infant and child with a lesion occurring in the middle and lower mediastinum may have no symptoms. The duplication may simply be noted incidentally on a chest roeutgenogram. Respiratory symptoms do occur, however, in 50–90 percent of reported cases (Table 3-2). Gastroesophageal complaints occur in ten-15 percent of cases and include epigastric pain, vomiting, hematemesis, gagging, and dysphagia (Table 3-2). It is of importance to note that chest pain, gastrointestinal hemorrhage, or hemoptysis may be the presenting feature, due to ectopic gastric mu-cosa within the duplication which may cause ulceration and hemorrhage. Significant hemorrhage occurred from peptic ulceration in an esophageal duplication cyst,[1] with death resulting from exsanguination in another patient.[23] Ordinarily, all neurenteric cysts and more than 80 percent of esophageal duplications do not communicate with the esophageal lumen. As these lesions are lined with a secretory epithelium, they may fill with fluid and attain a large size, causing compression symptoms. Respiratory symptoms, a mediastinal mass, and a vertebral anomaly form a triad present in 70 percent of patients with neurenteric cysts; lesions located in the upper thorax present earlier and more often have respiratory symptoms. The lower- and middle-third lesions are asymtomatic in 35 percent of patients. In the 65 percent of patients who were

**Table 3-2**

*Clinical Findings of Reported Cases of Esophageal Duplications and Neurenteric Cysts*

| Author | No. of Pts. | Ages | Respiratory Symptoms | GI Symptoms | True Duplication | Neurenteric Cyst | Vertebral Anomaly | Gastric Mucosa |
|---|---|---|---|---|---|---|---|---|
| Gans[20] | 2 | NB to 6 yrs. | 1 | 0 | 2 | 0 | 0 | 0 |
| Grosfeld[23] | 6 | NB to 14 yrs. | 5 | 1 | 3 | 3 | 1 | 2 |
| Favara[16] | 6 | NB to 2 yrs. | 3 | 3 | 4 | 2 | 1 | 3 |
| Ahmed[1] | 6 | NB to 5 yrs. | 5 | 1 | 1 | 5 | 5 | 3 |
| Pokorny[38] | 3 | > 1 yr. | 2 | 2 | 1 | 1 | 0 | 1 |
| Bower[9] | 16 | NB to 16 yrs. | 9 | 3 | not described | | 3 | 7 |
| Cohen[12] | 8 | NB to 18 yrs. | 6 | 3 | 6 | 2 | 0 | 2 |
| Superina[47] | 15 | NB to 18 yrs. | not described | | 0 | 15 | 11 | 9 |
| Total | 62 | NB to 18 yrs. | 31 | 13 | 17 | 28 | 21 | 27 |

[20] From: Gans SL, Lackey DA, Zukerbraun L: Duplications of the cervical esophagus in infants and children. Surgery 63:849, 1968. With permission.

[23] From: Grosfeld JL, O'Neill JA, Clatworthy HW: Enteric duplications in infancy and childhood: An 18-year review. Ann Surg 172:83, 1970. With permission.

[16] From: Favara BE, Franciose RA, Akers DR: Enteric duplications. Am J Dis Child 122:501, 1971. With permission.

[1] From: Ahmed S, Jolleys A, Dark JF: Thoracic enteric cysts and diverticulae. Brit J Surg 59(12):963, 1972. With permission.

[38] From: Pokorny WJ, Sherman JO, Idriss FS: Mediastinal masses in infants and children. J Thorac Cardiovasc Surg 68:869, 1974. With permission.

[9] From: Bower RJ, Sieber WK, Kiesewetter WB: Alimentary tract duplications in children. Ann Surg 188(5):669, 1978. With permission.

[12] From: Cohen SR, Geller KA, Birns JW, et al: Foregut cysts in infants and children: Diagnosis and management. Ann Otol Rhinol Laryngol 91:622, 1982. With permission.

[47] From: Case 33182. Congenital tracheobronchial cysts of the esophageal wall. N Engl J Med 236:172–172, 1947 With permission.

symptomatic, Arbona et al. reported that gastroesophageal complaints were most common.[3]

## Diagnosis and Differential Diagnosis

In the present era, there are several modalities available for the diagnosis of a mediastinal mass, beginning with the plain roentgenogram in the Posteroanterior (PA) & lateral projections. The chest radiograph demonstrates the mass, its effect on neighboring structures, whether or not there is an air fluid level within the mass, and whether or not associated vertebral anomalies coexist (Fig. 3-5). A barium esophagram may be helpful in delineating the course of the esophagus or a communication with the cyst. (Fig. 3-5).[52] In the evaluation of the posterior mediastinal mass, where a vertebral anomaly and respiratory symptoms are noted or an intra-abdominal duplication is suspected, myelography has been recommended. All six patients reported in one series who had a chest mass, vertebral anomaly, and neurologic symptoms had an abnormal myelogram.[47] Myelography was also carried out on three additional patients without neurologic symptoms; two of these patients had intraspinal masses. Overall, 25 percent of patients reported showed positive findings on myelography.[47] Ultrasonography is useful in determining whether the mass is solid or cystic.[49] Similarly, computerized tomography may yield information concerning anatomy, characterics of the mass, and extension of the mass below the diaphragm of extension into the intraspinal area, when combined with myelography.[50] A review of 62 patients reported in eight series indicated that 44 percent of the patients had duplications that contained histologically proven ectopic gastric mucosa (Table 3-2). This suggests that a radioisotopic technetium scan may be helpful in delineating cysts with gastric mucosa which have the potential for hemorrhage due to peptic ulceration. Recent experience indicates that magnetic resonance imaging may give additional noninvasive information concerning the diagnosis of mediastinal masses. Enteric and esophageal duplication account for ten percent posterior mediastinal masses and for ten percent of all gastrointestinal duplications. The differential diagnosis includes lymphoma, fibroma, hemangioma, and a variety of neurogenic tumors (e.g., neuroblastoma, ganglioneuroma, neurilemoma, or neurofibroma).[17,51]

## Treatment

As it may be impossible to arrive at a correct preoperative diagnosis in many cases, and since the risk of malignancy in a mediastinal mass in childhood is 40 percent, operative removal of these cysts is indicated. Complete removal of the cyst is advised; however, it should be understood that these lesions are benign and that vital structures should be preserved (Fig. 3-4). If complete resection is not possible, the mucosa may be stripped from the muscular wall if necessary in order to excise mucus-producing tissues and ectopic gastric mucosa.[45] During the operative procedure, the surgeon should be aware of possible transdiaphragmatic extension and/or attachments or communication with the spinal canal.[48] If there is an intraspinal extension, the symptomatic component should be removed first. If both portions of the mass are asymptomatic, then the intraspinal component should be removed first, as is done in dumbell neurogenic tumors in children to avoid neurologic sequelae (Fig. 3-4). Transdiaphragmatic extension of a neurenteric cyst may be excised at the time of the original

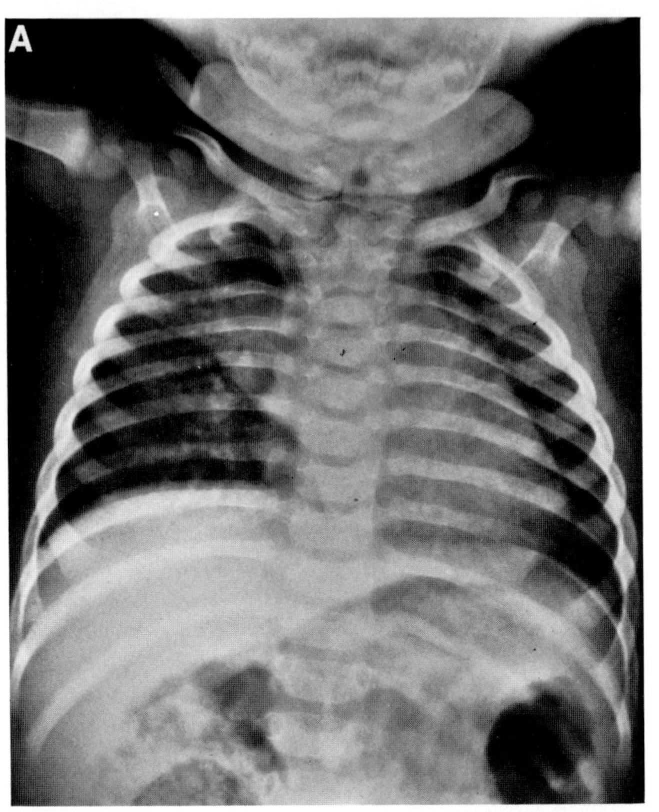

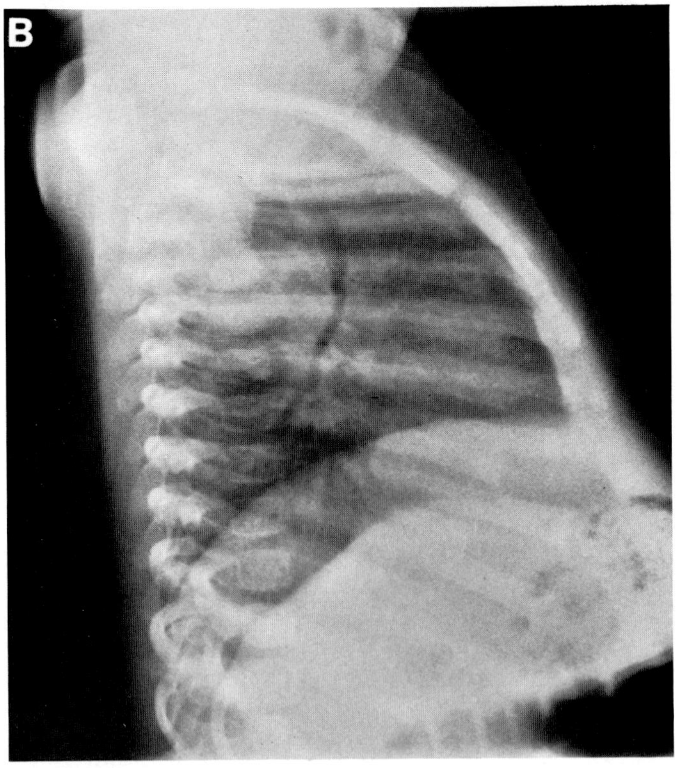

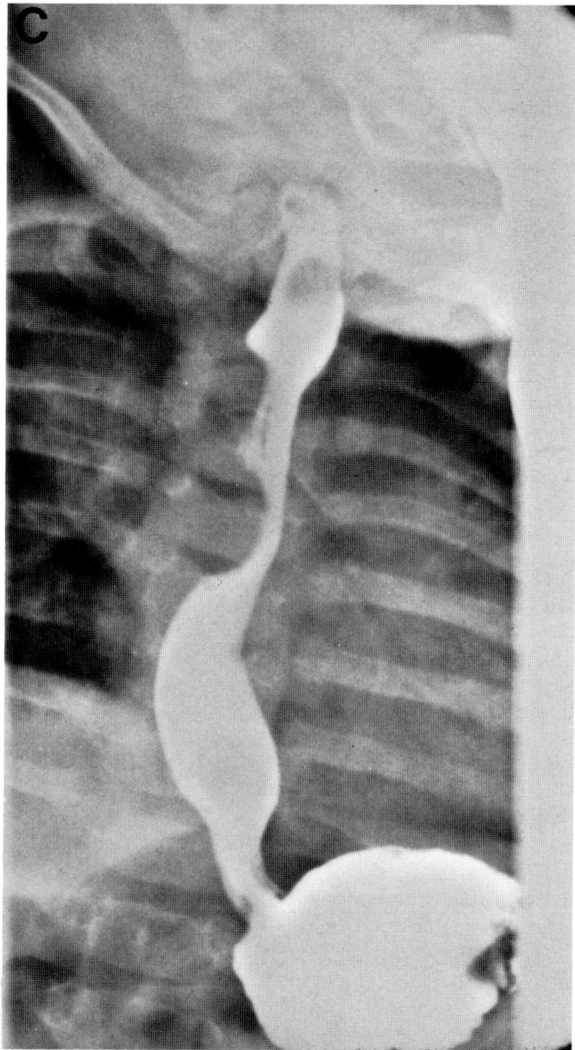

Figure 3-5. (A and B) Posteroanterior and lateral chest radiographs. Midposterior mediastinal mass and thoracic hemivertebrae. (C) Esophagram reveals a posterior mediastinal mass impinging upon the midesophagus.

procedure through a separate abdominal incision, or the lower extent may be oversewn and approached at a second procedure, depending on the intraoperative stability of the patient.

Mortality was evaluated from a review of 62 reported cases (Table 3-3). The cumulative data regarding postoperative mortality show three deaths related to sepsis and aspiration. Two other deaths occurred before operation could be carried out due to hemorrhage from a gastric mucosal-lined cyst and sudden respiratory obstruction. Among the 62 patients reviewed, there were six complications ranging from a wound

**Table 3-3**
*Complications and Deaths of Reported Cases of Esophageal
Duplications and Neurenteric Cysts*

| Author | No. of Cases | Complications | Deaths |
|---|---|---|---|
| Gans[20] | 2 | 1 (wound infection) | 0 |
| Grosfeld[23] | 6 | 0 | 1 (nonoperative hemorrhage) |
| Favara[16] | 6 | 1 (wound infection) | 0 |
| Ahmed[1] | 6 | 1 (respiratory failure) | 0 |
| Pokorny[38] | 3 | 0 | 0 |
| Bower[9] | 16 | 1 (aspiration) | 2 (nonoperative respiratory arrest) |
| Cohen[12] | 8 | 1 (aspiration) | 1 |
| Superina[47] | 15 | 0 | 1 (nonoperative respiratory arrest) |
| Total | 62 | 5 | 5 |

[20] From: Gans SL, Lackey DA, Zukerbraun L: Duplications of the cervical esophagus in infants and children. Surgery 63:849, 1968. With permission.

[23] From: Grosfeld JL, O'Neill JA, Clatworthy HW: Enteric duplications in infancy and childhood: An 18-year review. Ann Surg 172:83, 1970. With permission.

[16] From: Favara BE, Franciose RA, Akers DR: Enteric duplications. Am J Dis Child 122:501, 1971. With permission.

[1] From: Ahmed S, Jolleys A, Dark JF: Thoracic enteric cysts and diverticulae. Brit J Surg 59(12):963, 1972. With permission.

[38] From: Pokorny WJ, Sherman JO, Idriss FS: Mediastinal masses in infants and children. J Thorac Cardiovasc Surg 68:869, 1974. With permission.

[9] From: Bower RJ, Sieber WK, Kiesewetter WB: Alimentary tract duplications in children. Ann Surg 188(5):669, 1978. With permission.

[12] From: Cohen SR, Geller KA, Birns JW, et al: Foregut cysts in infants and children: Diagnosis and management. Ann Otol Rhinol Laryngol 91:622, 1982. With permission.

[47] From: Case 33182. Congenital tracheobronchial cysts of the esophageal wall. N Engl J Med 236: 172–172, 1947 With permission.

infection to respiratory failure secondary to aspiration. The two nonoperative deaths and the favorable results following surgical excision point out the importance of prompt diagnosis and early excision of these thoracic lesions before deleterious consequences occur.

## DIVERTICULUM OF THE ESOPHAGUS

Congenital true diverticulum of the esophagus is exceedingly rare. A true diverticulum must contain esophageal mucosa and submucosa with complete muscular walls. The embryonic origin is uncertain, but it may be related to either a persistent embryonic mucosal diverticulum[33] or to the presence of a small, blind duplication which subsequently enlarges by a mechanism similar to that noted with a pulsion diverticulum.

### Clinical Presentation

First described in 1926, esophageal diverticula usually present in late infancy and early childhood with signs and symptoms of recurrent respiratory infection and progressive dysphagia.[28] In contrast, lesions in the pharyngoesophageal area that occur in the newborn period present with symptoms similar to those of esophageal atresia. Excessive salivation, regurgitation of formula, and cough with feedings are the most common presenting findings. A rare patient presents with cyanosis. Even more rare is a diverticulum associated with either a tracheoesophageal fistula or a diverticulum proximal to an esophageal stenosis.

## Diagnosis

A barium esophagram is the method of choice in the diagnosis of congenital diverticulum of the esophagus. It is important to obtain two views of the esophagus to confirm the diagnosis. Endoscopy is also an important aid in the diagnosis of either a pharyngoesophageal or true esophageal diverticulum and may also detect an associated anomaly such as an associated tracheoesophageal fistula.

## Treatment

Several methods of treatment of esophageal diverticula have been described, however, surgical extirpation is the method of choice. A single-stage procedure is presently the preferred method.[13] The neck of the diverticulum should be allowed to develop prior to surgical repair, therefore allowing for adequate tissue for closure of the esophagus. The diverticulum should be freed to the level of its neck. Amputation of the diverticulum should allow for enough tissue to close the neck without causing esophageal stenosis. To assure this, the defect is closed in a transverse fashion.

Congenital diverticula are rare and adequate data are relatively unavailable to evaluate the results of surgical therapy. Repair of a similar acquired pulsion diverticulum, however, is associated with a postoperative mortality rate of less than one percent and a recurrence rate of less than five percent.

## REFERENCES

1. Ahmed S, Jolleys A, Dark JF: Thoracic enteric cysts and diverticulae. Brit J Surg 59(12):963, 1972.
2. Anderson LS, Shackelford GD, Mancilla-Jimenez R, et al: Cartilaginous esophageal ring: A cause of esophageal stenosis in infants and children. Radiology 108:665, 1973.
3. Arbona JL, Fazzi JGF, Mayoral J: Congenital esophageal cysts: Case report and review of literature. Am J Gastroenterol 79(3):177, 1984.
4. Azimi F O'Hara HE: Congenital intraluminal mucosal web of the esophagus with tracheoesophageal fistula. Am J Dis Child 125:92, 1973.
5. BarMaor JA, Posen JA, Hamilton DG, et al: Congenital oesophageal stenosis due to cartilaginous tracheobronchial remnants. South Afr J Surg 21(1):43, 1983.
6. Beardmore HE, Wiglesworth FW: Vertebral anomalies and alimentary duplications. Pediatr Clin N Amer 5:457, 1958.
7. Bergmann M, Charna RM: Tracheobronchial rests in the esophagus, their relation to some benign strictures and certain types of cancer of the esophagus. J Thorac Surg 35:97, 1958.
8. Bower RJ, Kiesewetter WB: Mediastinal masses in infants and children. Arch Surg 112:1003, 1977.
9. Bower RJ, Sieber WK, Kiesewetter WB: Alimentary tract duplications in children. Ann Surg 188(5):669, 1978.

10. Bremer JL: Diverticula and duplications of the intestinal tract. Arch Pathol 38:132, 1944.

11. Briceno LI, Grases PJ, Gallego S: Tracheobronchial and pancreatic remnants causing esophageal stenosis. J Pediatr Surg 16:731, 1981.

12. Cohen SR, Geller KA, Birns JW, et al: Foregut cysts in infants and children: Diagnosis and management. Ann Otol Rhinol Laryngol 91:622, 1982.

13. DeBakey ME, Heancy JP, Creech O: Surgical considerations in diverticula of the esophagus. JAMA 150:1076, 1952.

14. Deiraniya AK: Congenital oesophageal stenosis due to tracheobronchial remnants. Thorax 29:720, 1974.

15. Fallon M, Gordon ARG, Lendrum AC: Mediastinal cysts of foregut origin associated with vertebral anomalies. Br J Surg 41:520, 1954.

16. Favara BE, Franciosi RA, Akers DR: Enteric duplications. Am J Dis Child 122:501, 1971.

17. Filler RM, Simpson JS, Ein SH: Mediastinal masses in infants and children. Pediatr Clin N Am 26:677, 1979.

18. Fonkalsrud EW: Esophageal stenosis due to tracheobronchial remnants. Am J Surg 124:101, 1972.

19. Frey EK, Duschel L: Der Kardiospasmus. Ergeb Chirur Orthop 29:637, 1936.

20. Gans SL, Lackey DA, Zukerbraun L: Duplications of the cervical esophagus in infants and children. Surgery 63:849, 1968.

21. Goldman RL, Ban JL: Chondroepithelial choristoma of the esophagus associated with esophageal atresia. J Thorac Cardiovasc Surg 63:318, 1972.

22. Gray SW, Skandalakis JE: [bf]Embryology for Surgeons. Philadelphia: W.B. Saunders Co., 1972.

23. Grosfeld JL, O'Neill JA, Clatworthy HW: Enteric duplications in infancy and childhood: An 18-year review. Ann Surg 172:83, 1970.

24. Haller JA, Shermeta DW, Donahoo JS, et al: Life-threatening respiratory distress from mediastinal masses in infants. Ann Thorac Surg 19(4): 364, 1975.

25. Huchzermeyer H, Burdelski M, Hruby M: Endoscopic therapy of a congenital oesophageal stricture. Endoscopy 4:259, 1979.

26. Ibrahim NB, Sandry GJ: Congenital oesophageal stenosis caused by tracheobronchial strictures in the oesophageal wall. Thorax 36:465, 1981.

27. Ishida M, Tsuchida Y, Saito S, et al: Congenital esophageal stenosis due to tracheobronchial remnants, J Pediatr Surg 4:339, 1969.

28. Jackson C, Shallow TA: Diverticula of the esophagus: Pulsion, traction, malignant and congenital. Ann Surg 83:1, 1926.

29. Jewsberry P: An unusual case of congenital esophageal stricture. Br J Surg 58:475, 1971.

30. Johnson FT: The development of the mucous membrane of the esophagus. stomach and small intestine in the human embryo. Am J Anat 10:521, 1910.

31. Kumar R: A case of congenital oesophageal stricture due to a cartilaginous ring. Br J Surg 49:533, 1962.

32. Langman J: [bf]Medical Embryology. Baltimore: Williams and Wilkins, 1975.

33. Lewis FT, Thyng FW: The regular occurence of intestinal diverticula in embryos of the pig, rabbit and man. Amer J Anat 7:505, 1907.

34. McLetchie NG, Purvis JK, Saunders RL: The genesis of gastric and certain intestinal diverticula and enterogenous cysts. Surg Gynecol Obstet 99:135, 1954.

35. Nishina T, Tsuchida Y, Saito S: Congenital esophageal stenosis due to tracheobronchial remnants and its associated anomalies. J Pediatr Surg 16:190, 1981.

36. Ohkawa H, Takahashi H Hoshino Y, et al: Lower esophageal stenosis in association with tracheobronchial remnants. J Pediatr Surg 10:453, 1975.

37. Paulino F, Roselli A, Aprigliano F: Congenital esophageal stricture due to tracheobronchial remnants. Surgery 53:547, 1963.

38. Pokorny WJ, Sherman JO, Idriss FS: Mediastinal masses in infants and children. J Thorac Cardiovasc Surg 68:869, 1974.

39. Rahaney K, Barclay GPT: Enterogenous cysts and congenital diverticula of the alimentary canal with abnormalities of the vertebral column and spinal cord. J Path Bact 77:457, 1959.

40. Rose JS, Kassner EG, Jurgens KH, et al: Congenital esophageal strictures due to cartilaginous rings. Br J Radiol 48:16, 1975.

41. Saunders RL: Combined anterior and posterior spina bifida in a living neonatal human female. Anat Rec 87:255, 1943.

42. Sidaway ME: Duplication of the esophagus. Ann Radiol 7:400, 1964.

43. Sneed WF, LaGarde DC, Kogutt MS, et al: Esophageal stenosis due to cartilaginous tracheobronchial remnants. J Pediatr Surg 14:786, 1979.

44. Spath F, Ratzenhofer M: Ueber die angkborene Oesophagusstenose. Wien Klin Wochenschr 71:723, 1959.

45. Steinhagen RM, Pertsemlidis D, Feld HJ: Spontaneous perforation of intestinal duplications. Mt Sinai J Med 49:406, 1982.

46. Stephens HB: H-type tracheoesophageal fistula complicated by esophageal stenosis. J Thorac Cardiovasc Surg 59:325, 1970.

47. Superina RA, Ein SH, Humphreys RP: Cystic duplications of the esophagus and neuroenteric cysts. J Pediatr Surg 19(5):527, 1984.

48. Tarnay T, Chang CH, Nudget RG, et al: Esophageal duplication (foregut cyst) with spinal malformation. J Thorac Cardiovasc Surg 59:293, 1970.

49. Teele RL, Henschke CI, Tapper D: The radiographic and ultrasonic evaluation of enteric duplication cysts. Pediatr Radiol 10:9, 1980.

50. Weiss LM, Fagelman D, Warhit JM: CT demonstration of an esophageal duplication cyst. J Comput Assist Tomogr 7:716, 1983.

51. Whittaker LD, Lynn HB: Mediastinal tumors and cysts in the pediatric patient. Surg Clin N Am 53:893, 1973.

52. Youngblood D, Blumenthal BI: Enteric duplication cyst. South Med J 76:670, 1983.

Lucian L. Leape

# 4

# Chemical Injury of the Esophagus

Ingestion of caustic substances, whether accidental or in a suicide attempt, may result in serious injury to the oropharynx, esophagus, or stomach. The most corrosive and commonly ingested caustics are sodium or potassium hydroxide drain cleaners. These may be either liquid or granular in form. Less caustic alkalis which may be ingested are bleach (sodium hypochlorite), ammonia, laundry and dishwasher detergents (particularly trisodium phosphate), and disinfectants. Clinitest tablets contain concentrated lye and are capable of causing serious injury to the esophagus. Similarly, alkaline disk batteries used in calculators, cameras, hearing aids, and watches contain highly concentrated sodium or potassium hydroxide which is readily released on ingestion. Acid ingestion is less frequently seen and usually results from industrial products used carelessly or stored in the home.

There has been a significant decrease in the incidence of accidental ingestions as the result of stringent governmental regulation of commercially available drain cleaners since 1971. Caustic ingestion continues, nevertheless, to be a significant health problem; controversy still exists over details of optimal management, both of the acute injury and of later complications.

## LYE INGESTION

### History

Lye ingestion is a disease of the industrial era. Caustic ingestion was rarely seen before lye became available as a byproduct of the meat-rendering industry in the mid-19th century. It was then purchased by housewives for use as a cleaning agent and to make soap from fat. A white, granular substance which looked just like sugar, lye was an obvious target for inquisitive toddlers. When Chevalier Jackson began his pioneer-

Pediatric Esophageal Surgery
ISBN 0-8089-1776-5

ing work with the esophagoscope in the early 1900s, he quickly accumulated dozens of children with esophageal lye injuries who needed dilatations.

A compassionate and dedicated man, Jackson spent the rest of his professional lifetime beseeching state legislators to pass regulations requiring not that the substance be banned, but merely that it be labeled as a poison. After 20 years, 24 states had approved such legislation.

In the 1920s, two events changed the whole nature of the struggle: Meat packers began national distribution and Congress became interested in the regulation of interstate commerce (for which meat packers were now eligible). Jackson turned his attention to Washington. His efforts were successful when, in 1927, after several years of lobbying, the Federal Caustic Act was passed, requiring that all caustics containing more than ten percent hydroxide be labeled as poisons.

Direct sale of lye and the home manufacture of soap gradually declined, but lye-containing drain cleaners were developed. These were granular preparations of 50–60 percent sodium hydroxide mixed with other chemicals for stability and ease of use. Drano was the most widely distributed brand. The era of lye drain cleaner ingestion began. In 1969, more than 5,000 children under the age of five ingested lye, almost all of it labeled "poison".[12]

The currently used treatment protocols were developed in response to the problems presented by children who ingested granular lye in the postendoscopic, antibiotic, and steroid era. The risk of serious esophageal injury after granular lye ingestion is about 20–30 percent. About five percent of patients who ingest granular lye develop strictures. Almost all of these respond ultimately to repeated dilatations. Rarely, esophageal substitution is required.

In 1967, several manufacturers brought out concentrated (25–35-percent) sodium hydroxide solutions which were touted as being more effective than the granular lye drain cleaners. They were clearly easier to use. They were also clearly more hazardous. Experience rapidly accumulated demonstrating the devastating effects of liquid lye on the esophagus.[12] Instead of a 25 percent incidence of esophageal injury, when liquid lye was ingested the chance of esophageal injury was virtually 100 percent. Strictures developed in almost all of these patients, and most were refractory to dilatation, so that esophageal replacement was usually needed (Fig. 4-1).

Within three years, pressure from physicians and legislators led the FDA to invoke its new powers under the Hazardous Substances Act to ban these products. The 1971 regulations banned the sale of liquid lye preparations containing greater than ten percent sodium hydroxide unless packaged in a childproof container. The industry response was to reformulate the preparations in a lower concentration, add ingredients to give them an offensive smell, and also to put on child-resistant covers. As a result, there has been a significant decrease in the incidence of serious injuries from lye ingestion over the past decade.

In 1970, before the ban, 1,287 ingestions of corrosives by children under the age of five were reported to the National Clearinghouse for Poison Control Centers. Of these, 263 required hospital treatment and ten died (Table 4-1). It is estimated that only ten percent of ingestions are reported,[16] so the national total was probably about 13,000 ingestions and 100 deaths.

In 1982, while the total number of reported ingestions had only decreased by one-third, the number requiring hospital treatment had decreased by 87 percent to 35, and there were no fatalities reported.[18]

**Table 4-1**
*Corrosive Ingestion—Children Under 5 Years*[18]

|                          | 1970 | 1982 |
| ------------------------ | ---- | ---- |
| Total reported ingestions | 1287 | 868  |
| unspecified lye          | 47   | 9    |
| Drano                    | 297  | 22   |
| Liquid Plumr             | 122  | 7    |
| Plunge                   | 24   | 1    |
| Hospital visits          | 263  | 35   |
| Fatalities               | 10   | 0    |

[18] From: United States Department of Health and Human Services, Public Health Service, Food and Drug Administration. Bulletin, National Clearinghouse for Poison Control Centers, 1982. With permission.

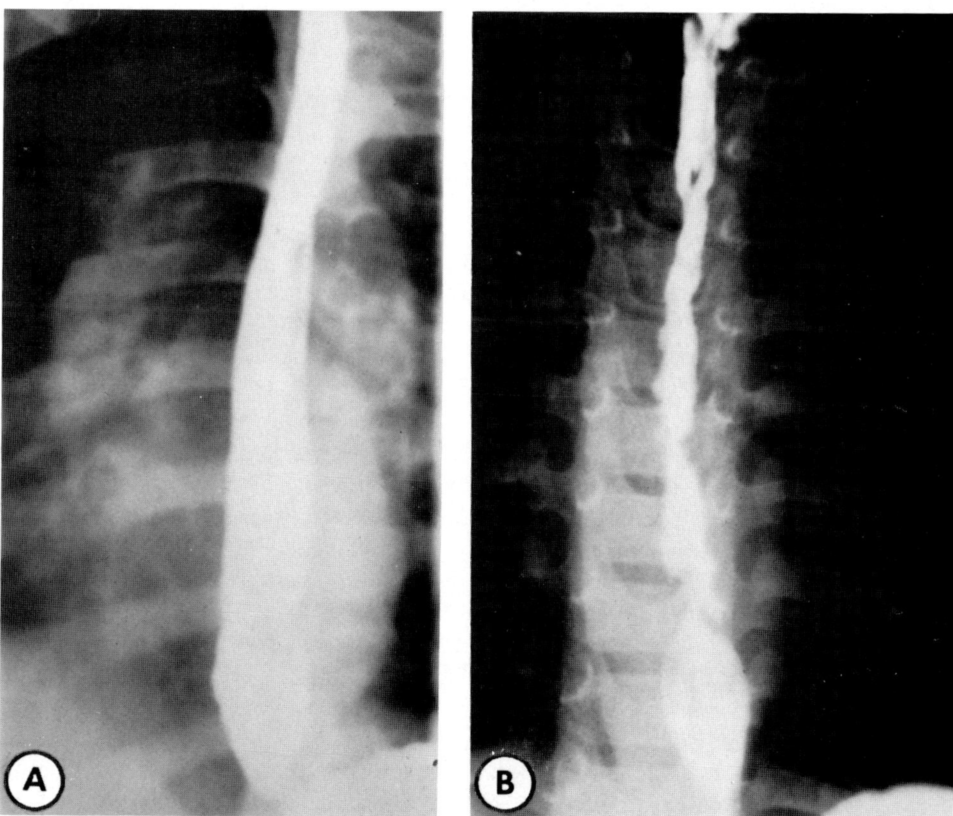

**Figure 4-1.** (A) Barium swallow two weeks following ingestion of the remains from an "empty" Liquid Plumr bottle. Patient taking Prednisone. (B) Esophagram at three months after ingestion showing severe extensive stricture despite repeated dilatations. Esophageal replacement was ultimately required.

## Epidemiology

Lye ingestion in older children and adults almost always results from a suicide attempt. Lye ingestion in young children is accidental—similar to the ingestion of other poisons. In both instances, the causes are usually psychosocial and difficult to control. Not only is it impossible to insulate toddlers from all of the hazards of life, but there is ample evidence that poisonings in children are not "accidental" but occur in situations of social stress.[16] Detailed histories of the circumstances surrounding accidental ingestions demonstrate a high frequency of social disturbances in the home or family at the time of the ingestion.

While educational programs will temporarily decrease poisonings, these behavioral patterns do not persist after the program is completed. Storage patterns are of questionable relevance. A controlled study failed to show any differences either in the knowledge about hazardous substances or in the storage practices of mothers with children who ingested poisons versus those whose children did not.[4] Similarly, it has not been possible to demonstrate clearly that "childproof" containers really are what they claim to be. The only *sure* way to prevent accidental lye ingestion is to make lye unavailable.

Although the present drain cleaners are demonstrably less hazardous than their predecessors, they still cause a significant number of injuries each year. Considering the questionable effectiveness of these agents and the ready availability of better methods (such as plungers and drain snakes), the time has long passed when they should be removed from the market altogether.

## Pathophysiology

Lye ingestion is most likely to result in injury to the esophagus, but in large quantities it can produce extensive damage to the entire upper gastrointestinal tract. Liquid lye burns have extended through the stomach to involve adjacent colon, pancreas, spleen, or small bowel.

Alkali rapidly penetrates into body tissues, probably because the hydroxyl radical rapidly binds the free hydrogen ion which is available on many essential intracellular particles: nucleic acids, proteins, and phospholipids. Tissue damage results in edema, infiltration of leukocytes, and an intense inflammatory reaction. Small-vessel thrombosis is characteristic of lye injury and extends its necrotizing effect. If the hydroxide concentration is high, transmural penetration rapidly occurs, with resultant destruction of the muscular wall of the esophagus. Perforation may result. Penetration into the periesophageal tissues may cause mediastinitis.

After several days, the necrotic tissue is sloughed and granulation tissue develops, followed by fibroblastic proliferation and collagen deposition. Cicatrization takes place over the next weeks to months as the collagen contracts and the scar matures. If the injury of the esophagus is circumferential, stricture results.

The extent and severity of injury results from three factors: (1) the concentration of caustic; (2) the quantity ingested; and, (3) the duration of contact. All of these factors are likely to be maximal in suicide attempts, while in accidental lye ingestion they vary considerably. Granular lye is slow to go into solution, so if only a small amount is ingested, the burns may be localized and not severe. In addition, the burning sensation in the mouth when granular lye is ingested often leads to its being spit out without much being swallowed. As a result, serious burns of the esophagus are not a common result of granular lye ingestion, and fewer than five percent of those who ingest granular lye develop stricture.

Concentrated liquid lye produces far more serious injury than do granular preparations. In part, this is because the liquid penetrates into the tissues almost instantly, whereas granular preparations must first dissolve in saliva before they are absorbed. This rapid penetration of liquid lye makes effective use of antidotes impossible, since injury occurs within seconds of contact.[12] Because liquid lye is easily swallowed, the injury to the esophagus is likely to be more severe than is the injury to the oropharynx. The area of contact is also much more extensive than is true of dry forms. If it is a concentrated preparation, full-thickness injury rapidly occurs. Even low-concentration liquid lye preparations will cause esophageal injury if the amount ingested is sufficient to result in prolonged contact.[3]

## Clinical Presentation

Granular lye is the most likely form of lye to cause severe oral burns because the particles stick to the mucosa. A few granules accidentally ingested may be spit out without swallowing, sparing injury to the esophagus. Liquid lye is easily swallowed, so it is possible to have little injury to the mouth, but serious esophageal damage. A few milliliters of concentrated liquid lye can cause serious esophageal injury.[12] The presence of oral burns thus confirms that ingestion has occurred, but it is not a reliable guide to the extent of esophageal damage. Conversely, 10–30 percent of patients with a history of lye ingestion have no apparent oral burns but have significant esophageal injury.

Lye ingestion in older children is usually the result of a suicide attempt. The amount ingested is likely to be large and the injury serious. The patient may be febrile and show signs of shock. Emergent treatment is indicated.

### Symptoms

Caustic injury often results in extensive edema and erythema of the lips and tongue with pain and drooling (Fig. 4-2). The child may be unable to swallow. Chest or back pain suggests mediastinitis and extensive esophageal injury. Abdominal pain may be present if large quantities of lye are swallowed. These patients may vomit blood. Abdominal tenderness and the development of signs of peritoneal irritation suggest full-thickness injury to the stomach with impending or actual perforation or necrosis. Immediate lapararotomy is indicated in these patients.

Fever and leukocytosis are rough guides to the extent of injury. If the white blood count is normal and there is no fever, it is unlikely that there is severe tissue destruction.

Dyspnea, stridor, or hoarseness suggest laryngeal injury. If there is progressive respiratory compromise, intubation or tracheostomy may be necessary. Respiratory signs may not develop for 24 hours, however, so overnight admission to the hospital is necessary for all patients suspected of lye ingestion.

Severe pain, tachycardia, or shock suggest sepsis, perforation, or extensive necrosis. Emergency resection of the stomach or esophagus may be needed.

In less severe cases, oral pain and dysphagia subside over three or four days and

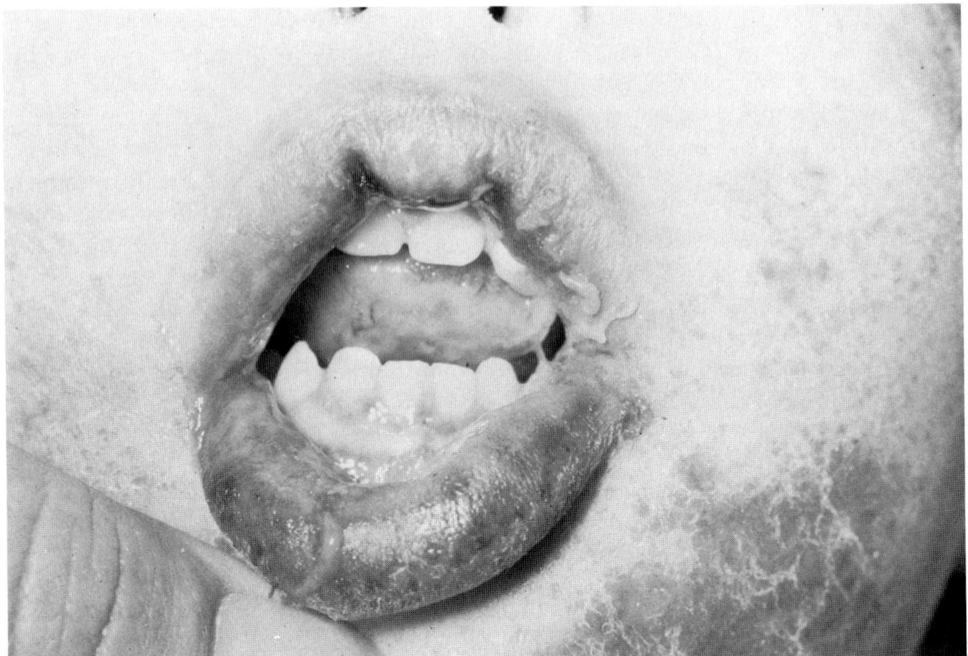

**Figure 4-2.**  Burns of lips and face from lye ingestion.

the patient can resume oral feedings. Dysphagia will return in two–six weeks if stricture develops.

Ammonia, bleach, and most detergents usually cause little or no injury unless very large quantities (200 ml or more) are swallowed. Stricture almost never occurs after ingestion of these substances.[9] Clinitest tablets, however, can cause severe injury; 50 percent of patients who have ingested these will have a deep burn. The tablet tends to stick in the esophagus, dissolve, and produce a full-thickness, localized necrosis (Fig. 4-3). Clinitest tablets also generate heat as they dissolve, adding thermal injury to other injury. Alkaline batteries can lodge in the esophagus or stomach and cause corrosive injury even without the outer casing having dissolved.[19]

## Diagnosis

### History

At times, it may be difficult to determine whether or not lye ingestion has actually occurred. Often the event was not witnessed. If burns of the lips or mouth are present, the issue is settled; otherwise, one is dependent on the history. There are few false alarms, however, so it is best to presume the parental concern is justified and treat the patient accordingly.

### Endoscopy

Endoscopic examination is necessary to determine whether or not there has been an esophageal burn. Studies have shown that signs and symptoms are unreliable guides to the presence or severity of an esophageal injury.[7] For this reason, esophagoscopy is

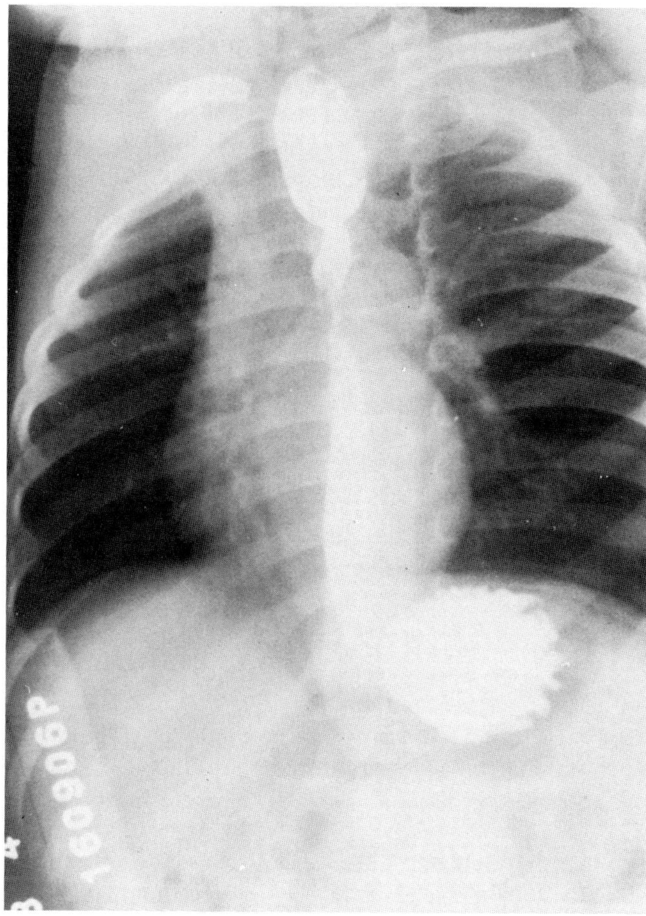

**Figure 4-3.** Esophagram showing severe stricture resulting from ingestion of a Clinitest tablet.

indicated. It should be performed the next day (12–24 hours after ingestion). Esophagoscopy should *not* be performed immediately because the extent of injury may be difficult to determine, and because if the patient has a full stomach, regurgitation of caustic may produce further injury. General anesthesia is essential in these terrified toddlers, both for humane reasons and to minimize the risk of injury.

The purpose of esophagoscopy is to establish whether or not there is a burn of the esophagus. If there is none, there is no need for further treatment, other than for the mouth burns, and the patient may be discharged. As many as 75 percent of patients will be found to have no esophageal injury. The most likely sites of injury are at points of natural narrowing of the lumen: the cricopharyngeus, the aortic arch, the left main stem bronchus, and the diaphragm.

It is not possible to accurately evaluate the depth of the burn at esophagoscopy. Although ulceration is usually associated with full-thickness damage, apparently mild mucosal changes may conceal a transmural injury. The risk of perforation is minimal if the examination is stopped when evidence of mucosal burn is seen. In instances of ingestion of large quantities of acid or liquid lye, some physicians have recommended gastroscopy to determine the extent of gastric or duodenal injury.

### Radiologic Evaluation

Radiologic evaluation should be performed after esophagsocopy. The introduction of contrast material will detect perforation if present, give some idea of the extent of involvement, and serve as a baseline for evaluating future changes. If there is marked atony of the esophagus, full-thickness injury and later stricture formation is probable. Except when severe changes are present, however, the esophagram is unreliable for predicting outcome.[17]

## Treatment

### First Aid

After any form of lye ingestion, it is imperative that the child *not* be given an emetic. Regurgitation of the lye doubles the exposure of the esophagus, increasing the chance of severe injury. Milk should be given in a moderate amount, or, if unavailable, water, to dilute and wash away residual lye. While these measures may help in the case of granular lye ingestion, the exceedingly rapid absorption of liquid lye makes it unlikely that anything can be given soon enough to alter the course of the injury.

### Mild or Moderate Injury

Admission to the hospital for overnight observation is necessary for all patients with suspected or actual caustic ingestion because of the risk of airway injury. Nothing should be given by mouth at first because of the tendency to vomit and increase the injury. Pain medication may be necessary. Intravenous fluids with additional blood or plasma should be given if the patient has signs of severe injury with reduced blood volume.

Ampicillin (Biocraft), 250 mg 4id, is given as prophylaxis for infection of the severely burned tissues. Prednisone, 2 mg/kg/day, is administered to decrease the extent of scar tissue formation and later stricture; experimental work[8] and one small clinical study[9] indicate its effectiveness. Steroids must be given early in the course of the injury, however, if they are to be effective.

Esophagoscopy should be performed the next day. If no burn is seen, treatment is stopped and the patient can be sent home. If a burn is discovered, antibiotics should be continued for ten days and Prednisone for three weeks. The patient may be fed when able, and discharged home when stable, to be followed closely for the development of signs of stricture formation. In patients who have circumferential esophageal burn, gastrostomy may be necessary for feeding and later management. Early passage of a string to guide dilators is advisable in these patients.

A follow-up barium esophagram is obtained at three weeks post-injury. If it is negative, but there has been significant injury, the study should be repeated in another three weeks—earlier if dysphagia develops.

In recent years, several investigators have advocated early placement of a Silastic (Dow Corning) stent to prevent stricture formation.[10,15] The value of this is still unproven, and since only five–ten percent of patients develop stricture, it is questionable which patients are candidates for this extreme treatment. If there is extensive tissue necrosis, neither stenting nor dilatation will prove effective.

Disk batteries which have been swallowed should be promptly removed from the esophagus or stomach by endoscopy or laparotomy.[19] Even if the battery is intact, strong alkali will leak out and can cause perforation after contact for as little as eight hours. If the battery has passed into the intestine, its passage through should be monitored by frequent X-rays (every six–eight hours). Purgatives are indicated to hasten its progress, and operative removal should be performed if there is no progress.

### Severe Injury

Early laparatomy or thoracotomy may be necessary as a life-saving measure in the case of severe injury. At laparotomy, necrotic stomach tissue should be removed and a gastrostomy established. If the stomach has sustained transmural lye injury, the esophagus almost certainly has been destroyed. Immediate total esophagectomy is indicated if the patient is to survive. Steroids are of no benefit and should be withheld because of the risk of further weakening the tissues and the favoring of infection.

## Outcome

The late complications of caustic ingestion include stricture of the esophagus or larynx, tracheoesophageal fistula, aortoesophageal fistula, and late development of carcinoma in the damaged esophagus.

### Esophageal Stricture

Esophageal stricture occurs in five–ten percent of patients with granular lye ingestion, and 50–100 percent of those who swallow concentrated liquid lye. If stricture is noted on follow-up barium swallow, esophageal dilatations are begun and

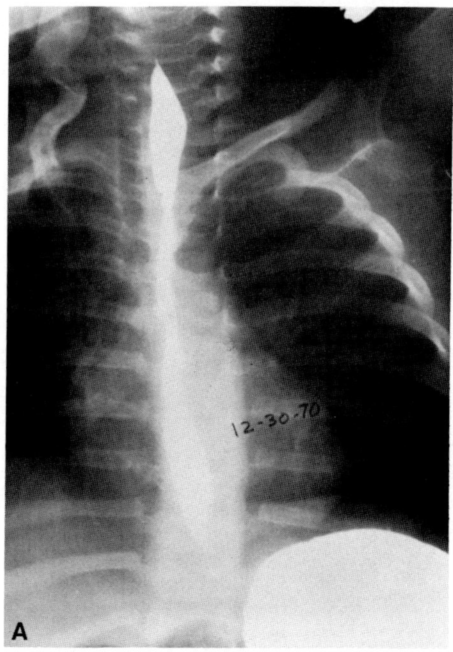
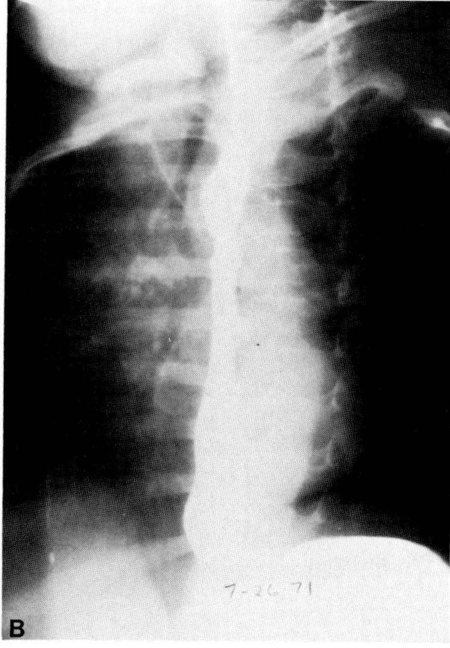

**Figure 4-4.** (A) Esophagram showing extensive stricture following ingestion of an unknown amount of liquid lye. (B) Barium swallow seven months later, after 33 weekly dilatations. Although an adequate lumen has been re-established, significant scarring and dysmotility remain.

repeated at seven–ten-day intervals until the stricture is eliminated. This may take several monhts (Fig. 4-4). Early and frequent dilatations are the optimal means to correct a stricture in the shortest time. Fortunately, most strictures will respond to dilatations and esophageal substitution is seldom required. The exception is the patient who has ingested concentrated liquid lye (Fig. 4-5).

Dilatation should always be performed under general anesthesia. Even though it is possible to carry out retrograde dilatation in the awake patient, it is cruel to do so and unnecessary with modern, safe anesthetic techniques. Esophageal dilatation is a safe surgical procedure. Antegrade dilatation with Maloney rubber dilators or filiform and followers is usually satisfactory, but patients with long, irregular strictures may require passage of a string and retrograde dilatation with Tucker dilators via a gastrostomy.

90 percent of esophageal strictures caused by granular lye ingestion will respond to serial dilatations. The response after concentrated liquid lye injury is much lower: ten–20 percent. The remainder will require esophageal substitution by colon or gastric tube. Early recognition and operation for the hopelessly damaged esophagus will spare the child repeated futile dilatations.

### Laryngeal and Tracheal Stricture

Laryngeal and tracheal stricture are fortunately rare. When present, however, they are very difficult to treat. Tracheal resection has been successfully employed in cases of severe lye stricture.[13] Arytenoidectomy may be required to maintain patency of the larynx if there is severe destruction. Tracheostomy is frequently required.

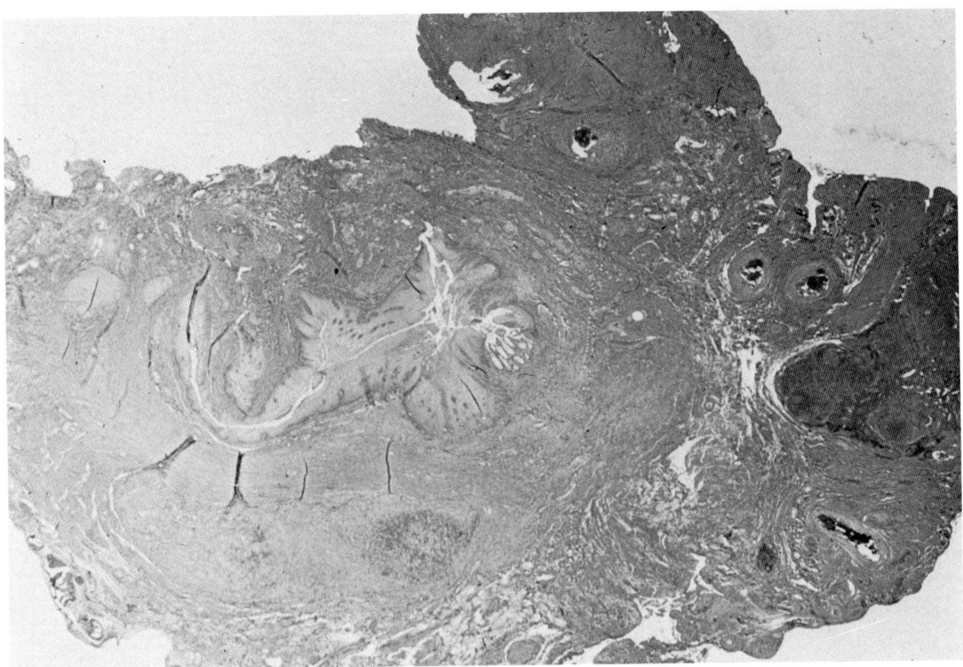

**Figure 4-5.** Liquid Plumr ingestion. Cross-section of esophagus removed at time of by-pass. This patient underwent 30 unsuccessful dilatations prior to replacement. Note the extent and thickness of scar tissue which has replaced the muscle layers. The mucosa has regenerated.

### Tracheoesophageal Fistula

Tracheoesophageal fistula may result from extension of the lye injury from the esophagus into the trachea.[1] This complication invariably results from a very severe esophageal injury in which the esophagus itself is not salvageable. The diagnosis is suspected if the patient develops cough and expectoration of gastric or esophageal contents or has signs of mediastinitis. Diagnosis can usually be established by contrast esophagram using a bronchographic medium (*not* water-soluble gastrointestinal contrast material, which is very irritating to the bronchi and lungs) or bronchoscopy.

Caustic tracheoesophageal fistula usually occurs in the acute phase of injury (first week), when the tissues are very friable and heal poorly. Attempts to patch the opening with local tissue are usually unsuccessful. Esophageal exclusion is the treatment of choice.[5] Both the upper and lower ends of the esophagus are closed, bringing out a proximal cervical esophagostomy. This is followed by gastrostomy. When the patient recovers, esophageal substitution is carried out.

### Aortoesophageal Fistula

Aortoesophageal fistula can occur, with prompt exsanguinating hemorrhage, if there has been penetration of the lye into the mediastinum or extensive esophageal necrosis and mediastinal infection (Fig. 4-6). It can be prevented only by prompt resection of the necrotic esophagus.

### Squamous Cell Carcinoma

Squamous cell carcinoma has been reported to develop in patients with long-standing esophageal stricture.[2,11] The risk of occurence is unknown, but may be from one to three percent. There is a long lag time (40–45 years) from the time of injury until the discovery of the tumor. These patients seem to have a somewhat higher rate of cure after resection or radiation than do patients suffering from other forms of esophageal cancer, but it is still only approximately 10 percent.[2,11] Because the risk of esophagectomy is probably greater than the mortality risk from later cancer development, most authorities do not recommend prophylactic esophagectomy for patients with lye injury. There are no reports of malignancy developing in the bypassed (unused) esophagus.

## ACID INGESTION

## Epidemiology

Accidental ingestion of acid occurs much less frequently than does lye ingestion because there are few strong acid products which are used in the home and available to the toddler. Lack of ready availability also limits the use of acid in suicide attempts. Toilet-bowl cleaners, battery acid, and industrial corrosives which are brought home for cleaning are the major offenders. Unfortunately, these are usually acids which are both strong (sulfuric or hydrochloric) and concentrated, so ingestion, whether accidental or deliberate, may result in serious injury.

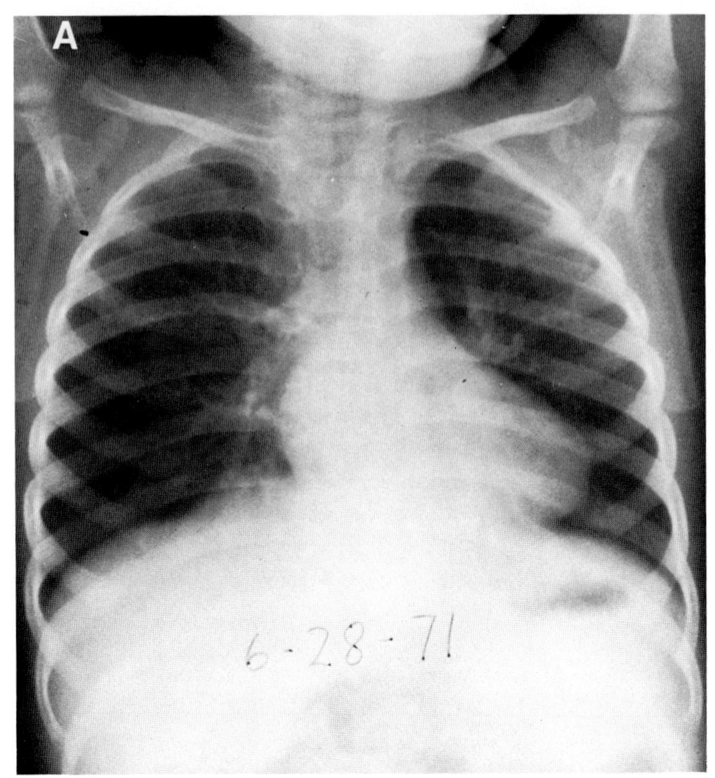
A
6-28-71

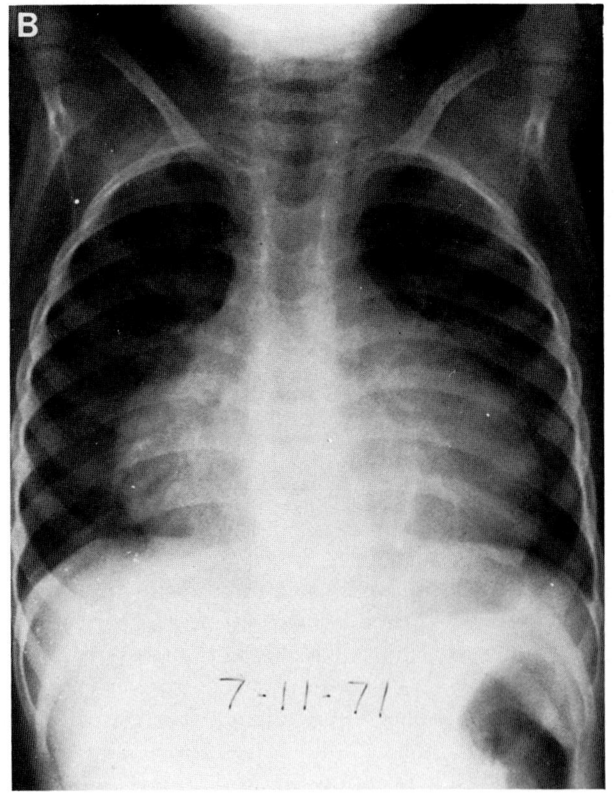
B
7-11-71

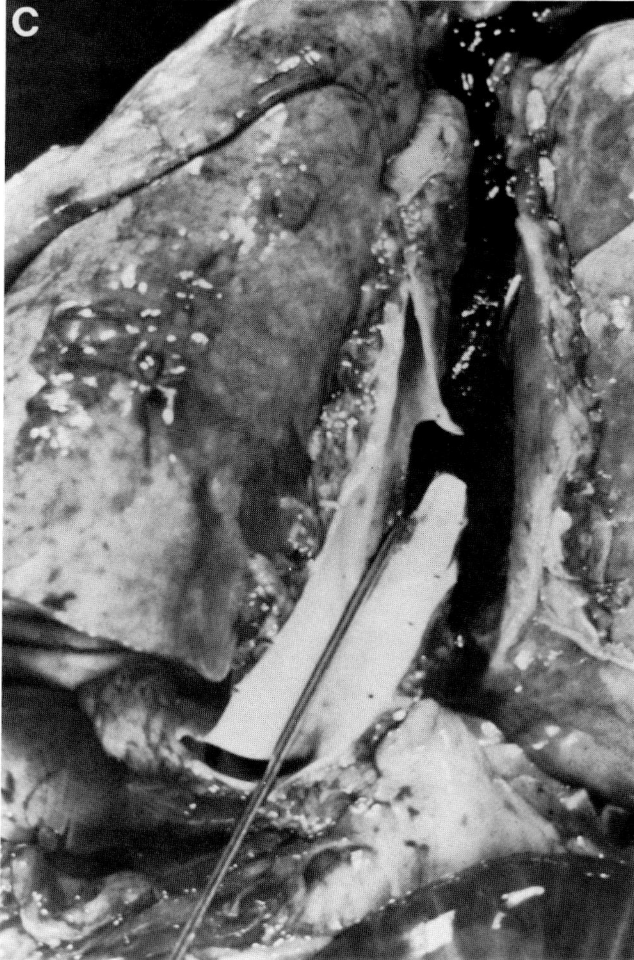

Figure 4-6. (A) Admission chest roentgenogram of a 21-month-old boy who ingested liquid lye. (B) Chest roentgenogram on the 13th post-injury day showing pericardial effusion secondary to severe mediastinitis. Patient suddenly exsanguinated later that day. (C) Autopsy specimen showing the aortoesophageal fistula which caused hemorrhage.

## Pathophysiology

In contrast to alkali ingestion, acid ingestion typically results in injury to the stomach or intestine rather than to the esophagus. The severity of acid injury is, like that of lye injury, proportional to concentration, volume, and duration of contact. Acid produces a coagulative necrosis on the surface of the area of contact which limits the degree of injury if small quantities are ingested. Larger doses result in full-thickness injury; necrosis and perforation may result, either acutely or when the necrotic eschar sloughs. If a small amount is ingested, the esophagus is usually spared, but the stomach may be injured because of pylorospasm which results in antral pooling, increasing the contact time with the acid. Food in the stomach may partially neutralize the acid and limit the damage. Ingestion of a large quantity of concentrated acid may result in necrosis of both the esophagus and stomach. The duodenum, and even the ileum, may be affected.

## Clinical Presentation

Acid causes immediate pain on contact in the mouth, so in cases of accidental ingestion the agent may be rapidly expelled and little actually swallowed. Large amounts are usually swallowed when the ingestion is part of a suicide attempt, but oral injury may be either mild or severe. As is true of lye ingestion, the extent of oropharyngeal damage is therefore a poor guide to the severity of internal injuries.

## Symptoms

Burning in the mouth and difficulty swallowing are the initial symptoms of acid ingestion. The mouth and lips may be red and edematous, or the mucosa may be white. Ulcerations and blood-tinged secretions may be present in the mouth.

Abdominal pain suggests gastric injury. If there is abdominal tenderness, full-thickness injury of the stomach may be present. Severe pain, fever, and tachycardia are signs of extensive necrosis or perforation and indicate the need for emergency exploration.

Dyspnea, stridor, or hoarseness may be noted if there is laryngeal injury.

## Diagnosis

### Endoscopy

Flexible fiberoptic esophagogastroscopy is the best way to assess the extent of injury from acid ingestion. It should be delayed until after initial treatment, however, and is inappropriate if there is obvious gastric necrosis requiring emergency operation.

### Radiologic Evaluation

Radiologic evaluation is also not appropriate initially, but may give valuable information after the patient has been stabilized.

## Treatment

### First Aid

If the patient is seen soon after ingestion, passage of a nasogastric tube and evacuation of residual acid can significantly reduce the dose and the duration of contact. Antacids should then be given in large amounts (200–300 ml) to neutralize any residual acid. In small-quantity ingestions, antacids alone should be given. Emetics are contraindicated for the same reason as in lye ingestion: these double the exposure of the esophagus and oropharynx.

### Mild or Moderate Injury

The patient should be given nothing to eat or drink until all abdominal symptoms disappear and there are no signs of toxicity. If peritoneal signs develop, early laparotomy is required. The value of steroids in the treatment of acid ingestion is unknown, but if there has been airway injury, corticosteroids may prevent laryngeal edema and the need for a tracheostomy. Antibiotics are indicated. Barium upper gastrointestinal examination should be performed when the patient is stable, and repeated at two and four weeks post-injury to search for antral scarring, the most common late effect.

### Severe Injury

Immediate laparotomy is necessary if there is evidence of peritonitis.[6] Nonviable or perforated tissue should be resected. Questionable areas should be left behind and re-evaluated at a second-look procedure 24–72 hours later. Although the prime target organ of acid ingestion is the stomach, when large quantities are ingested, the esophagus may also sustain significant injury and require emergency resection. In the past, many patients who ingested acid haven't survived, often because of delays in treatment; earlier operation will almost certainly improve the chance of survival.

## Outcome

### Gastric Stricture

Gastric stricture is the most common complication of nonfatal acid ingestion. Typically, this occurs in the antrum, where acid stasis results from pylorospasm after the ingestion. It may take three–four weeks for stricture to develop. Partial or total gastric resection is necessary.[14]

## REFERENCES


1. Amoury RA, Hrabovsky E, Leonidas J, et al: Tracheoesophageal fistula after lye ingestion. J Ped Surg 10:273, 1975.
2. Appelqvist P, Salmo M: Lye corrosion carcinoma of the esophagus, a review of 63 cases. Cancer 45:2655, 1980.
3. Ashcraft KW, Padula RT: The effect of dilute corrosives on the esophagus. Pediatrics 53:226, 1974.
4. Baltimore C Jr, Meyer RJ: A study of storage, child behavioral traits and mother's knowledge of toxicology in 52 poisoned families and 52 comparison families. Pediatrics (supplement 5) 44:816, 1969.
5. Burrington JD, Raffensperger JG: Surgical management of tracheoesophageal fistula complicating caustic ingestion. Surgery 84:329, 1978.
6. Chodak GW, Passaro E Jr: Acid ingestion, need for gastric resection. JAMA 239:225, 1978.
7. Gaudreault P, McGuigan M, Chicoine L, et al: Predictability of esophageal injury from signs and symptoms: A study of caustic ingestion in 378 children. Pediatrics 71:767, 1983.
8. Haller JA, Bachman K: The comparative effect of current therapy on experimental caustic burns of the esophagus. JAMA 186:262, 1963.
9. Hawkins DB Demeter M, Barnett T, et al: Caustic ingestion: Controversies in management, a review of 214 cases. The Laryngoscope 90:98, 1980.
10. Hill JL, Norberg H, Smith M, et al: Clinical technique and success of the esophageal stent to prevent corrosive strictures. J Ped Surg 11:443, 1976.
11. Hopkins RA, Postlethwait RW: Caustic burns and carcinoma of the esophagus. Ann Surg 194:146, 1981.
12. Leape LL, Ashcraft K, Scarpelli D, et al: Hazard to health—Liquid lye. New Engl J Med 284:578, 1971.

13. Leape LL, Ashcraft K, Mann C et al: Tracheal resection for lye stricture. Surgery 72:357–260, 1972.
14. Maull KI, Scher L, Greenfield L, et al: Surgical implications of acid ingestion. Surg Gynecol Obstet 148:895, 1979.
15. Mills LJ, Estrera A, Platt M, et al: Avoidance of esophageal stricture following severe caustic burns by the use of an intraluminal stent. Ann Thorac Surg 28:69, 1979.
16. Sobel R: The psychiatric implications of accidental poisoning in childhood. Ped Clin N Amer 17:653, 1970.
17. Stannard MW: Corrosive esophagitis in children. Am J Dis Child 132:596, 1978.
18. United States Department of Health and Human Services, Public Health Service, Food and Drug Administration. Bulletin, National Clearinghouse for Poison Control Centers, 1982.
19. Votteler TP, Nash J, Rutledge J, et al: The hazard of ingested alkaline disk batteries in children. JAMA 249:2504, 1983.

Alfred A. de Lorimier
Michael R. Harrison

# 5

# Esophageal Replacement

A normally functioning esophagus is a remarkable organ, for it very effectively propels ingested material aborally by coordinated peristalsis induced by the pharyngeal swallowing mechanism. At the same time, it inhibits reflux of the swallowed contents back into the pharynx at the cricopharyngeus. It has a sphincter at the esophagogastric junction which relaxes with the passage of a food bolus, but contracts and prevents reflux of gastric contents when the peristaltic wave subsides. Appreciation of these important functions becomes readily apparent when abnormal esophageal motility patterns occur. This is particularly evident in infants with dysmotility disorders associated with esophageal atresia or in patients with chalasia or achalasia and in those who have required a replacement of the diseased esophagus. With rare exception, a poorly functioning esophagus is usually better than any esophageal substitutes, and a decision to replace the esophagus must be considered very carefully.

## INDICATIONS

Indications for esophageal replacement might include:

1.  esophageal atresia
2.  chemical esophageal stricture or perforation
3.  Peptic esophageal stricture
4.  congenital lower esophageal stenosis
5.  mechanical or emetic esophageal perforation
6.  muscular hypertrophy
7.  esophageal varices
8.  esophageal epidermloysis bullosa
9.  esophageal tumors
10. severe motility disorders—achalasia, diffuse esophageal spasm, scleroderma
11. esophageal candidiasis

## Esophageal Atresia

In children one of the most common indications for esophageal substitution is esophageal atresia. The two esophageal ends may be so widely separated that an anastomosis would be under excessive tension or it would be impossible to bring the two ends together. This is unusual when there is an associated fistula between the trachea and the distal esophagus, which prevents the esophagus from retracting toward the diaphragm. In the past, however, there were many cases of this anomaly in which the anastomosis broke down and the survivors required an esophageal substitute. Esophageal atresia without a distal tracheoesophageal fistula usually is associated with a long gap between the two ends. This lesion occurs in six–eight percent of esophageal anomalies. In previous years, all of these infants had a cervical esophagostomy and gastrostomy. At a later time, various portions of bowel were interposed between the cervical esophagus and the stomach to establish continuity.

Recently, long-gap esophageal atresia has been aggressively treated to avoid esophageal substitution.[18] The proximal and distal esophageal ends can be approximated for primary anastomosis by a combination of techniques. Bougie stretching of the proximal esophagus alone or simultaneous stretching of the distal esophagus by passing the bougie through the gastrostomy into the distal esophagus have produced significant elongation of the two esophageal segments. When the proximal and distal ends can be approximated within one–three cm, the additional technique of circumferential esophageal myotomy can gain further length (Fig. 5-1). As many as three parallel myotomies have also been used on the proximal esophagus and one circumferential

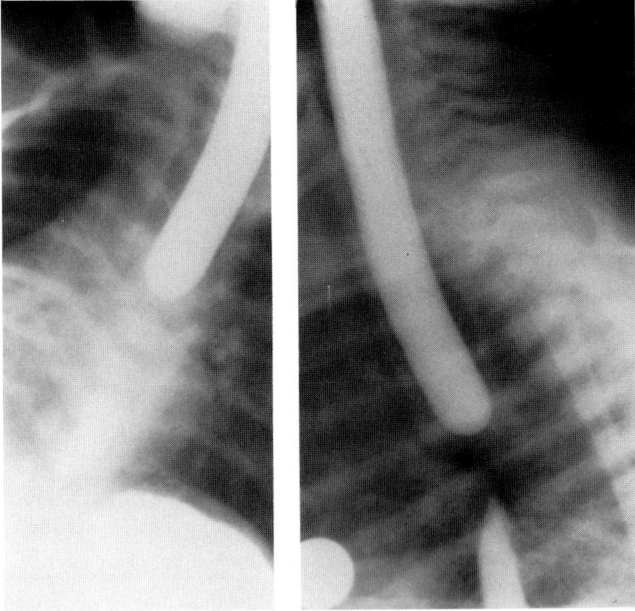

**Figure 5-1.** Radiograph of an infant with esophageal atresia after four weeks of esophageal elongation. A 24F Hurst bougie is pushing the proximal esophagus caudally and contrast placed in the stomach via gastrostomy is refluxed into the distal esophagus.

myotomy has been used between segmental vessels in the distal esophagus. Each myotomy allows elongation of the esophagus by about one cm to provide an anastomosis under acceptable tension. From 1975 through 1984, the authors have treated 11 infants with long-gap esophageal atresia, in whom an esophageal replacement would be considered necessary. Two of the 11 had distal tracheoesophageal fistulas and the others had atresia without fistulas. In nine infants, the esophageal ends were successfully approximated. In one infant, the distal esophagus did not elongate after weeks of attempted bougienage. It remained a very short diverticulum which did not project through the esophageal hiatus. In the other baby, six weeks of bougienage narrowed the gap from six to three cm, but the anastomosis still could not be completed because of excessive tension, in spite of three proximal esophageal myotomies. Perhaps a longer period of bougienage in this small infant would have resulted in satisfactory elongation of both esophageal segments.

Prior to 1980, esophageal atresia was the most common indication for esophageal substitution in children, accounting for one-half to two-thirds of the series reported. With bougienage and myotomy, the necessity for esophageal substitution for this diagnosis should become less frequent.

## Chemical Esophageal Stricture of Perforation

Chemical injury to the esophagus is now the most common indication for esophageal resection and replacement in children. Concentrated acid solutions produce a coagulative necrosis of tissue, thereby forming an eschar which prevents continued penetration of the substance into the deeper layers of the esophagus. Alkali agents such as sodium and potassium hydroxide, ammonia, and sodium hypochlorite are commonly used in the household for cleaning obstructed drain pipes, ovens, and floors and for bleaching. All of these agents have produced severe esophageal injury.[22,29,49,86] (See Chapter 4.)

Experimental work suggests that keeping the esophagus at rest, by feeding through a gastrostomy, allows more rapid healing with less inflammatory granulation and stricture than does continued swallowing by mouth.[46] The gastrostomy must be placed away from the greater curvature of the stomach in case a gastric-tube esophageal substitute becomes necessary at a later time.

Often, a burn involving the esophagus not only produces circumferential fibrosis and narrowing, but longitudinal contracture of the esophagus also develops. The shortened esophagus and direct injury to the gastroesophageal function will induce peptic reflux esophagitis. Continuous peptic inflammation enhances the fibrosis further. On two occasions, the authors have performed a Nissen fundoplication which stopped reflux due to a shortened esophagus, and repeated dilatation for mid- and lower-esophageal stricture could be discontinued (Fig. 5-2).

Excision of the esophagus is necessary, as an emergency, when full-thickness necrosis and mediastinitis have occurred. The decision to resect the esophagus might also be easy when an extensive perforation develops in the course of repeated dilatation of a refractory stricture. Aside from these two situations, the criteria for esophageal resection are not well defined. The variables to be considered include the extent of injury, the rigidity of the fibrotic area, and how frequently dilatations are required. Resection and replacement should not be performed if the area of fibrosis seems to involve a relatively short length, is soft and easily dilatable, and is perhaps confined to

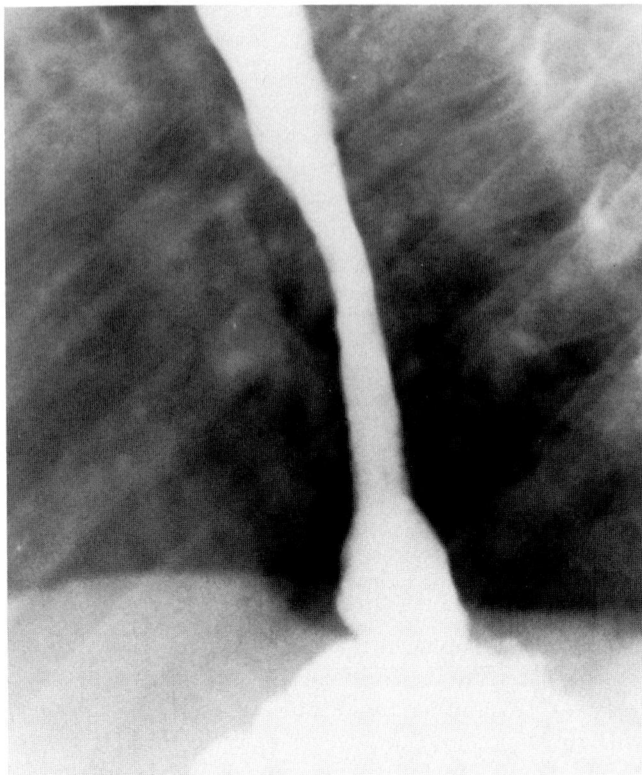

**Figure 5-2.**   Esophagram showing longitudinal shortening as well as circumferential fibrosis following caustic burn of the lower esophagus. This produced hiatal hernia and gastroesophageal reflux. Repeated esophageal dilatation was ineffective until repair of the hiatal hernia and a Nissen fundoplication were performed. Subsequently, the stenotic lower esophagus remained widely patent after several additional dilations.

the submucosal level, requiring dilatation at four–sex-week intervals. A deeper injury involving an extensive length of the esophagus with a thick, hard, nonyielding scar which contracts within days after dilatation makes the decision for esophageal resection easy (Fig. 5-3).

Brain abscess is a serious complication following esophageal dilitation, and such an incident would suggest that esophageal replacement is indicated in place of repeated dilatation.[48]

When esophageal interposition is performed, the proximal anastomosis must be accomplished in normal esophagus above any area of scar. The highest level of scarring should therefore be identified by esophagoscopy as well as esophagram.[8] Caustic burns which include the stomach may require gastrectomy along with esophagectomy (Fig. 5-4). Caustic injury of the esophagus is associated with a greatly increased incidence of carcinoma of the esophagus.[38] The mean interval for development of carcinoma following caustic injury is 40 years and the youngest patient reported was 15 years old—12 years after caustic ingestion.[43] The risk of carcinoma in the age group from 25 to 64

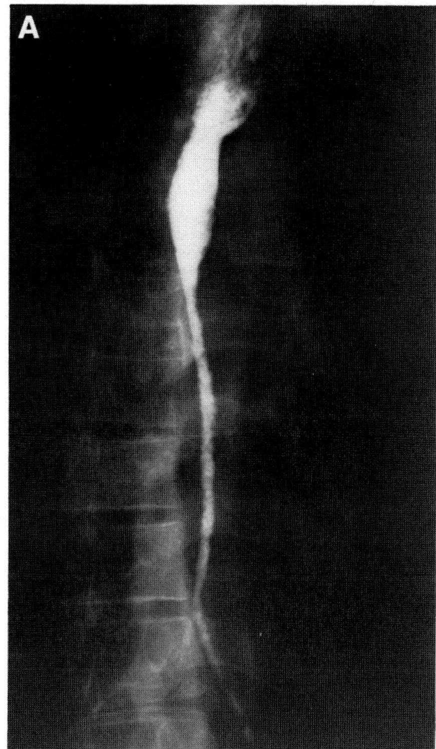
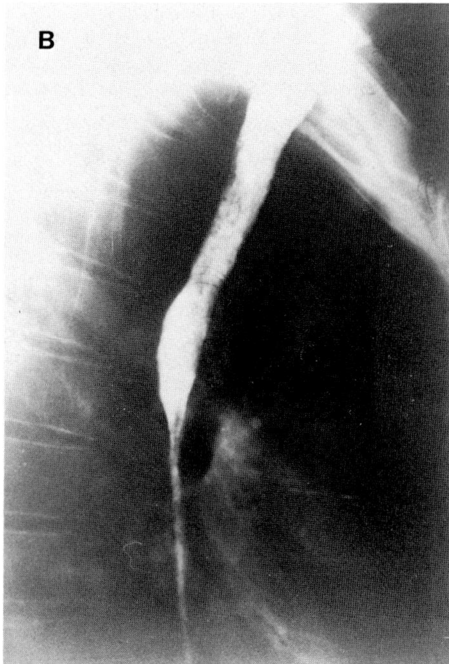

**Figure 5-3.** Anterior-posterior and lateral esophagram showing examples of severe and long stricture of the esophagus with mucosal ulcerations. Although the proximal esophagus appears to have an adequate lumen, it is also densely scarred and has to be replaced.

years, with an injury at least 24 years previously, is 1,000 times greater than in a noninjured population in the same age group[44] This conclusion is based upon nine cases of carcinoma in a follow-up of 381 caustic injuries. This experience does not justify routine esophagectomy for any caustic stricture. When caustic stricture becomes such a significant problem that an esophageal substitute is necessary, however, resection of the esophagus rather than bypass only would seem to be justified.

## Peptic Esophageal Stricture

Protracted gastric reflux and ineffective peristaltic stripping waves in the esophagus result in erosion of the esophageal mucosa and a penetrating injury similar to chemical burns. Usually, the stenosis is most intense at the gastroesophageal junction and extends a varying distance cephalad. In infants and young children, the narrowing is due to the inflammatory reaction and readily responds to an antireflux procedure. Following an antireflux operation, esophageal dilatation should be accomplished using very narrow bougies which will not disrupt the gastric fundal wrap.

Other children, usually teenagers, who have had life-long reflux will develop a long length of stricture with fibrotic retraction of the length of the esophagus and hiatal herniation of the stomach (Fig. 5-5). When the stricture of the esophagus does

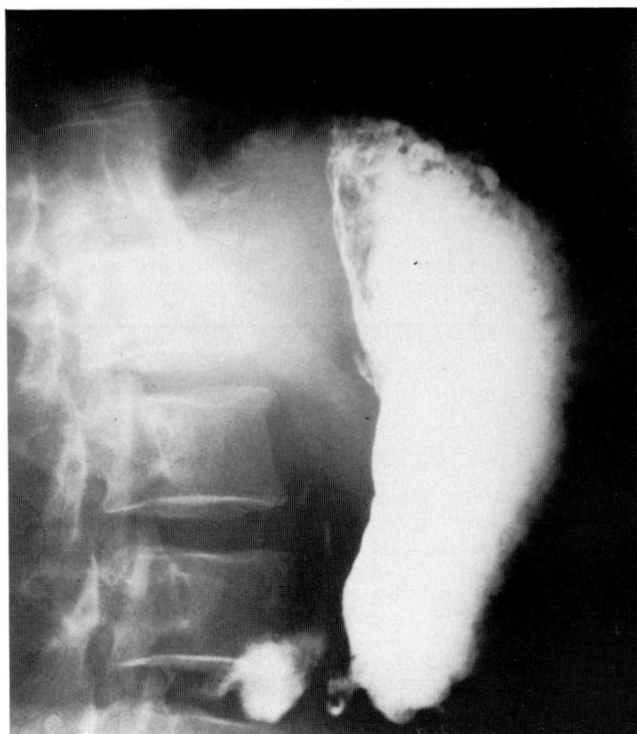

**Figure 5-4.** An upper gastrointestinal series shows stricture of the gastric antrum following caustic ingestion. In addition to esophagectomy, this patient required antrectomy and gastroduodenostomy. A gastric tube interposition would not be prudent because of the risk of infarction of the stomach and gastric tube.

not readily dilate with a bougie, it is unlikely that an antireflux procedure will reverse the hard, fibrotic stricture and esophagectomy and an interpositional replacement of the esophagus will be necessary.

Some patients develop a stricture at the midesophagus rather than at the gastroesophageal junction. This is usually the result of prolonged gastroesophageal reflux with metaplasia of the squamous epithelium to that of the gastric mucosa (Barrett's esophagus). Most of the metaplastic change is to columnar epithelium, but parietal and chief cells can also be found.[63] It is unknown why the stricture does not develop over a long length of the lower esophagus prior to the mucosal metaplasia. The stricture develops at the junction between the metaplastic lining and the squamous epithelium. Barrett's esophagus with stricture usually responds to bougie dilatation and an antireflux procedure. If there are a significant number of parietal cells in the metaplastic mucosa, however, acid reflux and recurring stricture or a penetrating esophageal ulcer may occur. An antireflux procedure does not result in reversion to squamous epithelium, but it can arrest the progression in a cephalad direction. Barrett's esophagus is associated with development of adenocarcinoma in ten–26 percent of patients followed.[58,66] Antireflux procedures do not seem to alter the propensity for the develop-

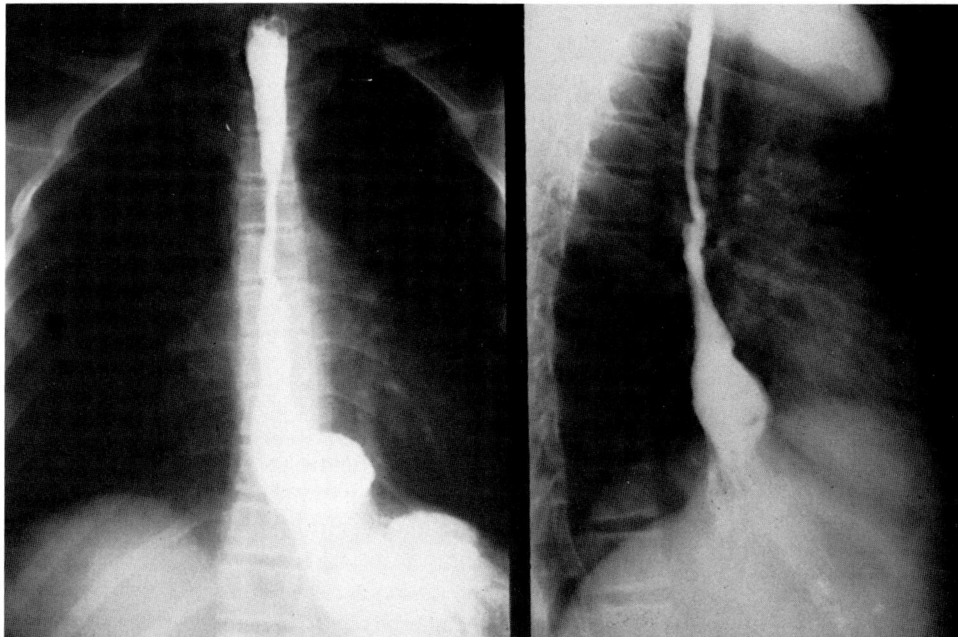

**Figure 5-5.** A,B. Anterior-posterior and later swallowing contrast radiogram showing esophagram in a 14-year-old male with life-long gastroesophageal reflux. The peptic esophagitis resulted in severe, hard fibrotic stricture, and shortening of the esophagus. An esophagectomy and whole-stomach interposition with Nissen fundoplication have been followed by no further morbidity.

ment of carcinoma. The duration of time required to develop carcinoma from the onset of Barrett's esophagus is unknown, but there are case reports of carcinoma developing in patients at age 30 years. Therefore, if an esophageal substitution is comtemplated, resection of the esophagus must be considered when Barrett's esophagus is present.

## Congenital Lower Esophageal Stenosis

Congenital narrowing of the esophagus is almost always located in the distal one-third of the esophagus, but there are reports of involvement in the upper and middle thirds.[81] Frequently, the patient will have been treated previously for esophageal atresia and tracheoesophageal fistula. The narrowing may be produced by a thin web, or it may be a long length of stenosis. The web is usually caused by submucosal fibrous tissue lined by squamous epithelium proximally and distally, and it is readily treated endoscopically with laser excision or by dilatation. Longer lengths of stenosis are usually produced by tracheobronchial remmants, consisting of mucous glands, respiratory epithelium and cartilage. This anomaly fails to yield to dilatation. Most of these patients are successfully treated by segmental resection and primary anastomosis. When a long length of esophagus must be resected, a primary anastomosis is likely to result in recurrent anastomic stricture and/or gastroesophageal reflux with esophagitis. Primary anastomoses may not be possible. In this instance, a segment of bowel may be interposed between the proximal and distal segments.

## Esophageal Perforation

Perforation of the esophagus occurs most commonly from dilatation of a stenotic area, but blunt or penetrating trauma, a swallowed foreign body, or vomiting (Boerhaave's syndrome) can cause a perforation.[73] Small cervical or upper mediastinal perforations heal with drainage and antibiotics. Long, linear perforations of the lower esophagus should be closed with polyglycolate sutures after debridement of the mediastinum and necrotic wound edges. A gastrostomy will minimize the risk of gastric reflux postoperatively. Nutrition should be sustained for 10 days postoperatively, either intravenously or by a feeding jejunostomy. When there is a delay of more than 24 hours before treatment, the widespread inflammatory reaction, tissue necrosis, and sepsis result in a very high mortality rate. If after extensive debridement there is little hope for primary repair, or if there is severe underlying esophageal pathology, the treatment should be esophagectomy with closure of the distal end, proximal cervical esophagostomy, and gastrostomy. A critically ill patient might be treated by chest-tube drainage, cervical esophagostomy (with or without ligating the cardioesophageal junction), and gastrostomy.[82] Controlled drainage of the perforation by using a T-tube and suture closure has also been advocated.[1,78] Following antibiotic treatment and replacement of fluid losses during the next 48 hours, intravenous alimentation should be provided until gastrostomy feedings are tolerated. After the interval of time required for complete resolution of the mediastinal inflammatory reaction (perhaps six months or more), an esophageal substitution will be indicated.

## Muscular Hypertrophy of the Esophagus

Nonobstructive, idiopathic hypertrophy of the esophagus is a rare cause for dysphagia. Some causes of hypertrophy are dysmotility and diffuse esophageal spasm.[23] Other cases seem to be isolated, segmental areas of muscular thickening, confined to the lower or midesophagus.[11] There are reports of congenital segmental hyperplasia primarily affecting the inner muscular layer which involves multiple segments of the gastrointestinal tract, including the esophagus, stomach, pylorus, duodenum, jejunum, ileum and/or colon.[15] The age at onset of symptoms varies from the newborn period to midadolescence. Todani et al. describe their experience with eight cases and summarize information on 36 reported patients.[80] Two-thirds of these cases involved the distal esophagus and the remainder involved with equal frequency the abdominal or midesophagus. Most patients responded very well to long esophagomyotomy similar to Heller's procedure, with the fibromuscular area splitting readily as in hypertrophic pyloric stenosis. Reflux esophagitis was a common postoperative complication. Short areas of involvement have been managed by segmental resection and anastomosis. A particularly thickened, fibrotic, and diffusely involved esophagus will require resection and esophageal substitution (Figs. 5-6 and 5-7).

## Esophageal Varices

Repeated bleeding from esophageal varices might be an indication for esophagectomy and esophageal substitution. In most instances, repeated bleeding from esophageal varices should be treated by lowering portal pressure by using some form of visceral-vein-to-systemic-vein shunt. About 25 – 30 percent of children with extrahepatic portal hypertension are unshuntable, however, because the thrombotic process

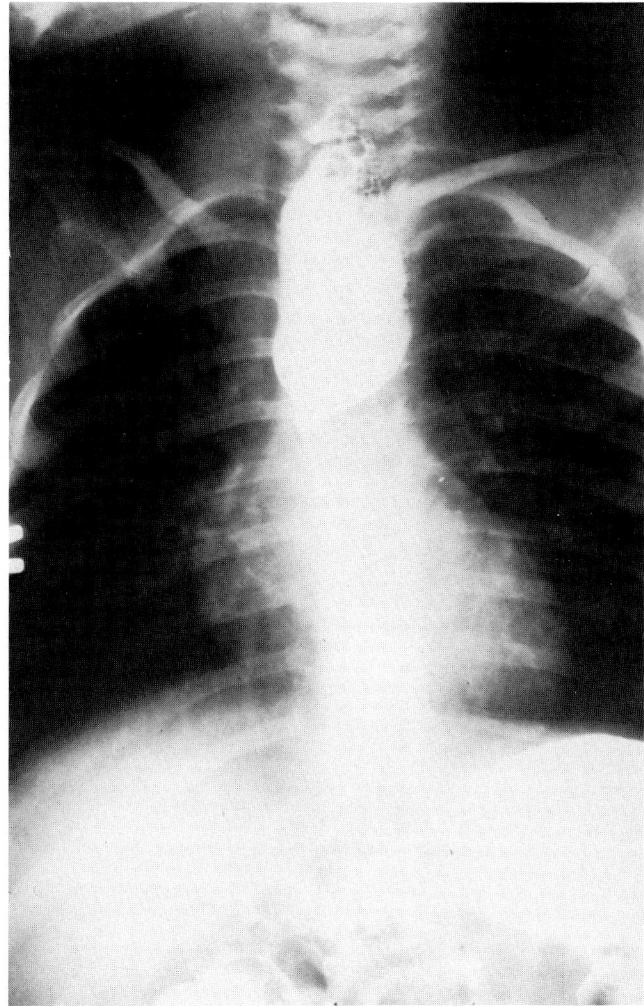

**Figure 5-6.** Esophagram of a three-year-old female with extensive idiopathic muscular hyperplasia of the distal two-thirds of the esophagus, producing obstruction. This lesion could not be dilated. Esophagectomy and colon interposition between the proximal thoracic esophagus and the cardio-esophageal junction resulted in no further symptoms.

obliterates the portal, splenic, and meseneric veins. The natural history of many children with extrahepatic portal hypertension is characterized by a diminishing frequency and severity of bleeding episodes over a period of years, presumably because of the development of effective collateral venous circulation other than esophageal veins. There are some children in whom a shunt is not possible, and who do not develop a diminishing frequency of bleeding.

Procedures which disrupt intramural esophageal collateral venous drainage may be an effective long-term alternative to portal decompression procedures.[77] Repeated endoscopic injections of sclerosing agents into the varices have been used. Most of

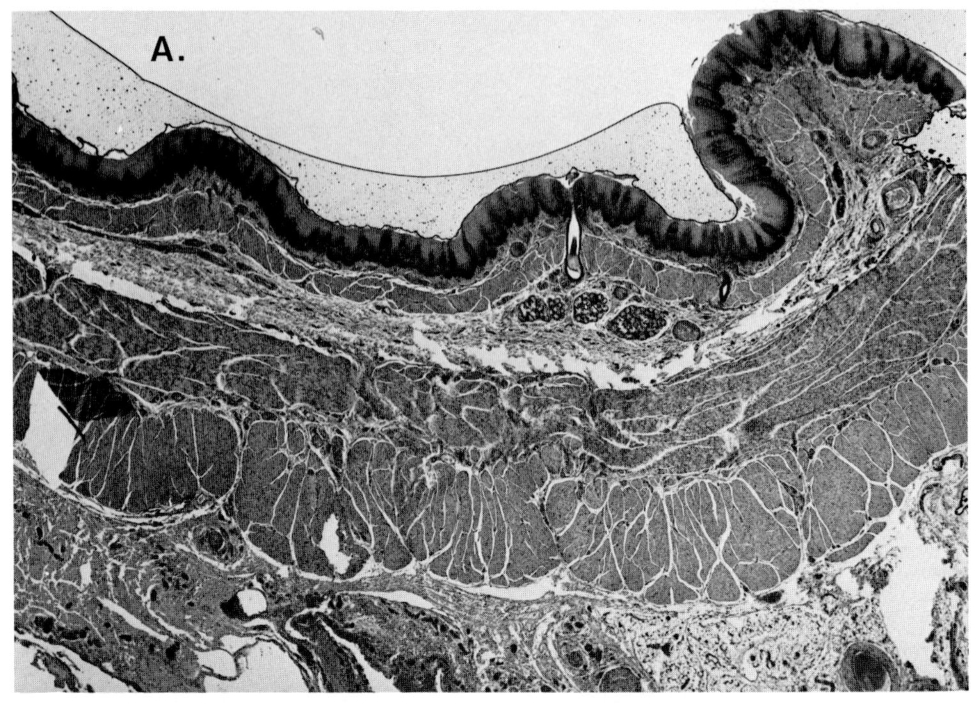

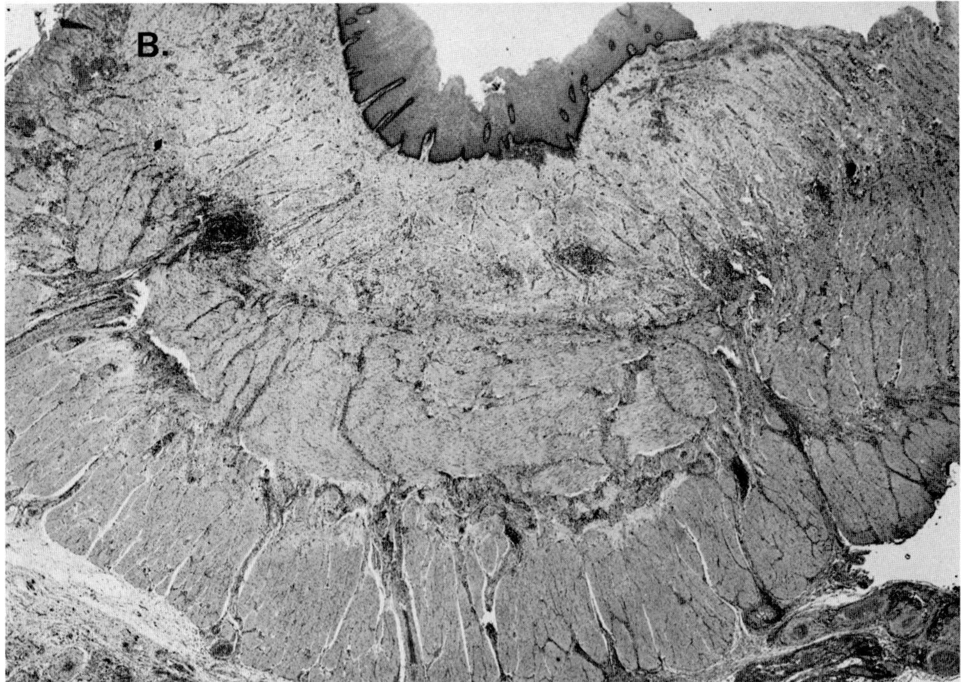

**Figure 5-7.** Patient in Figure 5-5 with muscular hyperplasia of the esophagus. (A) Microscopic cross-section of normal but hypertrophic esophagus proximal to the area of muscular hyperplasia. (B) Microscopic cross-section of distal esophagus showing idiopathic hyperplasis of the muscularis mucosa, circular, and outer longitudinal muscle of the distal esophagus with stenosis of lumen.

these patients develop recurrence of varices with return of extensive bleeding.[20,31,68] These operations in the lower esophagus may result in unyielding stenosis or necrosis, requiring resection and replacement of that portion of the esophagus. Repeated, life-threatening bleeding episodes (with or without liver disease acquired from transfusions) in a patient who lives in a region which is remote from emergency medical facilities might be an indication for esophagectomy with proximal gastrectomy and an esophageal substitute. This procedure does not completely eliminate occult bleeding and anemia, because some blood loss occurs from the small bowel. However, resection of the lower two-thirds of the esophagus and the proximal one-third of the stomach prevents massive, exsanguinating bleeding.

The esophageal substitute most commonly used is the colon interposition. Before this procedure is attempted, it is important to study the venous drainage of the proposed segment of bowel to be utilized. A splenoportogram or mesenteric arteriogram may be necessary (Fig. 5-8). If the venous drainage of the left colon is to the hemorrhoidal vessels, and not by way of the middle colonic vein, it is unlikely that the left colon can be mobilized into the chest without dividing the major venous outflow of that segment of bowel, resulting in infarction of the colon. Before resecting the esophagus, and before dividing the collateral blood supply to the segment of bowel which is selected as an esophageal substitute, it is particularly important to test the venous drainage by using gentle clamp occlusion of the collateral venous tributaries which have to be divided to ensure the viability of the bowel.

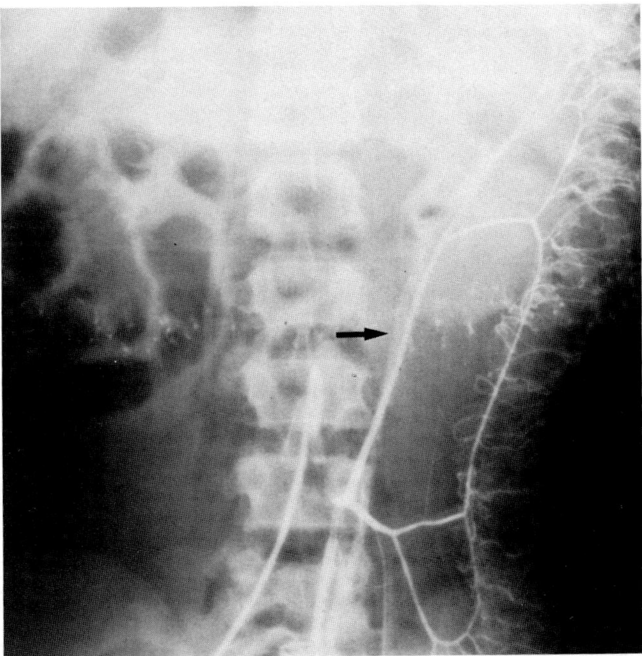

**Figure 5-8.** Selective inferior mesenteric arteriogram in a patient with unshuntable extrahepatic portal hypertension. The portal, splenic, and superior mesenteric veins were occluded. The venous phase of the arteriogram shows that the inferior mesenteric vein is patent (arrow), and, therefore, the left colon could be used for interposition following esophagectomy.

## Epidermolysis Bullosa

Some children with epidermolysis bullosa develop severe stricture of the esophagus[2,27] (Fig. 5-9) Whether the inheritance is of the recessive or dominant form, injury to any squamous epithelium may result in separation of the epidermis from the dermis and produce bullae, epithelial slough, and invasive infection and subcutaneous fibrous contractures. In addition to skin involvement, the oropharynx, esophagus, and anus may also develop stricture. The upper esophagus is affected in two-thirds of cases. The lower esophagus is involved in 25 percent of patients, which is an involvement probably due to mechanical injury from swallowed food.[38]

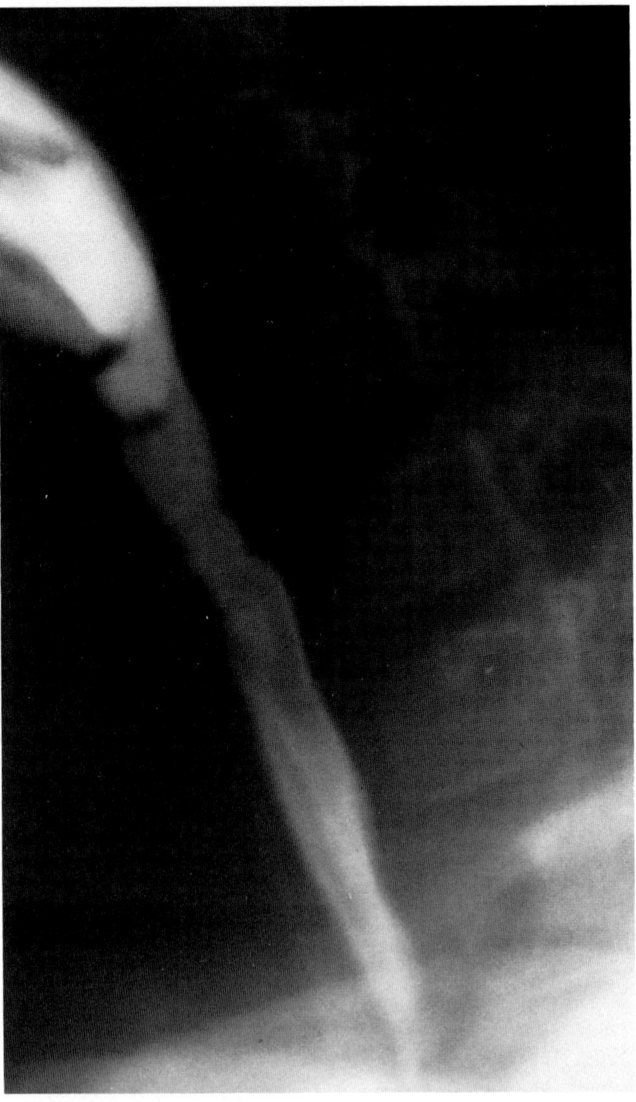

**Figure 5-9.** Esophagram of a patient with epidermolysis bullosa. Repeated trauma to the squamous epithelium of the esophagus has resulted in web formation in several areas of the cervical esophagus.

Treatment of these strictures by conservative measures can be successful. A mechanical soft diet prevents progression on long-term follow-up.[38] Esophageal dilatation and corticosteroids have been variably successful in preventing progression of the stenosis.[61] For isolated focal stricture, local excision of the scar has been useful.[45] Esophageal bypass using retrosternal colon interposition has been accomplished in four reported cases.[2,27,45]

Squamous cell carcinoma of the esophagus develops in about 15 percent of patients with epidermolysis bullosa.[2] Esophagectomy might be indicated rather than a bypass of the esophagus. In the two cases described by Absolon et al., however, in whom esophagectomy was performed three years after retrosternal colon bypass, there was little esophageal mucosa remaining, and there was nearly complete obliteration of the lumen.[2]

## Esophageal Tumors

Tumors of the esophagus in childhood are very rare. Of the benign tumors, leiomyoma is the most common in any age group. Of 167 cases collected from the English literature, only one male and 12 females were under the age of 20 years.[64] Almost all of these 167 cases were treated by local enucleation excision. Diffuse, multiple, nodular leiomyomas involving all of the esophagus have been successfully treated by longitudinal myotomy in four patients.[51] A 14-year-old girl with massive hematemesis from diffuse leiomyomatosis has been reported to have required a total esophagectomy and retrosternal colon interposition.[59]

Hemangiomas of the esophagus have been described more often in adults than in children. These hemangiomas are apparently of the noninvoluting, cavernous variety. In children, the involuting hemangioma is most common and, with current conservative treatment of these tumors, the indications for esophageal replacement should be very unusual.

Malignant tumors arising in the esophagus in children are extremely rare. Squamous carcinoma and malignant melanoma have been reported in children.[64] Adenocarcinoma arising in columnar mucosa of Barrett's esophagus is now well-known, and it has been reported in a 23-year-old.[64] As yet, rhabdomyosarcoma or leiomyosarcoma arising within the esophagus have not been described in childhood.

Esophagectomy may be necessary for tumors arising adjacent to the esophagus, at the hiatus, or in the mediastinum. The authors have resected the lower esophagus for retroperitoneal rhabdomyosarcoma in a four-year-old male. Esophagectomy to facilitate excision of an adjacent tumor should be deferred until a course of chemotherapy and/or radiotherapy has been utilized with the hope that the esophagus might be preserved.

## Severe Motility Disorders

Dysmotility of the esophagus may result in significant morbidity by contributing to aspiration pneumonia and/or inadequate nutrition. Of the many motility disorders, those of importance in pediatrics include achalasia, diffuse esophageal spasm, with or without associated esophageal atresia, and the dysmotility-of-collagen diseases, such as dermatomyositis and scleroderma. Achalasia and severe forms of diffuse esophageal spasm respond to a long esophageal myotomy, in which the esophageal muscle is widely separated longitudinally to avoid scar contracture and reapproximation of the muscle.[9,75] In the case of achalasia, the myotomy should extend through the cardioesophageal junction less than one cm on the gastric side to avoid inducing reflux. Following the long esophageal myotomy, the esophagus becomes a passive conduit— no different than an esophageal substitute. The dysphagia associated with the collagen diseases is not severe enough to warrant esophageal replacement. The motility disorders are therefore not an indication for esophageal replacement, except when complications of a myotomy or severe reflux esophagitis result in destruction of the esophagus.

### Esophageal Candidiasis

Esophagitis secondary to candida infection may be so extensive that esophageal substitution is required. This usually occurs in an immuno-compromised patient who is likely to have been on long-term steroid and antibiotic treatment. Mucosal ulceration may progress to invasive infection leading to scarring and stricture of the muscularis. Stricture formation and acute and chronic inflammatory reaction with bleeding which is unresponsible to Mycostatin (Squibb) and amphotericin would be indications for esophagectomy or bypass interposition.

## CHOICES AND POSITIONS FOR ESOPHAGEAL REPLACEMENT

The only practical esophageal substitutes are constructed from four viscera: stomach, jejunum, ileo-colon, and colon. There are no large series to compare the superiority of one or another procedure, and the preference is influenced by: (1) the length and segment of esophagus to be replaced; (2) anomalies or disease associated with the esophageal problem; and, (3) the adequacy of blood supply to the portion of bowel to be used as an esophageal substitute.

The use of a skin tube is only of historical interest, for this requires multiple operative procedures to construct, is cosmetically undesirable, and does not provide an adequate conduit. It is unlikely that conduits made from foreign material will ever be feasible, primarily because of infection and anastomotic disruption of the suture line.

When a conduit is to be constructed, it may be placed either: (1) by way of retrosternal route; (2) transpleurally behind the hilum of the lung; or, (3) by positioning along the mediastinum in the bed of the esophagus. The retrosternal route is favored by many surgeons because it is technically easiest to maintain the patient in a supine position with an abdominal and neck incision only, and a tunnel is readily developed behind the sternum by blunt dissection from an abdominal and neck incision.

In using the retrosternal route, the anomalous course for the conduit is responsible for dysfunctional problems. The upper connection requires that either the cervical esophagus or the bowel conduit must curve around the trachea from an anterior to a posterior position. The space between the clavicle-manubrium-sternomastoid muscle junction and the trachea can be very small. This contributes to a cosmetically undesirable bulge in the neck with each swallow of a bolus. Dysphagia results because ingested food is transiently arrested at that level, and, in younger children, aspiration commonly results. Some surgeons have advocated transecting the origin of the sterno-mastoid muscle or resecting the medial portion of the clavicle and part of the manu-brium to provide more space, but this produces a deformity which is cosmetically unsatisfactory. In the abdomen, the conduit extends over the liver and the anastomosis to the stomach is usually at the level of the antrum. Gastric peristalsis may push food back into the conduit, resulting in to and fro movement between the conduit and stomach, which delays gastric emptying. Theoretically, gastric reflux into a retros-ternal conduit would be minimized by compression between the liver and the abdomi-nal wall. Reflux is not, however, diminished in the authors' experience, and this area of compression usually produces impaired emptying of the conduit into the stomach. Not uncommonly, the colon dilates and becomes elongated above the liver (Fig. 5-10). The retrosternal conduit is longer than those placed posteriorly, and this added length is conducive to dysphagia.

The posterior mediastinal route, in the bed of the esophagus, requires a much shorter length of esophageal substitute, and the anastomosis can be accomplished between the distal esophagus or the fundus of the stomach. The proximal esophageal anastomosis in the neck or upper mediastinum will be in a normal posterior position, avoiding the problems presented by the retrosternal conduit at the thoracic inlet. The disadvantage of the posterior mediastinal position for an esophageal substitute is the

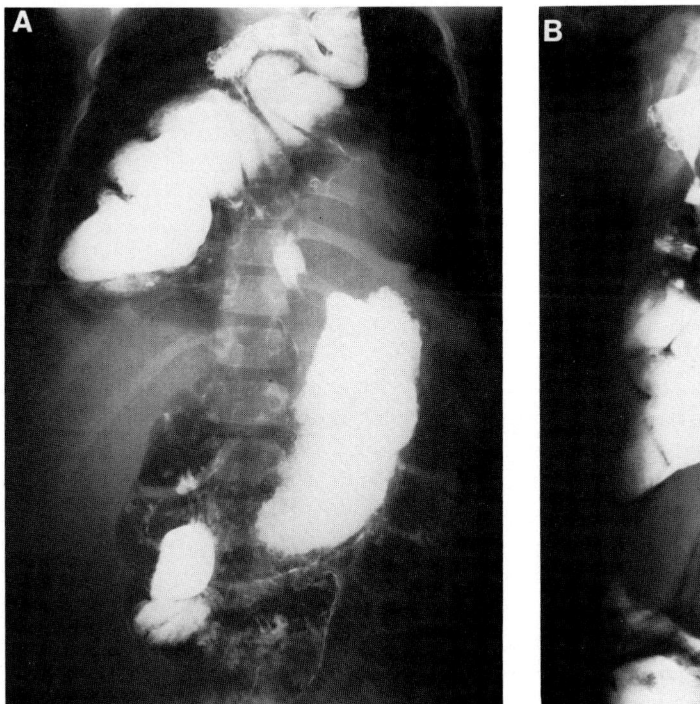
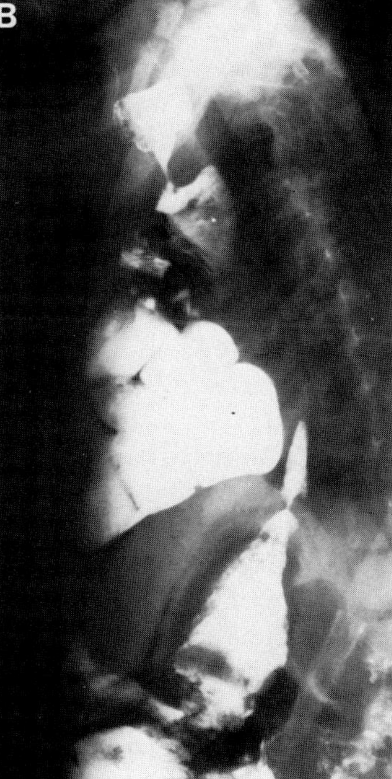

**Figure 5-10.**   Anterior-posterior and lateral radiograph showing a greatly dilated and elon-gated retrosternal colon interposition with compression of the colon segment between the liver and the anterior abdominal wall. Reflux into the distal esophagus may result in esophagitis with bleeding or perforation.

requirement of a thoracotomy, which results in a longer and a technically challenging operative procedure.

In the patient whose proximal and distal esophagus are intact, as in esophageal atresia or a midesophageal stricture, the authors prefer to use colon interposed between the two esophageal ends. The swallowing function with this reconstruction is associated with much less dysphagia than is true of the alternatives, such as a gastric tube or a retrosternal colon interposition. Anastomosis to the distal esophagus will minimize gastroesophageal reflux.

Other factors determine the choice of esophageal substitute. If there is a history of persistent diarrhea or loose stools, or if incontinence is present, as in patients with an associated high imperforate anus, use of a colon segment might not be appropriate. Lye stricture of the esophagus can be associated with gastric antral scarring and contracture which must be identified if whole stomach or a stomach tube replacement is being considered (Fig. 5-4). A high esophageal replacement might eliminate the use of jejunum because of the great difficulty in gaining a sufficient length of mesenteric blood supply. Small bowel is most susceptible to peptic ulceration if the interposition involves a gastric anastomosis in which reflux is inevitable. Further limitations involving the various choices for esophageal substitution are described below in the discussion of the bowel segment to be used.

## Stomach as an Esophageal Replacement

The entire stomach may be used as an esophageal replacement or a tube of stomach can be developed from the greater curvature. In teenaged children and adults, use of the entire stomach is probably one of the best esophageal substitutes.[12,33] It requires dividing the left gastric and short gastric vessels, but preserving the right gastric and gastroepiploic vessels. The duodenum should be mobilized by a Kocher manuever, so that when the stomach is passed through the esophageal hiatus, the pylorus will be positioned at the hiatus (Fig. 5-11). To leave a portion of the stomach below the diaphragm seems to exacerbate reflux, since a part of the stomach is subject to positive intra-abdominal pressure, while the intrathoracic portion is exposed to a negative pressure. This also tends to produce retention of food in the intrathoracic gastric pouch and may contribute to peptic ulceration of the stomach. To use the whole stomach, most of the esophagus should be removed so that the stomach will become an elongated, narrow pouch rather than an redundant bag in the chest. Since the anastomosis should be at or above the aortic arch, the authors like to mobilize the stomach, duodenum, and lower esophagus through a transverse upper abdominal incision. The esophageal anastomosis may be accomplished through a right (for a left-sided aortic arch) fourth intercostal space thoracotomy. When a left thoracotomy is used, the esophagus has to be mobilized between the carotid and subclavian arteries, providing very poor exposure and a risk of injuring the recurrent laryngeal nerve. It is ideal to retain at least four cm of intrathoracic esophagus to allow a Nissen fundoplication about the proximal esophageal remnant, which will minimize gastroesophageal and pharyngeal reflux. The anastomosis can be at the original gastroesophageal junction or in any convenient area on the body of the stomach which allows a fundoplication to be performed. If there is a problem with adequate length of stomach, the gastroesophageal junction should be oversewn and the fundus of the stomach will have to be the area for anastomosis. Since a vagotomy inevitably occurs in this proce-

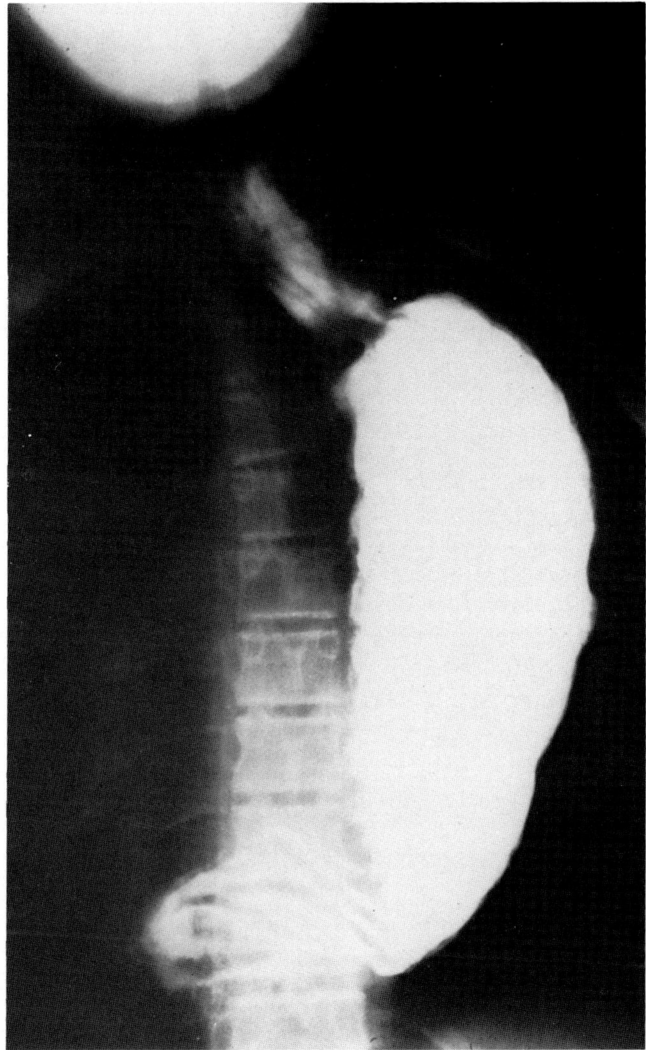

**Figure 5-11.**    Contrast radiograph showing whole-stomach replacement of the esophagus. The pylorus is positioned at the esophageal hiatus to minimize stasis in gastric emptying and to avoid reflux of duodenal contents. A Nissen fundoplication at the upper thoracic esophagus effectively prevented reflux into the pharynx.

dure, impaired gastric emptying from pylorospasm will develop in a significant number of patients. A pyloroplasty might therefore be considered at this stage, or it could be done later when gastric retention is an established problem. It is possible to preserve the hepatic and celiac branches of the right vagus nerves to minimize post-vagotomy diarrhea syndrome. A nasogastric tube should be placed for postoperative decompression, to avoid overdistention of the initially atonic stomach.

Use of the whole stomach in infancy and early childhood is not advised, because the gastric capacity following a feeding results in crowding of the lungs and compression of the trachea, and because there is an impressive incidence of reflux (Fig. 5-12).[5] In a one-year-old baby, the total lung volume is less than 1000 ml, and a feeding of eight ounces (240 ml) encroaches significantly on the lung capacity. Reflux of gastric contents is also a very great hazard in young infants because of their greater propensity to aspirate than is true of older patients.

The large gastric reservoir could be reduced in size by resecting the lesser curvature and the esophagogastric junction.[85] There is a risk of necrosis because the blood supply of the remaining stomach is dependent upon the integrity of collateral blood flow between the right and left gastroepiploic vessels. The same result could be accomplished by resecting the greater curvature, but the length of the gastric tube available would be short. These techniques have not been popular, probably because it seems wasteful to sacrifice normal stomach. In addition, it is desirable to have a reservoir, as well as an esophageal conduit, to facilitate digestion and absorption and to minimize dumping syndrome.

## Gastric Tube Interposition

The complications of a large gastric reservoir in the thorax and of a vagotomy can be avoided by using a gastric tube developed from the greater curvature of the stomach. This is an effective conduit in any age beyond the first year. The gastric tube can be based at the fundus or from the antrum of the stomach.[3,4,13,19,30,35,50] When the tube is to placed in the bed of the esophagus, the fundus becomes the base for the blood

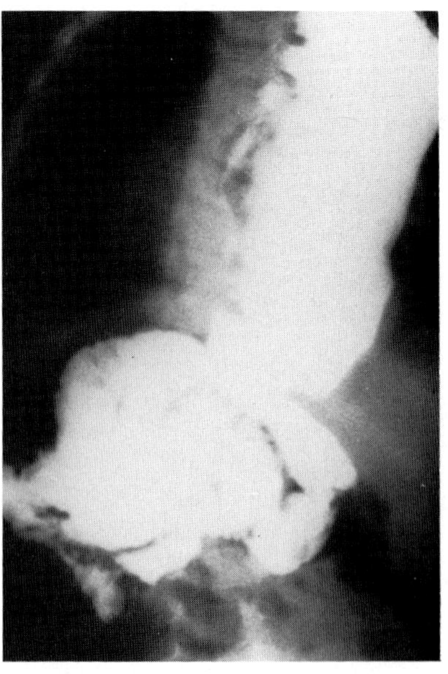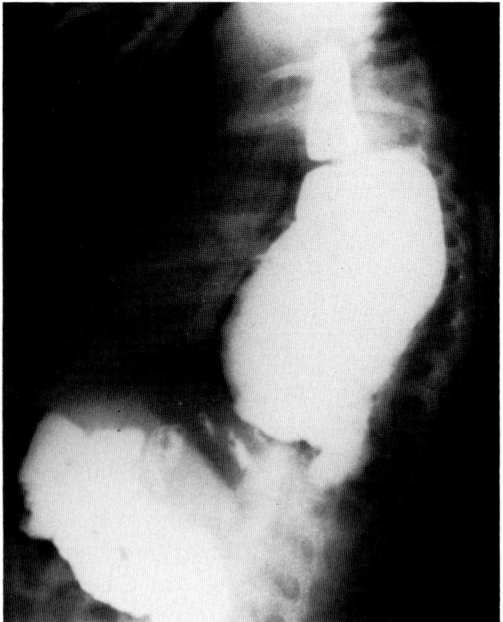

**Figure 5-12.** Anterior-posterior and lateral radiograph with contrast in an infant with esophageal atresia, in whom a whole-stomach interposition was performed. The stomach, large relative to the thoracic capacity, contributed to significant dyspnea. Reflux into the pharynx resulted in recurrent aspiration.

supply. Many pediatric surgeons prefer using a retrosternal tunnel in which case the blood supply for the tube originates at the antrum.[13,50]

For a retrosternal placement of the gastric tube, the patient is placed in a supine position with a rolled towel under the shoulders to extend the head and neck. The abdominal incision may be midline or transverse. The omentum is resected, preserving the gastroepiploic vessels. An incision is made across the anterior and posterior wall of stomach on the greater curvature close to the fundus of the stomach. A size 20–26 French red rubber catheter is then passed into the lumen and along the greater curvature of the stomach to outline the proposed line for incision along the anterior and posterior walls of the stomach. Mattress sutures placed adjacent to the tube, through and through the anterior and posterior walls, help to mark the line of incision and to align the gastroepiploic vessels. A marking pen can also be used to ink the line of incision. The gastro-intestinal anastomosis (GIA) stapler facilitates incision and suture closure of the stomach and the tube. The short gastric vessels must be divided but the spleen should be preserved. The authors prefer to reinforce the stapled suture line with 4-0 seromuscular silk sutures to minimize the risk of leakage. The tube is then passed over the left lobe of the liver and through a tunnel developed behind the sternum to a incision above the manubrium in the neck. There has usually been a cervical esophagostomy previously created. Most surgeons delay the cervical esophageal anastomosis until two–four weeks later, to ensure viability of the end of the tube. In this procedure, the main body of the stomach will become rotated so that the posterior surface faces anteriorly. A gastrostomy is therefore placed in the posterior wall of the stomach for feeding.

For posterior, intrathoracic placement of the gastric tube, the fundus becomes the base of the tube (Fig. 5-13). A thoracoabdominal or separate abdominal, thoracic, and neck incisions will be required. In this instance, the short gastric vessels and the spleen are preserved. An incision is made across the greater curvature in the antrum of the stomach, after dividing the right gastroepiploic vessels. The most distal area for this incision must provide for an adequate lumen at the antrum to allow unimpaired gastric emptying. After development of the tube, the end of the tube is passed into the chest through a new opening in the posterior diaphragm, which is placed to the left of the esophageal hiatus. Twisting and distortion of the origin of the tube with the fundus should be avoided to prevent peptic ulceration or tube ischemia from an impaired blood supply.[4] The gastric tube should not be used to replace only a short length of distal esophagus because significant reflux and esophageal stricture seems to be most common when the tube is short.[19,35] Theoretically, it is desirable to have several centimeters of gastric tube within the abdomen, in the hope that intra-abdominal pressure will compress the tube and minimize reflux, as opposed to having a wide-funneled, stomach-to-tube junction positioned at the diaphragm or in the chest. Although construction of the tube in this manner is antiperistaltic, there has been no report that retrograde peristalsis occurs to impair swallowing.

Vagotomy is unnecessary unless it was performed in the course of an esophagectomy. If a vagotomy has been done, a pyloromyotomy or a small pyloroplasty is necessary to facilitate gastric emptying and we perfer to perform a pyloromyotomy to minimize dumping syndrome. The authors have not experienced impaired drainage from performance of a pyloromyotomy rather than a pyloroplasty. Decompression of the stomach is accomplished by a gastrostomy to avoid possible erosion from a nasogastric tube.

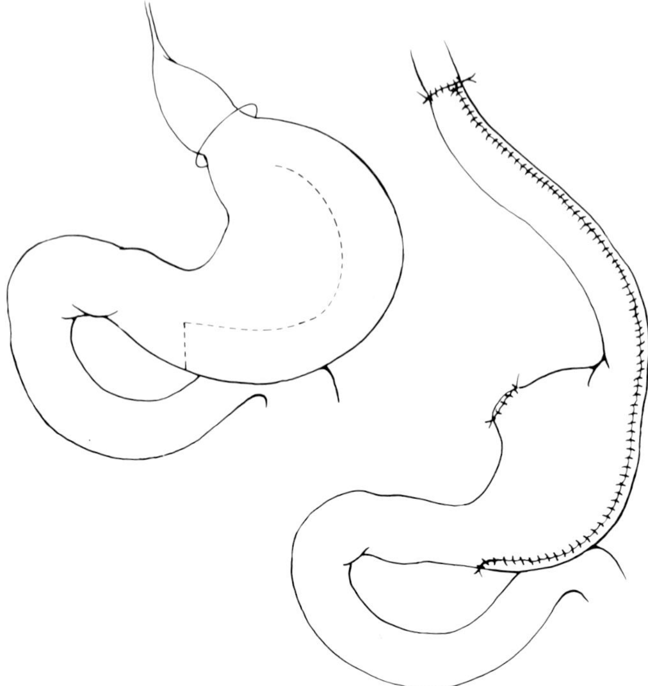

**Figure 5-13.**   A gastric tube operation. The drawing on the left shows a dashed line on the greater curvature of the stomach which outlines the plan for incision. The drawing on the right shows the completed gastric tube mobilized to the proximal esophagus.

Advantages of a gastric tube, as compared to use of other bowel segments, include: (1) the fact that it is a straight, thick-walled conduit which does not become elongated, redundant and dilated; and, (2) a presumed better blood supply with a lesser risk of ischemia at the esophageal anastomosis. The use of stomach might be preferred in children who have long-gap esophageal atresia and a high imperforate anus anomaly or a known diarrhea syndrome where incontinence is expected. Use of the stomach is also an option when the blood supply to the colon is compromised, or when there is an intrinsic disease of the colon. Impairment in growth has been a concern in infants and very young children who have esophageal substitutes. There are limited, long-term, follow-up reports on gastric interpositions, but so far retarded growth and development have not been described.[3,20,50,52]

Potential complications in using the stomach include: (1) gastric reflux; (2) small gastric reservoir; (3) gastric outlet obstruction; (4) leakage from the prolonged suture line of the greater curvature and gastric tube; (5) peptic ulcer or stricture at the junction of the stomach reservoir and gastric tube; and, (6) leakage and stricture at the esophagogastric anastomosis.

Reflux from the gastric tube interposition has been a troublesome problem. Surgeons who perform a preliminary cervical gastrostomy have noted reflux of gastric contents to the level of the neck.[20] This complication might be diminished by using a long tube and by leaving a five-cm length of tube within the abdominal cavity. However, reflux is present in all patients with either the retrosternal or transthoracic gastric tube.[10,20] Reflux esophagitis and stricture have occurred when the gastric tube is too short.[20,35] The authors find that reflux of gastric contents to the level of the pharynx is just as significant as with any other esophageal substitute, and it is a severe problem to some patients. The reflux probably contributes to the high incidence of esophageal anastomotic leakage and stricture. The Nissen fundoplication principle has been attempted in an effort to minimize reflux, although without success (Fig. 5-14).

Depending upon the size of the stomach, the gastric tube does diminish the gastric capacity to some extent. Gastric outlet obstruction might occur if the gastric tube extends into the antrum sufficiently far to compromise the lesser curvature lumen. The risk of leakage could be considered in proportion to the length of the suture-line closure. Obviously, the stomach wall closure has to be carefully performed. Although the stomach has a presumed superior blood supply, leaking of the esophageal anastomosis and necrosis at the end of the tube with stricture seems to be as common as with other esophageal substitutes.[19,20,50,52]

A splenectomy has been a part of the gastric tube procedure performed by some surgeons. There is no reason to remove the spleen, for if the gastrosplenic ligament limits mobilizing the tube into the chest, the short gastric vessels can be divided without impairing splenic blood flow.

A gastric tube procedure should not be attempted if a previous gastrostomy has been placed within the greater curvature area which would be used to form the tube, because the blood supply will be compromised.

Although the gastric tube is currently a very popular esophageal substitute for use

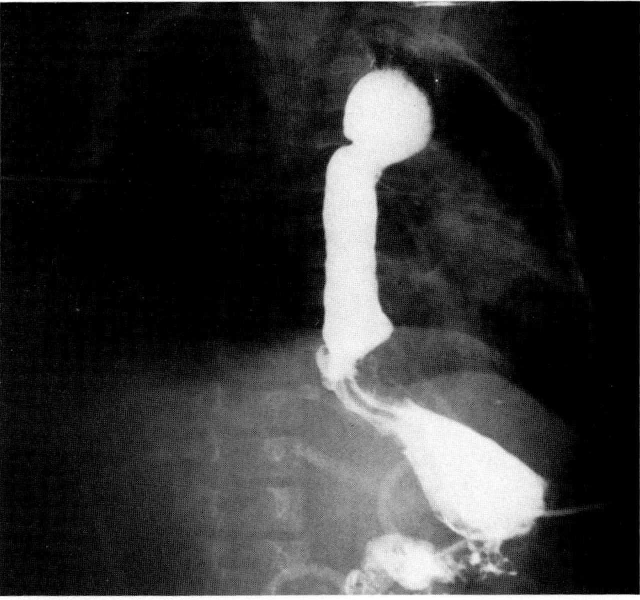

**Figure 5-14.**   A contrast radiograph demonstrates gastric tube interposition in the bed of the esophagus. A partial wrap of the fundus is evident by the narrowing at the lower end of the gastric tube, which was ineffective in preventing reflux. Note the reduced size of the intra-abdominal reservoir.

in pediatric surgery, it has not been shown to be clearly superior to the colon interposition. In the authors' opinion, preferential use of the gastric tube should be considered when there are clear *contraindications* for use of the colon.

## Small Bowel Substitutes

Jejunum has been used as an esophageal substitute but it is not a bowel segment preferred by most surgeons.[10,16,24,33,52] The blood supply to the jejunum limits the length of jejunal tube which can be constructed. The vasculature to the jejunum is composed of numerous short primary, secondary, and tertiary arcades repeatedly branching from the origin of the superior mesenteric vessel to form a fan-shaped mesentery.[7,24] This results in the bowel assuming serpentine coils attached to the mesentery, so that isolation of any length of jejunum results in an elongated, tortuous, and redundant segment. The mesentery is very short and usually cannot span any great length of the chest. Infarction of the jejunal segment commonly occurs because pulling the bowel through the chest produces stretching of the mesenteric vessels and because of variation in the blood supply.[7] Use of the jejunum has therefore usually been confined to replacing short lengths of the lower esophagus (Fig. 5-15).

An experience with 34 consecutive cases of successful anterior interpositions of jejunum between the cervical esophagus and the antrum of the stomach has been reported.[26,32] All patients underwent cervical esophagostomy and gastrostomy. Because of concerns about blood supply, the procedure was staged by first isolating the desired length of jejunum and passing it along a subcutaneous tunnel over the sternum to form a cervical jejunostomy proximally with an end-to-side Roux Y jejunostomy distally. The vascular pedicle is brought through an opening in the transverse mesocolon and gastrocolic ligament. The second stage is a take-down of the esophagostomy and the cervical jejunostomy with esophagojejunostomy. At the second, or as a third-stage, procedure, the Roux Y is converted to a jejuno-antrostomy, at which time there is an attempt to eliminate redundancy of the jejunal interposition. The final stage consists of placing the jejunal limb in a retrosternal position by way of a median sternotomy. Surgeons are gradually reducing the number of operative stages by more direct approaches, but remain concerned about serious complications should the jejunal limb necrose.

The technique for achieving adequate length of jejunum consists of: (1) identifying and preserving the third dominant jejunal artery and vein originating from the superior mesenteric vessels; (2) incising the peritoneal cover of mesentery, including the lymphatics and autonomic nerves in a radial direction from the base of the mesentery; and, (3) dividing two or three minor secondary arcades while ensuring that continuity of the blood supply is intact.[26]

Unlike other esophageal substitutes, this long length of jejunum is not just a conduit. Swallowing is achieved by jejunal peristalsis. Initially, these patients have to eat very slowly, but eventually they apparently can achieve a normal eating time.[32] In an 18–33-year follow-up, one-half of the patients were unable to vomit, and only 31 percent were described as having a redundant jejunum.[32] Cervical fistulas occurred in 23 percent and stricture developed in ten percent. These problems are about the same as those reported with other types of esophageal substitutes. The jejunum is susceptible to peptic ulceration. In spite of vagotomy and pyloroplasty, reflux of gastric juice through the jejunal conduit can produce peptic jejunitis and ulceration. If the jejunal

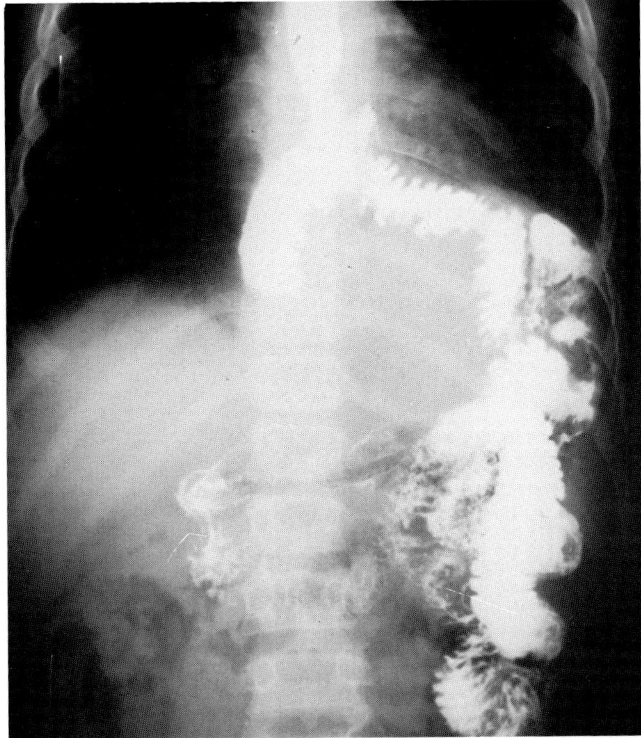

**Figure 5-15.** An esophagram shows jejunum interposed between the midesophagus and the stomach. The lower half of the esophagus and proximal half of the stomach were resected for recurrent bleeding in a 14-year-old boy with extrahepatic portal hypertension. The redundancy of the jejunum was necessary in order to maintain the blood supply to the level of the esophageal anastomosis.

segment is short, reflux peptic esophagitis above the esophagojejunal anastomosis may also occur.[45] Jejunal ulceration has not, however, developed in series of 32 and 12 cases.[26,32]

The terminal ileum has a blood supply which arborizes less extensively than does the jejunum, and the long marginal branch of the ileo-colonic vessels makes it possible to provide a long length for esophageal substitution without the redundancy of the jejunum.[26,33,67] The addition of the ileo-cecal valve with a short length of right colon has been advocated as a means of gaining a greater length of conduit and to provide an antireflux mechanism.[33,39] The cecum and right colon tend, however, to become widely dilated and produce a sense of fullness in the neck, palpitations, and a foul breath related to slow emptying of the bowel.[33] Ileum is more resistant to peptic ulceration than is jejunum, but less so than the colon.[33] Isolation of the ileum and ileo-cecal valve may contribute to malabsorption, particularly when post-vagotomy diarrhea and dumping syndrome might occur if an esophagectomy has been performed. Ileo-colon should probably be reserved for a retrosternal interposition to avoid the consequences of vagal nerve transection associated with esophagectomy. The use of the small bowel has not been popular because the use of stomach or colon to replace the esophagus is technically easier.

## Colon Interposition

The colon can be used in either a retrosternal or posterior mediastinal position. The long vascular branches from the superior or inferior mesenteric vessels and the elongated solitary vessels coursing along the mesenteric border of the bowel allow mobilization of long sections of the colon, which can extend to the level of the hypopharynx, if needed. The disadvantage of using the right and transverse colon is the very wide diameter and thin wall, as compared to the left colon. The colon frequently becomes greatly dilated, redundant, elongated, and a poorly functioning conduit (Fig. 5-16). The right and transverse colon are usually placed in an isoperistaltic position, while the left colon is usually passed through the chest in an antiperistaltic direction. The motility of the colon is very desultory, and clinical studies do not suggest that antiperistaltic left colon interferes with swallowing more than does the isoperistaltic transverse or right colon.[21,26,39,40,62,67]

In patients with severe caustic injury above the cricopharyngeus, a sufficient length of colon must be selected to bring it to a very high level in the neck. The colon can be withdrawn and anastomosed to a level as cephalad as the inferior and middle constrictors of the pharynx with satisfactory swallowing function. These patients are likely to have caustic injury which also involves the larynx, and a tracheostomy will

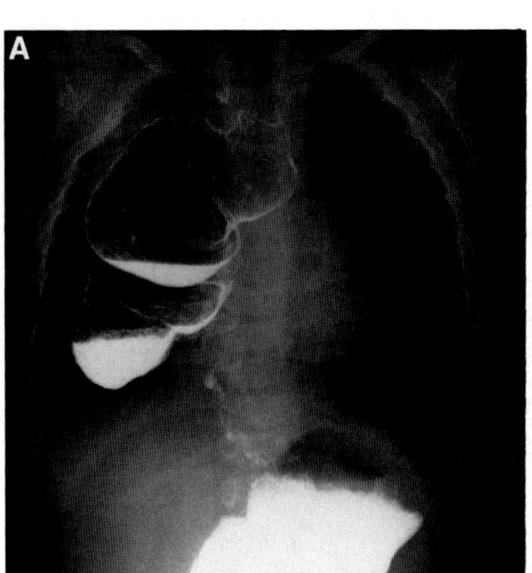
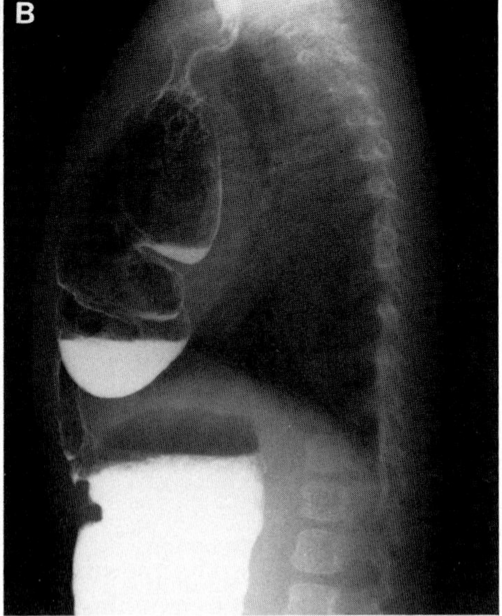

**Figure 5-16.** Anterior-posterior and lateral contrast esophagrams demonstrate a greatly dilated right colon interposition placed retro-sternally for treatment of long-gap esophageal atresia. Stagnation of swallowed contents in the dilated segments resulted in impaired swallowing of solids and reflux into the pharynx.

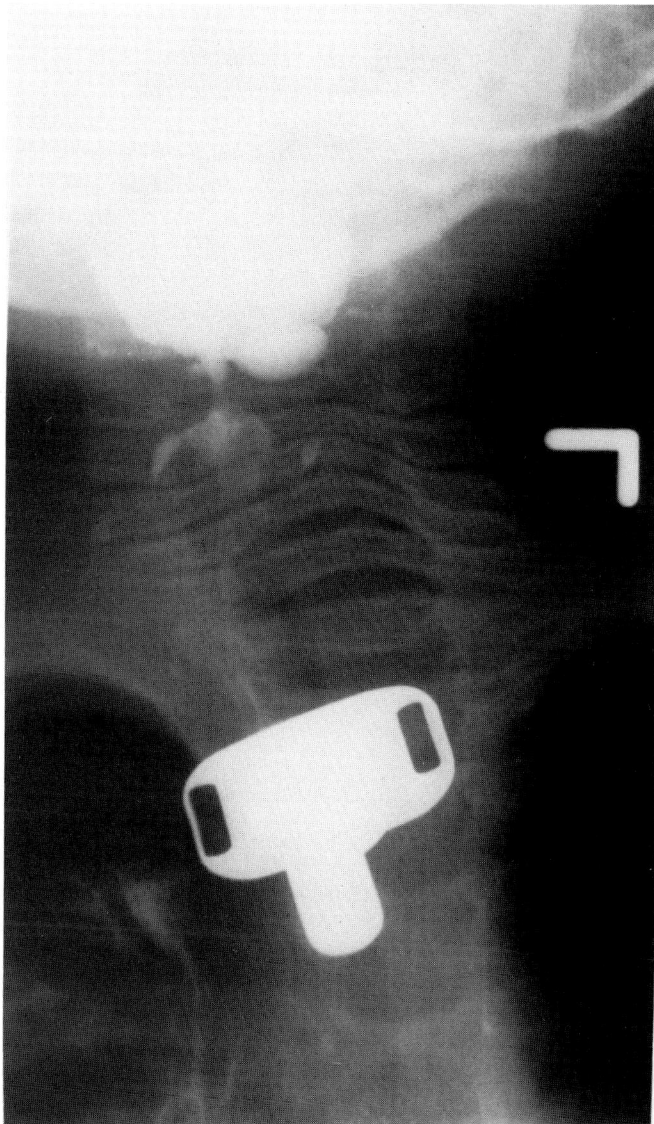

**Figure 5-17.** An anterior-posterior radiograph of the neck and upper chest shows almost-complete occlusion of the pharynx, above the level of the larynx, following lye ingestion. A tracheostomy was necessary because the larynx was severely burned.

probably have already have been performed. (Fig. 5-17)[38] The laryngeal and pharyngeal branches of the vagus nerves should nevertheless be preserved. Sensation to the larynx will be impaired and impending aspiration of food will not be perceived. If scarring of the laryngeal closure mechanism allows repeated aspiration and if phonation is impossible because of the very fibrotic laryngeal muscles, a laryngectomy may be necessary to protect the lungs from infection.

### Operative Technique

Beginning two days preoperatively, the colon is cleansed of stool by feeding the patient clear liquids only, and by repeated saline enemas. An effective alternative mechanical bowel preparation which the authors prefer is the passing of a nasogastric tube and infusion of 100–1000 ml Golytely/hour (depending upon the patient's size) until the diarrhea fluid is clear.[17] The Golytely (Braintree Labs) preparation can cleanse the bowel within three–four hours. The authors do not use oral antibiotics. Two–five mg vitamin K is given intramuscularly because the depletion of bowel flora may result in prolonged prothrombin times. Prophylactic antibiotics are started intravenously in the operating room. The authors use ampicillin, 50 mg/kg q6h, and gentamicin, 2 mg/kg q8h. A central venous catheter is placed in the subclavian vein on the side opposite the neck incision or thoracotomy. An arterial cannula placed percutaneously helps to monitor blood gases. A Foley catheter is passed into the bladder to follow the urinary output.

### Retrosternal Colon Interposition

This has been a procedure favored by many surgeons.[3,10,14,21,40,42,50,52,60,62,71] For a retrosternal interposition, the patient is placed in a supine position with the head and neck hyperextended by a soft roll placed under the shoulders. The skin of the jaw and the entire anterior chest and abdomen are scrubbed with antiseptic solution. In children, any segment of the colon is readily exposed through a transverse upper abdominal incision. After mobilization of the selected segment of colon, the neck is dissected. The cervical esophagus is exposed through a transverse incision in the right side of the neck two centimeters above the suprasternal notch and clavicle. Dissecting the right side avoids potential injury to the major lymphatic ducts which are present on the left side. The cervical esophagus is exposed between the carotid sheath and the trachea. The recurrent laryngeal nerve must be preserved on both sides when dissecting the esophagus. The cervical esophagus is mobilized so that it courses around the lateral side of the trachea. The anastomosis is most commonly at the level of the suprasternal notch.

In the development of a retrosternal tunnel, a large hiatus must be formed in the diaphragm posterior to the xyphoid process. Blunt dissection in the anterior mediastinum from the abdomen and from the transverse incision above the suprasternal notch develops a channel to withdraw the bowel to the neck. Theoretically, by avoiding entry into either pleural space, the confines of the retrosternal tunnel prevent subsequent distention and redundancy of the colon. The retrosternal bowel interposition necessitates a course over the left lobe of the liver, and the distal anastomosis is usually beyond the mid-anterior body of the stomach. If the colon, with its blood supply, is passed anterior to the stomach, there is a risk of compressing the lumen and causing gastric outlet obstruction. It is preferable to bring the blood supply behind the stomach and through the gastrohepatic omentum (Fig. 5-18). The colon is carefully brought through the tunnel and out the neck incision, avoiding traction on the blood vessels. A median sternotomy is indicated if the blood supply to the colon seems to be compromised by tunneling it blindly. The excess length of proximal colon is excised and the anastomosis must be with normal, unscarred esophagus, using a single layer of interrupted polyglycolate suture. The neck incision is drained and closed.

The anastomosis of colon to the stomach is accomplished after the cervical esoph-

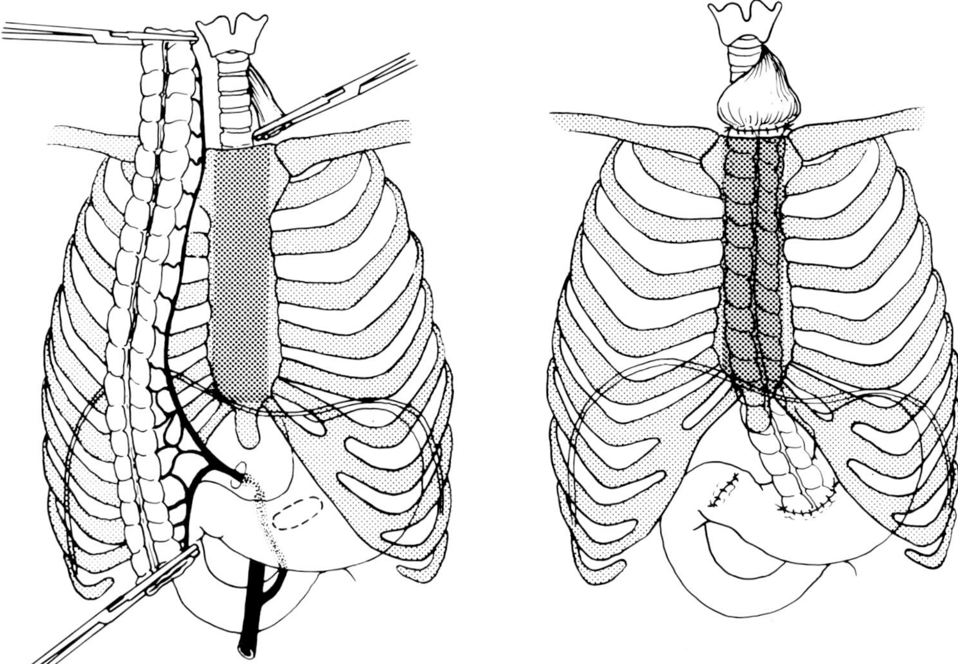

**Figure 5-18.**   Drawing depicts a retrosternal colon interposition. The vascular supply is based upon the middle colonic vessels. The colon, along with the vessels, is drawn behind the stomach, through the gastrohepatic ligament, over the liver to the retrosternal tunnel. The anastomosis in the neck is usually at the level of the suprasternal notch. The distal anastomosis is to the antrum or midanterior body of the stomach. A pyloroplasty may be required if impaired gastric emptying develops.

ageal anastomosis has been performed. Most authors describe making the gastric anastomosis initially, but this prevents the opportunity of removing redundancy in the interposition and providing as straight a conduit as possible. After the proximal esophageal anastomosis is completed, the amount of redundant colon is readily apparent. By dividing the mesenteric vessels immediately adjacent to the bowel wall, the excess bowel can be excised without compromising the viability of the remaining segment.

The anastomosis to the stomach is usually placed in the anterior mid-body of the stomach. To minimize reflux back into colon interposition during a gastric peristaltic wave, it is desirable to anastomose the colon as cephalad on the stomach as possible. If the lower esophagus is absent or if it has been resected, the fundus of the stomach can be mobilized for anastomosis by dividing the left gastric vessels. Some surgeons believe that compression of the colon between the liver and the anterior abdominal wall prevents gastric reflux, but the authors find that this probably accounts for impaired emptying of the colon and contributes to elongation and dilatation of the interposition (Fig. 5-16).

The retrosternal approach for esophageal bypass is favored by many surgeons because it is technically the easiest operation. The authors believe, however, that the functional and cosmetic results are not as favorable as are those of other approaches.

### Posterior Colon Interposition

The shorter the esophageal substitute the less dysfunctional swallowing occurs. The restrosternal conduit is necessarily an elongated one, while a posterior interposition is much shorter. This is particularly the case when only a short segment of intrathoracic esophagus is to be replaced. The authors prefer the posterior colon interposition because it functions better, even though it is technically a more difficult and time-consuming procedure than is the retrosternal esophageal bypass.

The colon interposition can be passed through the left pleural space or it may be placed in the bed of the esophagus. The operation may be accomplished three ways: (1) through a left postero-lateral thoracotomy; (2) through a left thoraco-abdominal incision; or, (3) by separate right or left thoracotomy and an abdominal incision.

When using the thoracotomy only, the patient is placed in a right lateral decubitus position. This approach is usually used for patients who already have had a cervical esophagostomy.[83,84] If the anastomosis is required in the neck, the sterile preparation of the skin should include the entire left arm, the neck, and the chest. The left arm is draped with tubular stockinette so that it can be moved freely to give good exposure to the neck. The incision for the thoracotomy has been placed by various surgeons from the sixth to the tenth intercostal space.[28,36,83,84] The abdomen is entered by dividing the left diaphragm at the costal margin from the parasternal area to approximately the posterior or mid-axillary line. The lower intercostal incisions provide the best exposure to mobilize the transverse and proximal descending colon. Visualization of the proximal esophagus in the mediastinum is, however, poor. The lower incision is therefore used when the esophageal anastomosis is to be placed in the neck. A sixth intercostal space incision is a compromise for simultaneous exposure below the diaphragm and the upper esophagus. To have access to the abdomen and the mediastinal esophagus, the authors have used a standard postero-lateral thoracotomy, over the fifth rib, through the chest wall muscles, and a seventh intercostal space incision has been used to enter the abdomen through the diaphragm. After mobilizing the colon, the third or fourth intercostal space is then incised in order to allow the surgeon to perform an anastomosis in the upper mediastinum. The left thoracotomy has been a popular approach for colon interposition, but it provides less than optimal visualization of the colon and its blood supply in the abdomen.

Because of the limited abdominal exposure through the diaphragm, some surgeons advocate a thoraco-abdominal approach by extending a seventh, eighth, or ninth intercostal incision through the costal margin; this incision is then continued across the midline of the upper abdomen.[28] The authors find that this incision is also a compromise which does not provide an optimal view of either the thoracic or abdominal contents, but it is better than the thoracotomy alone. Postoperatively, the area of the incised costal arch from the thoraco-abdominal incision usually becomes unsightly because of overgrowth and bulging or the rib cartilage. This can be minimized by trimming away several centimeters of rib cartilage before suturing them together with the chest wall closure.

It is the authors' preference to use a separate, transverse upper-abdominal incision to mobilize the selected bowel segment, with the patient in a supine position. The child can then be rolled in a right or left lateral decubitus position to place the thoracotomy at a level which is optimal for resecting the diseased portion of the esophagus and for esophageal anastomosis. This approach may require both a lower-seventh and an upper-third intercostal incision, as described above. To obtain access to the entire abdomen, the left or right chest, and the neck, the skin is prepared with antiseptic solution from the jaw to the groin, including the chest from the mid-axillary line of one side to a level across the midline of the vertebral spine on the other side. The arm of the same side as the thoracotomy is also scrubbed with the skin-sterilizing solution, and it is included in the sterile operative field. This requires suspending the child away from the operating table until sterile towels can be applied, using skin staples. Then the child is placed on the table and two split sheets complete the draping.

A right thoracotomy provides the best exposure to the proximal 80 percent of the esophagus, particularly if the anastomosis is desired above the level of a left aortic arch. To use this approach, a wide channel must be established through the diaphragm, usually to the left of the esophageal hiatus. The blunt dissection to develop a tunnel behind the stomach and through the diaphragm has to be carefully done and it is "blind". The colon has to be guided and not pulled through to avoid kinking or spasm of mesenteric vessels.

The chief limitation in using a left thoracotomy is gaining access to the esophagus at the level of a left-sided aortic arch and above. When the bowel interposition is to be passed through the thoracic inlet from a left thoracotomy, it may be tunneled lateral to the aortic arch, between the carotid and left subclavian arteries, with care taken to avoid injury to the recurrent laryngeal nerve.[84] An alternative route is to develop a tract in the bed of the esophagus from the level of the inferior pulmonary vein to the neck, using careful blunt dissection from the mediastinum and the neck incision.[28]

If a cervical esophagostomy was required as a first-stage procedure, it can be brought out through the right or left side of the neck. There is no preference as to whether a left or a right thoracotomy is used to anastomose to the cervical esophagus. A right thoracotomy is important only for proximal, intrathoracic esophageal anastomosis; consequently, a left thoracotomy is used more often to bring a colon interposition to the level of the neck. Because many surgeons are concerned about the tenous blood supply to the colon resulting in necrosis, anastomotic leakage, and infection, they perform only cervical esophageal anastomosis. The authors are convinced that the shorter the interposition, the less dysphagia and other complications develop. If the cervical and proximal intrathoracic esophagus is normal, the anastomosis should be in the chest.

### The Intra-abdominal Procedure

The blood supply to the right colon and the transverse colon is usually based upon the middle colonic vessels, but, occasionally, the right colic or the ileo-colic vessels are long enough to serve as the major blood supply (Fig. 5-19). When the left colon is desired, vascularization is derived from either the middle colic or the left colonic vessels. If either the middle colic or the left colic artery and vein are to be divided, it is important to establish the integrity of the collateral marginal vessels at the splenic flexure. The success of operations for esophageal substitutes is most dependent upon preserving the blood supply. The distance between the proximal esophagus and the distal anastomosis (esophagus or stomach) is measured, and the required length of colon is surveyed, with particular emphasis on an adequate vascular supply. The vessels to be divided should be compressed with soft, rubber-shod clamps to insure

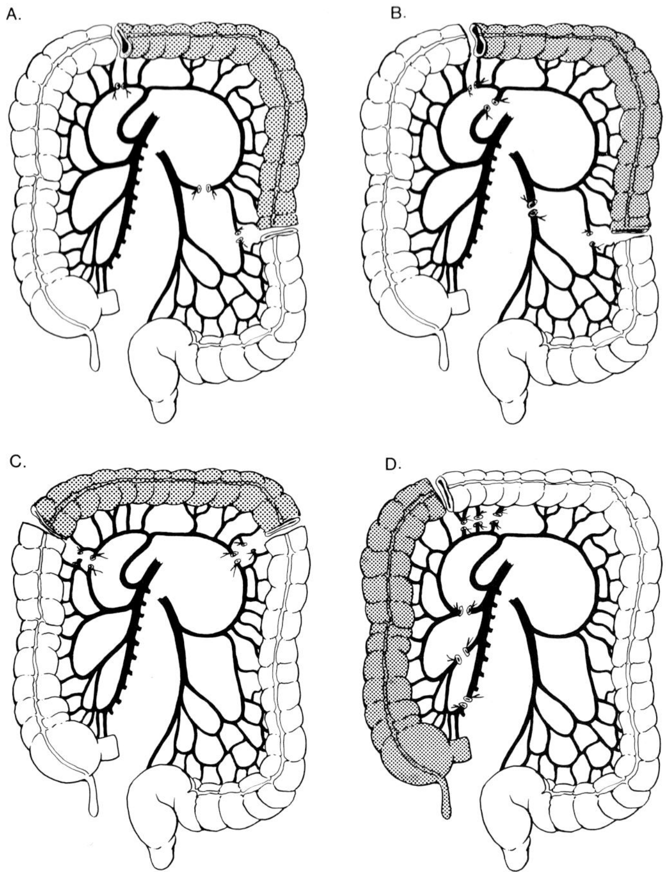

**Figure 5-19.** Drawing of the colon and the most common pattern of vascular supply. (A) The left transverse and descending colon can be supplied by the middle colic artery, and the distal bowel would be used for proximal esophageal anastomosis in an antiperistaltic direction. (B) The transverse and descending colon may be supplied by the ascending branches of the left colic artery. In this case, the transected end of the transverse colon would be anastomosed to proximal esophagus isoperistaltically. (C) The transverse colon is based upon the middle colic artery. (D) The right colon may be supplied by the middle colic, right colic, or ileo-colic vessels. The terminal ileum may be included as part of the interposition.

that the vessel to be preserved will perfuse the entire section of colon. The adequacy of blood flow is usually identified by noting whether the color of the bowel wall is normal and equivalent to that of the adjacent intestine. It is important to select a longer length of bowel than seems necessary to reach the proposed area for the proximal esophageal anastomosis. This is the most important segment to bridge the chest, because it is excessive tension on the mesenteric vessels to reach the proximal esophagus which contributes to vascular compromise.

The integrity of the blood supply is usually excellent until the intestine is mobilized to span the thorax. The manipulation and elongation of mesentery commonly result in impaired perfusion, either from kinking within the mesentery or at the origin from the superior mesenteric vessels curving around the pancreas, or from stretch-narrowing of the vessel, or from vascular spasm. The presence of ischemic bowel should be corrected by examining the course of the blood supply for areas of kinking or torsion. If there is a question of bowel ischemia, staging the procedure might help. The colon conduit is aligned in the abdomen or chest where the blood flow seems to be adequate and the operation is terminated. One or two days later, the operation resumes, and it is to be hoped, the time interval will have allowed improved mesenteric perfusion. Some have advocated only dividing the appropriate mesenteric blood vessels as a first-stage procedure to allow the selected dominant vessels to enlarge and compensate for the loss of collaterals. In this instance, the patient is reoperated several months later and the bowel is divided for interposition.

The use of staplers has greatly facilitated transection of the colon. Long, 4-0 silk sutures are used to oversew the end of the bowel to be anastomosed to the proximal esophagus. The ends of these sutures are then used only as a guide and must not be utilized to drag the bowel through the diaphragm or thoracic inlet. Anastomosis of the intra-abdominal proximal and distal colon ends should be anterior to the mesenteric vessels supplying the interposition and oriented without twisting. The colon interposition with its mesentery should be passed behind the stomach. On many occasions, the mesenteric vessels will be less likely to be compressed and will have a shorter course if interposition is passed behind the pancreas. This can be readily accomplished by gentle blunt dissection or by reflecting the spleen and pancreas to the right.

The proximal anastomosis to the esophagus should be completed initially. The authors recommend use of single-layer, interrupted polyglycolate suture because it seems to be associated with a small incidence of stricture formation. The proximal esophageal anastomosis should be positioned above or below the thoracic inlet so that, if severe stricture develops, it will not be a great problem to revise the anastomosis.

Sometimes there is insufficient colon to reach the proximal esophagus without excessive tension. This may occur either because an insufficient length of colon was mobilized or because the end of the bowel became ischemic and had to be resected. A very valuable technique to gain considerable length on the colon is to make multiple transverse incisions through the taenia at 1.5-cm intervals.[55]

Almost invariably, the distal colon length is excessively long. To avoid redundancy, the distal end is resected by dividing the mesenteric blood supply closely adjacent to the bowel wall to avoid devascularizing the entire graft. The authors use interrupted, single-layer polyglycolate suture to anastomose to the distal esophagus. If the anastomosis is to the stomach, a two-layer suture is preferred, in which the inner row is for hemostasis. The hiatus in the diaphragm, through which the interposed colon passes, should be narrowed to avoid another viscus from herniating into the chest.

## Free Revascularized Intestinal Grafts

The use of free, revascularized segments of small or large bowel is increasing in popularity. This technique is used primarily to replace the cervical and upper thoracic esophagus.[25,57,79] It is also a valuable procedure to bridge an area of ischemic necrosis following a standard interposition based upon intra-abdominal blood supply.[25,79] The operation consists of selecting a segment of jejunum or colon and isolating the major artery and vein branches of the superior mesenteric vessels. In adults, the length of free jejunal graft is limited to 18–22 cm before the conduit becomes unduly tortuous. Pedicled jejunal grafts of 50 cm have, however, been possible.[79] After dividing the major vessels, some surgeons perfuse the vessels with cold Ringer's lactate or Sack's solution containing heparin and a vasodilator, such as lidocaine. Other surgeons do not wash out the vessels. The artery is anastomosed to the carotid artery or superior thyroid artery and the vein is anastomosed to the jugular vein. The technique requires the use of microvascular instruments, 10-0 monofilament suture, and magnification lenses or an operating microscope. The blood vessels in young children are very small, and when they are less than one–two mm in diameter, there is a great risk of bowel infarction. This procedure may therefore be limited to use in older children. The youngest reported patient was five years old.[79]

## Postoperative Care

The postoperative recovery can be very difficult because of the very extensive dissection. Large "third-space" fluid loss should be anticipated and it must be adequately replaced with Ringer's lactate and/or colloid solutions for 24–48 hours postoperatively. The authors find that hetastarch six-percent solution seems to maintain the blood volume with less capillary "leakage" than does crystalloid alone, and it is cheaper and less hazardous than are blood products. The authors do not give blood transfusions if the hematocrit is above 25 percent. Rheologically, the increased rate of blood flow from a lower hematocrit seems to be more important than is the presumed superior oxygen-carrying capacity of a blood hematocrit greater than 35 percent. It is important to maintain normal blood volume and visceral perfusion to avoid infarction of the esophageal substitute.

Vasoconstrictors such as norepinephrine are released with anesthesia, hypovolemia, and pain. The vessels of the skin and mesentery are more intensely constricted than are vessels in other areas of the body. Although renal perfusion may be adequate, as identified by a urine output greater than one ml/kg/hour, cutaneous blood flow may be a better endpoint to reflect mesentric visceral perfusion. The rate of capillary refill after compression of the nail bed should be within one–two seconds. Use of a transcutaneous $pO_2$ and $pCO_2$ monitors can be helpful. Maintenance of normal arterial pH, $pO_2$, and $pCO_2$ is imperative. The base deficit should be calculated; the presence of metabolic acidosis identifies inadequate blood volume replacement.

Dissection in the neck and upper mediastinum contributes to impaired swallowing and edema of the airway. The pain from the thoracic and abdominal incisions results in shallow breathing and retained tracheobronchial secretions. It might therefore be advisable to maintain the endotracheal tube in place to assist ventilation and to aspirate airway secretions for 24–48 hours postoperatively. The viability of the interposition is dependent upon adequate blood volume replacement and prevention of hypoxia.

Intravenous antibiotics are continued for five days postoperatively. After 48 hours, the patient is given nutrition by intravenous alimentation solutions. When ileus has resolved, nutrition can be maintained by continuous drip infusion through a gastrostomy if there is little probability of reflux or vomiting, which would interfere with healing of the suture line.

Oral feedings are deferred for 10 days postoperatively to minimize the risk of leakage from the interposition anastomosis. If there is no drainage from the neck incision, an esophagram is performed on the tenth postoperative day. Oral feedings are begun when no leakage has been documented from either anastomosis. Initially, thick-ened, puree-consistency feedings are easier to swallow than are liquids or solids. Oral feedings are not given for several weeks if an anastomotic leak is present, until the fistula tract is walled off, with little risk of infection spreading in the neck or medias-tinum.

## COMPLICATIONS

Complications of esophageal substitution might be somewhat arbitrarily sepa-rated into anatomical problems and functional disorders. Anatomical complications are related to the technique of the operation or else they are correctable by an opera-tion. Functional disorders are complications of the operations which do not have a surgical solution. The complications might include:

*Anatomical Problems*

1.  impaired blood supply
2.  anastomotic leakage
3.  anastomotoc stricture, lodged foreign body
4.  laryngeal nerve palsy, Horner's syndrome, phrenic paralysis
5.  dilation and elongation of the substitute
6.  impaired gastric emptying
7.  peptic ulcer or reflux esophagitis
8.  excessive intraoperative bleeding
9.  thoracic duct injury
10. cosmetic deformity

*Functional Disorders*

1.  major infection—pneumonia, sepsis
2.  dysphagia—reflux
3.  dumping syndrome
4.  diarrhea
5.  malabsorption—growth failure

## Anatomical Problems

### Impaired Blood Supply

Vascular compromise of the esophageal substitute is one of the greatest hazards of esophageal substitution and accounts for most of the mortality reported. Necrosis of the entire interposition has been described by surgeons with a very large experi-ence.[6,34,50,52,70] Adequate venous drainage is equally as important as arterial supply. In the construction of the gastric tube, perfusion of the conduit is dependent upon collateral blood flow from the right and left gastroepiploic vessels. It is probably advantageous to preserve the short gastric vessels which supply the left gastroepiploic vessels when performing a reversed gastric tube operation. Selection of the optimal segment of small or large bowel is primarily dependent upon identifying a dominant artery and vein to preserve blood flow, and by demonstrating that temporary occlusion of collateral mesenteric vessels at the proposed site for bowel transection does not compromise circulation. Some surgeons suggest that the operation should be staged. In the initial operation, the collateral vessels would be divided, and, following a delay of several weeks or months to allow maximum distention and blood flow in the dominant vessels, the bowel segment would be mobilized. The dominant artery and vein must also course along the bowel conduit sufficiently far so that the proximal area of the esophagus is approximated without excessive tension on the vascular pedicle. The smaller the patient, the smaller the vessels and the less the tolerance for kinking or spasm. As the conduit is mobilized toward the proximal esophagus, it must be manipu-lated very gently. Traction or pulling the conduit produces stretch-narrowing and/or spasm of the vessels which may not regress.

That portion of the conduit to be anastomosed to the proximal esophagus is almost invariably at greatest risk for ischemia, since it is most distal from the origin of the blood supply. Before performance of the anastomosis, the adequacy of blood supply can be identified by the color of the bowel wall and the color and vigor of bleeding when the end of the bowel is incised.

Fluorescein can be used to monitor perfusion. After the operating team has become dark-adapted in the darkened operating room, fluorescein, 15–30 mg/kg is given intravenously and an ultraviolet light is projected over the bowel interposition to observe whether there is a difference between the green fluorescence of the nor-mally perfused intestine and the conduit. The disadvantages of this technique are that it can be used one time only because of the time lag in washout of the tissue and that there is only a qualitative difference in color changes.

A sterile Doppler flow probe can also be placed along the path of the arteries to identify the point where pulsatile flow is impaired. Venous flow can be identified by venous hum in the large proximal veins. When impaired perfusion of the conduit is recognized, the site of obstruction should be identified. The Doppler probe will reveal the area of obstruction, and the mesenteric tissues surrounding these vessels should be dissected away, since nerve trunks and fibrous bands are occasionally kinking the vessels.[60]

Frequently, vascular spasm occurs, and it seems to be relieved by dissecting the adventitia off the vessel. Vasodilators such as lidocaine (0.5 percent or longer-acting bupivacaine (0.5 percent) can be infiltrated into the tissues around the vessels or dripped topically on the vessel to relieve spasm. When used topically, the addition of sodium bicarbonate to neutralize the hydrochloride salt of the local anesthetic agent might help release the active cationic form of the drug. Papaverine solution is also used topically as a local vasodilator. Application of sponges soaked with warmed Ringer's lactate or normal saline may help relieve spasm.

Systemic drugs to enhance perfusion of the ischemic bowel have not been shown to be clearly beneficial. Obviously, the blood volume must be maintained close to normal to prevent release of vasoconstrictors such as norepinephrine or angiotensin. Use of inhibitors of platelet aggregation and blood coagulation, such as acetylsalicy-late, dipyridamole, and low-molecular-weight dextran 40 or heparin, is hazardous because of the risk of producing pathological bleeding.

When the blood supply remains precarious, it is wise to abandon the attempt at anastomosis, to place the segment of bowel in a position which is compatible with optimal perfusion, and to close the wounds. About 48 or more hours later, the bowel segment can be re-examined to assess the viability and feasability of completing the operation. Otherwise, another segment of intestine will have to be mobilized.

If the bowel has been mobilized to the neck and it appears dusky, the level of normal perfusion should be observed to consider whether there is sufficient length to excise the marginal area. If the length of the colon is inadequate (e.g., when it becomes necessary to resect the ischemic end, or when it has retracted following a staged operation) multiple transverse incisions in the taenia are an effective method for elongating the bowel.[55]

### Anastomotic Leakage

When a cervical esophageal anastomosis has been performed, the incidence of anastomotic leakage is 20–63 percent.[3,6,13,20,31,34,52,70] This complication occurs in all age groups. It develops as commonly with the colon as with a gastric tube interposition, and it occurs with equal frequency in the cases of a single-layer and a two-layer anastomosis. Undoubtedly, it is related to impaired blood flow in the cephalad end of interposition. Curiously, many surgeons prefer to make the anastomosis in the neck, with the expectation that it will leak. Leakage is, however, unusual in the chest, and it is rare at the distal anastomosis.

Delaying the anastomosis has been advocated in order to help identify ischemic bowel and to allow the collateral blood flow to develop.[19,32,52] The end of the bowel and the cervical esophagus are brought out to the skin as fistulas, and several days to weeks later the anastomosis is accomplished. Unfortunately, this technique does not lessen the incidence of leakage following the subsequent anastomosis.[52]

To avoid the risk of disrupting a tenuous suture line, the patient is not fed until an esophagram on the tenth postoperative day verifies the integrity of the anastomosis. Because leakage of a cervical esophageal anastomosis occurs frequently, the neck should always be drained. It is advisable to avoid placing the anastomosis at the thoracic inlet where leakage might produce severe mediastinitis, and where, if a subsequent hard stricture should occur, it would be very difficult to revise surgically. Most of the cervical anastomotic leaks will heal within one–two weeks, unless there has been extensive necrosis of the interposition with disruption.

When a leak has occurred, the patient should be given nothing by mouth until drainage stops or until approximately two weeks have passed, by which time a well-walled-off tract will have formed. After two weeks, oral feedings can be given without impairing the subsequent closure of the fistula. Nutrition is maintained by gastrostomy or jejunostomy feedings or by intravenous alimentation.

An extensive anastomotic disruption should be reoperated with an attempt to mobilize the bowel and esophagus for a possible reanastomosis. If this is not feasible, a cervical esophagostomy will be necessary. The stoma of the interposition will have to be either exteriorized or oversewn.

If the proximal anastomosis is within the thorax and it leaks, an emergency thoracotomy will be necessary. Closure of the leak might be attempted, or a cervical esophagostomy and closure of the interposition will be necessary. Extensive necrosis of the graft will require resection to the area of viability. The mortality rate with intra-thoracic leakage is very high because of delay in recognizing and treating the perforation which produces mediastinitis and empyema.

Following a prolonged period of recovery, three options are available to re-establish continuity of the esophagus. The first is direct reapproximation of the two ends which will require mobilization of the interposition sufficiently to accomplish the anastomosis without tension. Second, extensive necrosis and fibrotic contracture of the interposition may have occurred, and it is necessary to resect the substitute and use another segment of colon. Third, the defect between the esophagus and the interposition could be bridged with a free graft of jejunum or colon with microvascular anastomosis to the neck vessels.[25]

**Anastomotic Stricture**

Stricture is described in 15–100 percent of reported series.[3,6,13,20,31,34,52,70] It usually occurs at the proximal esophageal anastomosis, but it can also develop in a distal esophageal or gastric anastomosis. When the interposition is performed for caustic injury, it is important to be certain that the anastomosis is accomplished in normal, unscarred esophagus and that there is no risk of an area of fibrous contraction developing in a segmental area of injury more proximally, as in the hypopharynx. In most instances, the stricture is related to ischemia and/or leakage of the anastomosis with a surrounding inflammatory reaction.[20,52] The incidence of stricture may be greater in the case of gastric tube interposition than in the case of colon interposition.[32,52] The fibrous contracture may not be confined just to the circle of suture line; it may extend into the muscularis of the interposition for a distance of several centimeters.

Depending upon the extent of collagen reaction, the stenosis may respond very readily to just a few antegrade dilatations. Some surgeons believe that a string should be passed down the esophagus and interposition and out the gastrostomy for retrograde dilataion. Prompt contracture within a short interval after dilatation is usually due to severe fibrotic reaction.

If the stricture is a relatively narrow ring of fibrosis, a trial of triamcinolone acetonide injections into the scar might soften and atrophy the stricture.[37] The injections could be repeated three or four times. The authors have found that the fibrous ring is easiest to identify before dilatation, which is done in order to ensure that the triamcinolone is injected directly into the scar tissue.[37] There are several cautions to be considered before using steroid injections. Although triamcinolone acetonide is a crystalline suspension which theoretically does not become absorbed systemically, patients treated with this steroid can develop Cushing's syndrome. The risk of brain abscess is a possibility with the use of corticoids and dilatation.[48] Finally, if there is a likelihood that the anastomosis will have to be revised, it should be recognized that it will not heal with a deposit of steroid in the tissues. The use of corticoids should therefore be employed with caution.

A stricture which does not respond to dilatation will have to be excised and a new anastomosis will be necessary. Usually, the new anastomosis heals very well because the blood supply will have improved by this time. The risks of recurrent nerve, phrenic nerve, and major vascular injury are, however, great because there will be significant scarring in the surrounding neck structures from the previous dissection and inflammatory reaction.

As in any esophageal operation, the ring of healed suture line will not distend and accommodate to a swallowed object which is larger than the diameter of the anastomosis. Lodgement of ingested foreign bodies and food particles will acount for a sudden onset of dysphagia.

## Nerve Injury

There are four nerves which have been injured because of their proximity to the cervical and upper mediastinal esophagus. These are the superior and recurrent laryngeal nerves, the phrenic nerve, and the inferior and middle cervical ganglia.[20,75] Superior laryngeal nerve injury may occur when the dissection extends above the area of the cricoid cartilage. The internal laryngeal branch of the superior laryngeal nerve is sensory to the laryngeal mucosa above the vocal cords, while the external branch innervates the cricothyroid muscle.

The recurrent laryngeal nerves innervate all of the laryngeal muscles except the cricothyroid, and they provide sensation below the vocal cords. Both nerves could be impaired by injury to the vagus nerve during its descent in the neck and chest. The left recurrent laryngeal nerve is vulnerable from the level of the ligamentum arteriosum and the medial side of the aortic arch. The right recurrent laryngeal leaves the vagus nerve to curve beneath the right subclavian artery. Both recurrent nerves are close to the esophagus throughout their course. Injury to the nerve on the side ipisilateral to the neck incision is probably less common than on the contralateral side, because the opposite nerve is not visualized during circumferential mobilization of the esophagus.

The incidence of recurrent nerve injury is probably underestimated because palsy of one side may be undetected unless routine visualization of the vocal cords is performed. Following injury, the voice may be normal, or it may become slightly raspy or whispered. Bilateral recurrent nerve injury usually results in severe inspiratory obstruction because the vocal cords do not abduct, while the voice may remain relatively normal or hoarse. Several series describe the necessity for performing postoperative tracheostomy.[20,31,36]

The phrenic nerve is laterally placed in the neck, but if dissection of the esophagus is approached lateral to the carotid artery, it becomes vulnerable. In the thoracic inlet and upper mediastinum, it is also subject to traction or compression injury resulting in paralysis of the diaphragm.

Compression or transection of the cervical sympathic nerves, particularly the inferior cervical ganglion, will produce Horner's syndrome.

Injury of the vagus nerves below the recurrent laryngeal branches may produce gastric outlet obstruction.

## Dilatation and Elongation of the Substitute

This complication is not a problem in the case of gastric interpositions. When jejunum is selected as a bowel substitute, it is characteristic for it to be elongated and redundant because of the mesenteric vascular supply. The technique of dividing secondary arcades in the jejunal mesentery while maintaining the collateral tertiary branches helps to straighten the jejunal conduit.[26] Redundancy and distention of colon can be minimized by: (1) selecting the left transverse and proximal descending colon, which has a narrow diameter; (2) avoiding compression of the colon at any point between the esophagus and the stomach; and (3) performing the proximal esophageal anastomosis initially so that the excessively redundant distal portion of the conduit can be resected.

Dysphagia, delayed emptying of the conduit, reflux of ingested food with recurrent aspiration and pneumonia, and foul breath are consequences of dilated and elongated colon interpositions. These complications are justification for revising the conduit. Simple resection of an intra-abdominal segment of the interposition may be all that is necessary. More commonly, the entire conduit may have to be mobilized and shortened. The authors have reduced the diameter of a widely dilated colon segment by placing staples along the antimesenteric half of the circumference, using a large tube within the lumen as a guide for an appropriate diameter. Occasionally, attempted mobilization of the conduit disrupts the integrity of the bowel so extensively that it has to be resected, and a new interposition must be developed.

### Impaired Gastric Emptying

Truncal vagotomy results in significant pylorospasm in 15 percent of patients. For this reason, pyloroplasty is usually performed. The consequence of this may be dumping syndrome, which is difficult to treat in these patients. The authors try to preserve the vagus nerves, if possible. For example, if the intrathoracic esophagus is to be resected, the nerves are dissected free while mobilizing the esophagus. If truncal vagotomy is necessary, as in whole-stomach interposition, the authors prefer to perform a pyloromyotomy rather than a pyloroplasty. This can be technically difficult because the pyloric muscle is soft and does not readily split and separate from the underlying mucos. If a pyloroplasty is necessary, a very limited Heineke-Mikulic procedure is desirable.

### Peptic Ulcer and Reflux Esophagitis

Peptic ulcers following colon interposition have been described in 10 adults and one six-year-old child.[56] The ulcers were produced symptous of pain, bleeding, or perforation. Symptoms developed within one year of the operation in most of the cases. The ulcers in the colon interpositions were located within four cm of the cologastric anastomosis. There were no apparent differences, whether the anastomosis was at the fundus, mid-body, or antrum of the stomach. Most of these patients seemed to have had an ulcer diathesis with high gastric secretion. None had had bilateral vagotomy. Significant gastrointestinal bleeding from presumed peptic ulceration of colon interpositions have been reported in children by others.[10,50,75,76] The ulcer may also develop in the stomach instead of the colon interposition.[60]

Reflux of gastric juice into the interposition is the source of peptic ulcer. Some surgeons have attempted to minimize reflux by techniques such as an anastomosis to the posterior body of the stomach to create a valve-like effect, or by everting the end of the colon, similar to maturing an ileostomy, prior to anastomosis.[6,42,47,54] When the distal esophagus is not diseased and is not subject to significant gastroesophageal reflux, the risk of ulceration of the interposition can be reduced by making the anastomosis to the distal esophagus, rather than to the stomach.

Ulceration of jejunal, gastric tube, and whole stomach interpositions also occur (Fig. 5-20).[4,16,20,33,52,69] Confirmation of the diagnosis by contrast radiography is not very productive in children because the ulcers tend to be obscured by mucosal folds and to be relatively shallow. Huge ulcers several centimeters in diameter have, however, been described in adults. Flexible endoscopy should be used to establish the presence of an ulcer when contrast radiologic studies fail.

Little is known about gastric physiology following interposition procedures in which the vagus nerves and stomach are intact. However, following whole-stomach interposition, in which vagotomy is inevitable, typical findings are: (1) atrophic gastric mucosa; (2) basal and pentagastrin-stimulated maximal acid production is below nor-

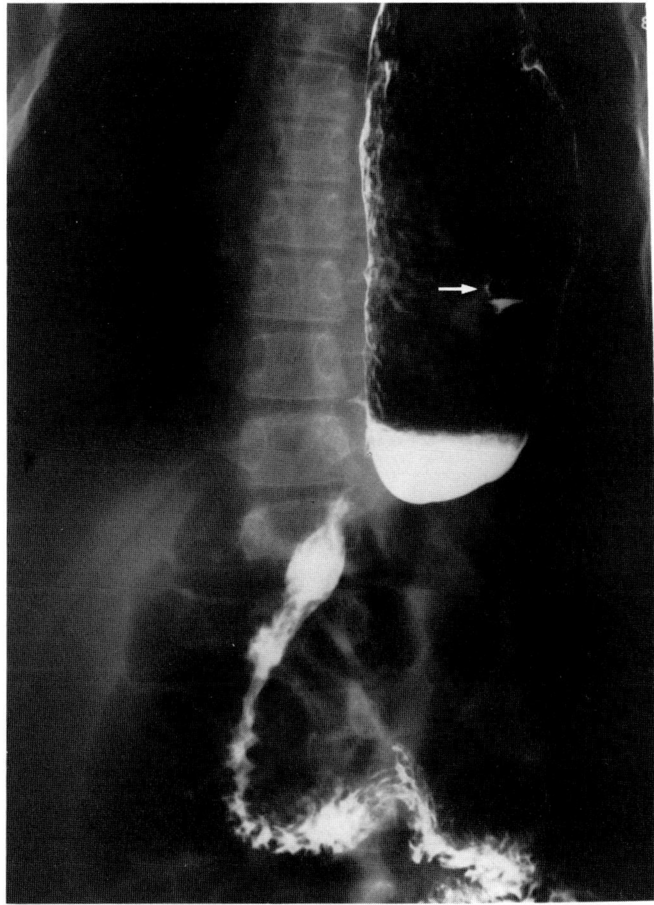

**Figure 5-20.**   A barium swallow demonstrates whole-stomach replacement of the esophagus. In spite of vagotomy and pyloroplasty, a symptomatic ulcer (arrow) developed in the mid-posteior body of the stomach, which responded to hydrogenion blockers.

mal, while, (3) basal and postprandial gastrin levels are abnormally high; (4) the stomach responds in only 40 percent of patients with increased peristaltic emptying following feeding; and, (5) following intravenous administration of metoclopramide, increased gastric peristalsis is very transient.[41]

An ulcer diathesis in a given patient is obviously a cause for development of an interposition ulcer. There has been much speculation regarding other causes. The lack of complete vagotomy, impaired gastric emptying, and mucosa susceptible to ulceration are most commonly considered. Ulcers also tend to form in areas of the interposition where there may be marginal focal blood flow from extrinsic compression, such as at the edge of the diaphragm or a twist of the bowel.

The treatment of interposition ulcer will depend upon the presenting symptoms. If the patient fails to respond to hydrogen blockers and the vagus nerves are intact, a selective or truncal vagotomy and pyloroplasty might be required. A perforation of recent onset or hemorrhage is usually treated by excision of the ulcer and a vagot-omy.[56] A patient with an intact lower esophagus and retrosternal or posterior interpo-sition anastomosed directly to the stomach might be treated by taking down the gastric anastomosis and rerouting the bowel to utilize the distal esophagus.

Bleeding and perforation due to gastric reflux into the retained esophagus have been described following a substernal bypass.[65]

### Extensive Intraoperative Bleeding

When full-thickness injury of the esophagus extends to involve surrounding mediastinal structures, esophagectomy may be associated with exaggerated bleeding. The inflammatory reaction and friability of tissue may extend to major vascular struc-tures, such as the aorta, with exsanguinating hemorrhage.[24] (See Chapter 4.)

### Thoracic Duct Injury

Esophagectomy or dissection to develop a plane for a bowel interposition can readily result in transection of major lymphatic ducts. The position of the lymhatics must be considered, and dissection immediately adjacent to the esophagus will help to prevent this complication. The authors favor mobilizing the esophagus on the right side of the neck to avoid the dominant lymphatic duct which drains into the left subclavian and jugular vein confluence.

### Cosmetic Deformity

Unlike the adults, almost all of the indications for esophageal replacement in children are for benign lesions. The intent of treatment in these children is to provide a good quality of life for many decades, and cosmetic effects of the operation should be considered. Transverse incisions should be in normal skin lines and are cosmetically preferable to vertical incisions. A significant disadvantage of the substernal interposi-tion is the bulge which develops in the neck upon swallowing a bolus. Cutting the sternomastoid muscle or resecting the clavicle and manubrium is not cosmetically an answer to the problem. Use of a thoraco-abdominal incision, in which the costal cartilages are transected, results in overgrowth of the ribs to produce a promient and unsightly bulge at the costal margin. To minimize this defect, the cartilage should be resected two–three cm on either side of the rib incision before wound closure. The curious posturing of the head and neck in Sandifer's syndrome has been described in a child following the reverse gastric tube interposition.[74] Some patients develop loud borborygmi in the chest, which is a source of embarrassment. The cosmetic conse-quences of the operative procedures must be considered in concert with the great technical challenge of achieving satisfactory swallowing function.


## Functional Disorders


### Major Infections

Two major infections following esophageal replacement are pneumonia and sep-sis. Children are particularly susceptible to infection because of immaturity of the immune system and because of depleted nutritional status. Infants are particularly susceptible to pneumonia and sepsis, and this is reflected in the significantly high mortality rate when interpositions are attempted in those under one year of age, compared to older children.[60] Patients with esophageal atresia who are staged by esophagostomy and gastrostomy commonly do not follow a normal growth curve in spite of the opportunity to force calories by the gastrostomy. Older children with chemical esophageal strictures usually are nutritionally depleted as well. The magnitude of the operative procedure for esophageal interposition produces an extreme catabolic state which readily exhausts the energy reserves of a marginally nourished patient.

Pneumonia is a particular hazard. Infants with cervical esophagostomy must be encouraged to swallow food while being fed by gastrostomy in order to maintain a swallowing reflex, so that when the interposition is accomplished, episodes of aspiration will be minimized. It is advisable to delay esophageal substitution in infants until an age when they assume an upright position and can avoid pooling of swallowed contents in the interposition which will reflux back into the pharynx and then into the tracheobronchial tree.

### Dysphagia

Dysphagia becomes a problem when narrowing and stricture of the anastomosis occur. Except for jejunum, other esophageal substitutes are passive conduits and the passage of food requires vigorous swallowing effort in order to entrain food aborally. An upright position is important during feeding to provide gravitational pull on swallowed materials traveling into the stomach. The lack of peristalsis and reflux from the stomach into the conduit and from the conduit into the pharynx contributes to anorexia, poor feeding, aspiration with chronic cough, and feelings of fullness, gaseous eructations, pneumonia, and foul breath. The retrosternal interpositions seem to produce dysphagia at the thoracic inlet more frequently than do conduits in a posterior position. The severity of dysphagia seems to be in direct porportion to the length of the conduit.

### Dumping Syndrome

The intact stomach and pylorus are important for reservoir function and to slowly advance feedings into the small bowel. Significant dumping syndrome occurs in any series where pyloroplasty is performed. For this reason, pyloromyotomy is advocated. The normal pyloric sphincter can be difficult to split without entering the mucosa of the bowel. If a pyloroplasty is required, it should not be made widely patent.

Treatment of dumping can be very difficult in these patients. The principle of treating dumping by feeding dry foods and reserving the swallowing of liquids between meals is almost impossible in these patients. Most children have to swallow large volumes of liquids with the ingestion of solids to convey the feeding aborally. Children are particularly desirous of eating foods with a high sugar content such as soft drinks and candy, which can produce profound dumping symptoms. Even a sound diet, however, may induce dumping and the dietary constraints can become confining and contribute to impaired nutrition and failure in growth.

### Diarrhea

Diarrhea is a frequent problem in most reported series. There is no apparent relationship of the incidence of diarrhea to the segment of bowel used for esophageal substitution. The diarrhea may occur without a vagotomy, but post-vagotomy diarrhea can be especially troublesome. The diarrhea persists for several months and will then resolve in most children. About one-third of the children have intermittent diarrhea for many years. The authors have not encountered frequent, mushy, or runny stools in patients who have had a short segment of esophagus replaced without vagotomy or pyloroplasty. Although the diarrhea is a significant nuisance, it is not usually associated with malabsorption.

### Malabsorption and Growth Failure

Malabsorption has been described in adults and in children who have had colon interposition, and the malabsorptive state was attributed to the operative procedure.[53,74] Vagotomy and pyloroplasty are well-established causes for malabsorption, but the etiology of malabsorption for isolated esophageal substitution is unknown. It is speculated that stagnation of food in the conduit and delayed gastric emptying contribute. Presumably, bacterial overgrowth, as in a blind loop syndrome, induced the malabsorption. The authors have not identified bacterial overgrowth in their interposition patients by means of the hydrogen breath test. In circumstances in which ileum is utilized for interposition, it would be expected that bile salt and fat absorption might be particularly affected.[39]

In most reported series of children, growth failure is a common problem. A number of series demonstrate that most of the children follow growth curves well below the third percentile.

Of particular interest, however, is the fact that most of these patients had esophageal atresia and were growing poorly before the interposition procedure.[28,42,50,53,62,84] Impaired growth does not seem to be a problem in patients who have undergone interposition for caustic stricture of the esophagus. During the period prior to the interposition, the esophageal atresia patients underwent esophagostomy and gastrostomy. In spite of the opportunity to force feed all the required nutrients, these infants usually do not grow very well. The cause for this is unknown, but impaired absorption does not seem to be present. Following interposition, these patients do not swallow effectively, even though they have preconditioned by swallowing with a cervical esophagostomy. Many do not seem to express hunger, and therefore they require gastrostomy supplementation of the oral feeding. Some of the children have repeated aspiration of feedings during swallowing and, as a result of recurring reflux, have repeated pulmonary infections. Although the pulmonary infections induce a catabolic state, these are transient episodes which do not account for the persistent poor growth. Endocrine studies have been normal, in the authors' patients, and no deficiency in growth hormone is present. It would appear that growth failure is a part of the anomaly package. Over a period of years, however, growth seems to accelerate into the range between the third and 50th percentiles.

## SUMMARY

Esophageal substitution is associated with serious technical hazards and complications. The procedure is uncommonly performed in children, and there is a considerable learning curve in executing the operation which will provide optimum swallowing function with a minimum of complications. The authors prefer to use colon to replace only the diseased portion of the esophagus. The shortest segment of bowel substitute possible should be used. Every effort should be made to preserve the cricopharyngeal

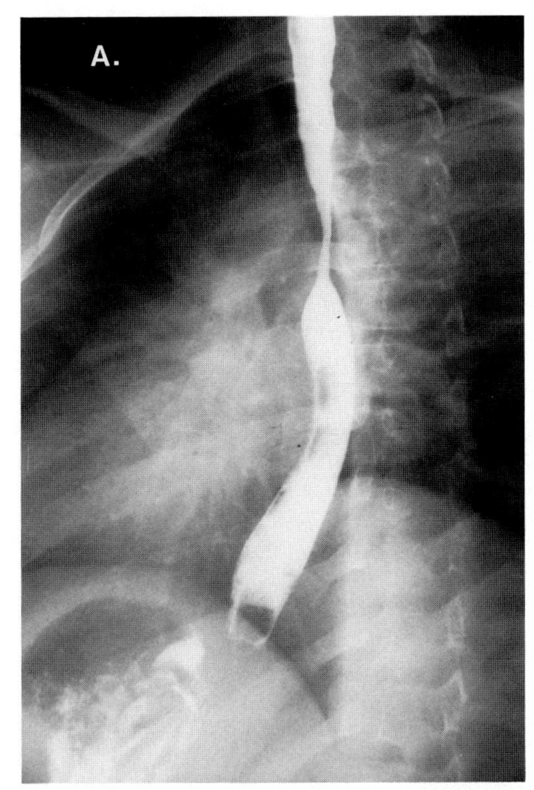

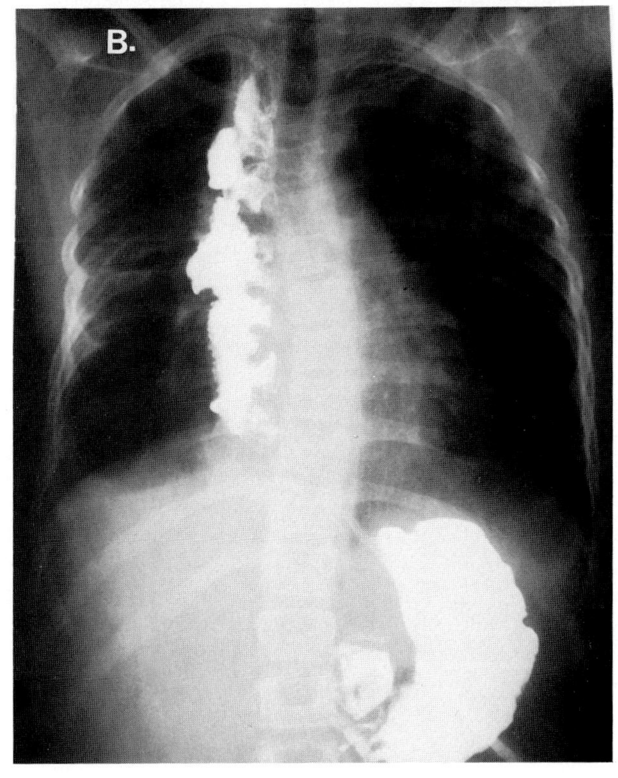

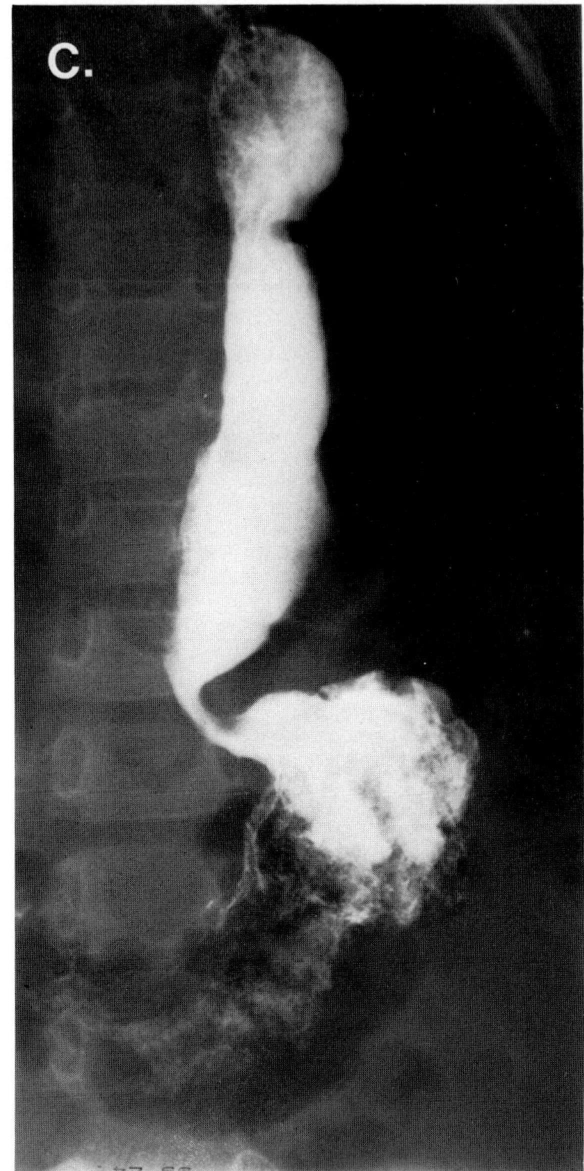


**Figure 5-21.** (A) Esophagram showing midesophageal stricture and a normal distal esophagus. (B) Esophagram of a colon
interposition between the proximal and distal esophagus performed through a right thoracotomy. (C) Esophagram of a colon
interposition replacing a segmental midesophageal stricture
from a left thoracotomy.

and cardioesophageal sphincters. Although it is technically the most demanding approach, the authors prefer the abdominal and right or left thoracotomy with interposition in the posterior mediastinum (Fig. 5-21). Alternative procedures such as gastric
tube, whole-stomach, and small bowel interpositions may be required in some clinical
circumstances.

## REFERENCES


1. Abbott OA, Mansour KA, Logan WD, et al: Atraumatic so-called "spontaneous" rupture
   of the esophagus: A review of 47 personal cases with comments on a new method of
   surgical therapy. J Thorac Cardiovasc Surg 59:67–83, 1970.
2. Absolon KB, Finney LA, Waddill GM, et al: Esophageal reconstruction—Colon trans-
   plant in two brothers with epidermolysis bullosa. Surgery 65:832–836, 1969.
3. Anderson KD: Esophageal substitition. In Holder TM, Ashcraft KW (Wds.): Pediatric
   Surgery. Philadelphia: W.B. Saunders Company, pp. 284–291, 1980.
4. Anderson KD, Randolph JG, Lilly JR: Peptic ulcer in children with gastric tube interposition. J Pediatr Surg 10:701–707, 1975.
5. Atwell D Jr, Harrison GSM: Observations on the role of esophago-gastrostomy in infancy
   and childhood with particular reference to long-term results and operative mortality. J
   Pediatr Surg 15:303–309, 1980.
6. Azar H, Crispin AR, Waterston DJ: Esophageal replacement with transverse colon in
   infants and children. J Pediatr Surg 6:3–9, 1971.
7. Barlow TE: Variations in the blood supply of the upper jejunum. Brit J Surg 43:473–475,
   1955–1956.
8. Berkowitz WP, Roper CL, Spector, GJ, et al: Surgical management of severe lye burns of
   the esophagus by colon interposition. Ann Otol Rhinol Laryngol 84:576–582, 1975.
9. Berquist WE, Byrne WJ, Ament ME, et al: Achalasia: Diagnosis, management and clinical course in 16 children. Pediatrics 71:798–805, 1983.
10. Blanchard H, Roy CC, Perreault G, et al: Retrosternal esophageal replacement in 18
    children. Canad J Surg 15:137–145, 1972.
11. Blank E, Michael TD: Muscular hypertrophy of the esophagus: Report of a case with
    involvement of the entire esophagus. Pediatrics 32:595–598, 1963.
12. Boyd AD, Cukingnan R, Engleman RM, et al: Esophago-gastrostomy. J Thorac Car-
    diovasc Surg 70:817–825, 1975.
13. Cohen D, Middleton AW, Fletcher J: Gastric tube esophagoplasty. J Pediatric Surg
    9:451–459, 1974.
14. Corazziari E, Mineo TC, Anzini F: Functional evaluation of colon transplants used in
    esophageal reconstruction. Am J Digest Dis 22:7–11, 1977.
15. Crocker J, Thompson RM: Multiple smooth muscle hypertrophies in a newborn infant.
    Arch Dis Child 41:514–518, 1966.
16. Dane KS, Wooler GH, Holden MP, et al: Esophageal replacement with jejunum for non-
    malignant lesions: 26 years' experience. Surgery 72:466–476, 1972.
17. Davis GR, Santa Ana CA, Morawski SG, et al: Development of a lavage solution associ-
    ated with minimal water and electrolyte absorption or secretion. Gastroenterol 78:991–
    995, 1980.
18. de Lorimier AA, Harrison MR: Long gap esophageal atresia—Primary anastomosis after
    esophageal elongation by bougienage and esophagomyotomy. J Thorac Cardiovasc Surg
    79:138–141, 1980.
19. Ein SH, Shandling B, Simpson JS, et al: A further look at the gastric tube as an esophageal
    replacement in infants and children. J Pediatr Surg 8:859–868, 1973.

20. Ein SH, Shandling B, Simpson JS, et al: Fourteen years of gastric tubes. J Pediatric Surg 13:638–641, 1978.

21. Elkins RC, Jones EL, De Meester TR: Functional evaluation of the colonic interposition operation for benign esophageal stricture. Rev Surg 28:376–380, 1971.

22. Ernst RW, Leventhal M, Luna R, et al: Total esophago-gastric replacement after ingestion of household ammonia. N Engl J Med 15:815–818, 1963.

23. Ferguson TB, Woodbury JD, Roper CL, et al: Giant muscular hypertrophy of the esophagus. Ann Thorac Surg 8:209–216, 1969.

24. Ferrer JM, Bruch HM: Jejunal and colonic interposition for non-malignant disease of the esophagus. Ann Surg 169:533–543. 1969.

25. Fisher J, Payne WS, Irons GB: Salvage of a failed colon interposition in the esophagus with a free jejunal graft. Mayo Clin Proc 59:197–201, 1984.

26. Foker JE, Ring WS, Varco RL: Technique of jejunal interposition for esophageal replacement. J Thorac Cardiovasc Surg 83:928–933, 1982.

27. Fonkalsrud EW, Ament ME: Surgical management of esophageal stricture due to recessive dystrophic epidermolysis bullosa. J Pediatr Surg 12:221–226, 1977.

28. Freeman NV, Cass DT: Colon interposition: A modification of the waterston technique using the normal esophageal route. J Pediatr Surg 17:17–21, 1982.

29. French RJ, Tabb HG, Rutledge LJ: Esophageal stenosis produced by ingestion of bleach. South Med J 63:1140–1144, 1970.

30. Gavriliu D: Aspects of esophageal surgery. In: Current Problems in Surgery. Chicago: Year Book Medical Publishers, 1975.

31. German JC, Waterston DJ: Colon interposition for the replacement of esophagus in children. J Pediatr Surg 11:227–234, 1976.

32. Goring WS, Varco RL, L'Heureux PR, et al: Esophageal replacement with jejunum in children. J Thorac Cardiovasc Surg 83:918–927, 1982.

33. Grimes OF: Replacements of the esophagus. Amer J Surg 100:278–290, 1960.

34. Gross RE, Firestone FN: Colonic reconstruction of the esophagus in infants and children. Surgery 61:955–964, 1967.

35. Heimlick HJ: Esophagoplasty with reversed gastric tube. Review of fifty three cases. Amer J Surg 123:80–92, 1972.

36. Hendren WM, Hendren, WG: Color Interposition for esophagus in children. J Pediatr Surg 20 1985.

37. Holder TM, Ashcraft KW, Leape LL: The treatment of patients with esophageal strictures by local steroid injection. J Pediatr Surg 4:646–653, 1969.

38. Hopkins RA, Postlethwait RW: Caustic burns and carcinoma of the esophagus. Ann Surg 194:146–148, 1981.

39. Jezioro Z, Kus H: Experiences with the retrosternal esophageal replacement employing jejunum and ileum. Surgery 44:275–286, 1958.

40. Jones EL, Booth DJ, Cameron JL, et al: Functional evaluation of esophageal reconstructions. Ann Thorac Surg 12:331–346, 1971.

41. Karen G, Frand M, Jonas A, et al: Sandifer's syndrome following reverse gastro tube operation (Gavrilim's operation). J Pediatr Surg 18:632–633, 1983.

42. Kelly JP, Shackelford GD, Roper CL: esophageal replacement with colon in children: Functional results and long-term growth. Ann Thorac Surg 36:634–641, 1983.

43. Kinninan J, Shin HI, Witteland P: Carcinoma of the esophagus after lye corrosion: Report of a case in a 15 year old Korean male. Acta Chir Scand. 134:489–493, 1968.

44. Kiviranta UK: Corrosion carcinoma of the esophagus-381 cases of corrosion and nine cases of corrosion carcinoma. Acta Otolaryngol 42:89–95, 1952.

45. Kralik J, Rapant V: Radical surgical treatment of esophageal stenosis due to epidermolysis bullosa. J Thorac Cardiovasc Surg 69:790–802, 1975.

46. Krey H: Treatment of corrosive lesions in the esophagus. Acta Oto-laryngologica (supplement) 102: 1–49, 1952.

47. Lamm KH, Lim STK, Wong J, et al: Gastric histology and function in patients with intrathoracic stomach replacement after esophagectomy. Surgery 85:283–290, 1979.

48. Leahy WR, Toyka KV, Fischbeck KM: Cerebral abscess in children secondary to esophageal dilatation. Pediatrics 59:300–301, 1977.

49. Leape LL, Ashcraft KW, Scarpelli DG, et al: Hazard to health—Liquid lye. N Engl J Med 284:578–581, 1971.

50. Lindahl M, Louhimo I Virkola K: Colon interposition or gastric tube? Follow-up study of colon-esophagus and gastric tube-esophagus patients. J Pediatr Surg 18:58–63, 1983.

51. Lortat-Jacob JL: Myomatoses localisées et myomatoses diffuses, de l'oesophage. Arch Mal Appl Dig 39:519, 1950.

52. Lortat-Jacob JL, Giuli R: Esophageal replacement. Prog Surg 12:77–95, 1973.

53. Louhimo I, Pasila M, Visakorpi JK: Late gastrointestinal complications in patients with colonic replacement of the esophagus. J Pediatr Surg 4:663–673, 1969.

54. Lynn HB: Colon interposition in pediatric patients with esophageal varices. Ann Surg 173:706–713, 1971.

55. Lynn HB: Simple method of elongating a colonic segment for esophageal replacement. J Pediatr Surg 8:391–393, 1973.

56. Malcolm JA: Occurrence of peptic ulcer in colon used for esophageal replacement. J Thorac Cardiovasc Surg 55:763–772, 1968.

57. Meyers WC, Seigler HF, Hanks JB, et al: Postoperative function of "free" jejunal transplants for replacement of the cervical esophagus. Ann Surg 192:439–448, 1980.

58. Naef AP, Savary M, Ozzello L: Columnar-lined lower esophagus: An acquired lesion with malignant predisposition J Thorac Cardiovasc Surg 70:826–835, 1975.

59. Nahmad M, Clatworthy HW: Leiomyoma of the entire esophagus. J Pediatr Surg 8:829–830, 1973.

60. Neville WE, Najem AZ: Colon replacement of the esophagus for congenital and benign disease. Ann Thorac Surg 36:626–633, 1983.

61. Orlando RC, Bozymski EM, Briggaman RA, et al: Epidermolysis bullosa: Gastrointestinal manifestations. Ann Int Med 81:203–206, 1974.

62. Othersen HB, Clatworthy HW: Functional evaluation of esophageal replacement in children. J Thorac Cardiovasc Surg 53:55–63, 1967.

63. Paull A, Trier JS, Dalton MD, et al: The histologic spectrum of Barrett's esophagus. N Engl J Med 295:476–480, 1976.

64. Postlethwait RW: Surgery of the Esophagus. New York: Appleton-Century-Crofts pp. 415–438, 1979.

65. Postlethwait RW, Sealy WC, Dillon ML et al: Colon interposition for esophageal substitution. Ann Thorac Surg 12:89–109, 1971.

66. Radigan LR, Glover JL, Shipley FE, et al: Barrett esophagus. Arch Surg 112:486–491, 1977.

67. Raffensperger JG: Esophageal substitution. In Raffensperger JG (Ed.): Swenson's Pediatric Surgery (4th ed.). New York: Appleton-Century-Croft, 1980.

68. Raffensperger JG, Shkonlik AA, Boggo JD, et al: Portal hypertension in children. Arch Surg 104:249–256, 1972.

69. Rapant V, Kralik J, Doubravsky J: Peptic ulcer in the jejunum or colon following esophageal replacement. Int Surg 54:126, 1970.

70. Schiller M, Frye TR, Boles ET: Evaluation of colonic replacement of the esophagus in children. J Pediatr Surg 6:753–760, 1971.

71. Seiber AM, Seiber WK: Colon transplants as esophageal replacement: Cineradiographic and manometric evaluation in children. Ann Surg 168:116–122, 1978.

72. Shaw A, Garvey J, Miller B: Lye burn requiring total gastrectomy and colon substitution for esophagus and stomach in a two-year-old boy. Surgery 65:837–844, 1969.

73. Shepard RL, Raffensperger JG, Goldstein R: Pediatric esophageal perforation. J Thorac Cardiovasc Surg 74:261–267, 1977.

74. Shils ME, Gilat T: The effect of esophagectomy on absorption in man. Clinical and metabolic observations. Gastroenterol 50:347–357, 1966.

75. Soulier Y, Lefort J, Borde J, et al: Le mega-oesophage idiopathique de l'enfant. Chir Pediatr 20:311–316, 1979.

76. Stanley-Brown EG: Massive hemorrhage after colon interposition: Early and late. J Pediatr Surg 9:235–237, 1974.

77. Sugiura M, Futagawa S: Further evaluation of the Sugiura procedure in the treatment of esophageal varices. Arch Surg 112:1317–1324, 1977.

78. Symbas PN, Hatcher CR, Harlaftis N: Spontaneous rupture of the esophagus. Ann Surg 187:634–639, 1978.

79. Ti-Sheng C, Oi-ling H, Wang-Wei: Reconstruction of esophageal defects with microsurgically revascularized jejunal segments: A report of 13 cases. J Microsurg 2:83–94, 1980.

80. Todani T, Watanabe Y, Mizuguchi T, et al: Congenital esophageal stenosis due to fibromuscular thickening. Z Kinderchir 39:11–14, 1984.

81. Tubino P, Maronelli LF, Alves E, et al: Choristoma: Esophageal stenosis, due to tracheobranchial remnants. Z Kinderchir 35:14–17, 1982.

82. Urschel HC, Razzuk MA, Wood RE, et al: Improved management of esophageal perforation: Exclusion and diversion in continuity. Ann Surg 179:587–591, 1974.

83. Waterston DJ: Colonic replacement of esophagus (intrathoracic) Surg Clin N Amer 44:1441–1447, 1964.

84. Waterston DJ: Reconstruction of the esophagus. In Mustard WT, (Eds.): Pediatric Surgery (vol. I). Chicago; Year Book Publishers, 1969.

85. Yamato T, Hamanaka Y, Hirata S, et al: Esophagoplasty with an autogenous tubed gastric flap. Amer J Surg 137:597–602, 1979.

86. Yarington CT: ingestion of caustic: A pediatric problem. J Pediatr 67:674–677, 1965.

Ronald J. Sharp

# 6

## Esophageal Foreign Bodies

Foreign body of the esophagus is not a modern disease by any means. Aesop was one of the first to report such a case in 600 b.c.:

"A wolf devoured his prey so ravenously that a bone stuck in his throat, giving him great pain. He ran howling up and down, and offered to reward handsomely anyone who would pull it out. A crane, moved by pity as well as by the prospect of the money, undertook the dangerous task. Having removed the bone, he asked for the promised reward. "Reward!" cried the wolf. "Pray you greedy fellow, what reward can you possibly require? You have had your head in my mouth, and instead of biting it off I have let you pull it out unharmed. Get away with you, and don't come again within reach of my paw." [The Wolf and the Crane. The Fables of Aesop, 600 b.c.]

The lethal nature of esophageal foreign body is epitomized in a poem by Mathew Arnold in *Light of Asia.*

> "Then came—who knows?—some gust of jungle wind,
> A stumble on the path, a taint in the tank,
> A snake's nip, half a span of angry steel,
> A chill, a fishbone, or a falling tile,
> And life was over and the man is dead." [55]

Of historical interest is the tradition in many tropical countries of crushing the head of a fish in one's teeth while using both hands to rebait the hook. A native of India practiced this technique with an eel-like fish that slipped into his esophagus and could not be withdrawn because of its short fins. The man died in great agony within the hour. He was buried with the creature still lodged in his esophagus as his friends were unable to remove it even after his death.[13]

Prior to 1854, esophageal foreign bodies were treated with some form of bougie in an attempt to force the object into the stomach. This dangerous practice is unfortunately still in vogue today. Gross, in 1854, advocated the use of various instruments, some designed by himself (Gross Probang and Graefe Coin Catcher), to retrive esopha-

Pediatric Esophageal Surgery
ISBN 0-8089-1776-5

geal foreign bodies.[13] Esophagoscopy was first attempted in 1795 by Bozinni, who was undoubtedly inspired by the facility of sword swallowers. Max Einhorn was the first to suggest use of an auxiliary illumination tube in the esophagoscope in order to illuminate the distal end of the scope.[13]

## INCIDENCE AND EPIDEMIOLOGY

It is estimated that between 1500 and 3000 Americans die each year as a result of foreign bodies in the air and food passages. It is the most common cause of death in children less than six years of age in the home.[13,19,46] The portion of these deaths caused by esophageal foreign bodies is small, but nonetheless a concern. A child instinctively examines objects with the mouth. Any object that a child can get into the mouth is at risk of being aspirated or swallowed (Fig. 6-1).[44] Foreign objects swallowed vary from culture to culture, as one would expect. The coin, however, is an international favorite, with the copper penny taking first place in the USA. In China, coins are only slightly exceeded by fish bones as a leading source of esophageal foreign bodies in children.[18] One of the largest series reported, consisting of adults and children in China,[2,32] had bones at the top of the list, followed by coins and food as the next most common foreign bodies.[25]

In the author's recent ten-year experience involving 122 children with esophageal foreign bodies, the coin was the most frequently encountered foreign body. Food foreign bodies were the next most common. Toys, pins, buttons, etc. account for the remainder (Table 6-1). Ages of patients ranged from two months to 12 years, with a median of 18 months of age. The male:female ratio was 1.6:1. Unlike the data reported for many series which include all age groups, 39 percent of these children had some type of pre-existing esophageal abnormality. Esophageal atresia (67 percent), lye stricture (12 percent), and recent distal esophageal surgery (21 percent) accounted for most of these abnormalities. In a recently reported series, 21 percent of esophageal foreign body patients had some type of pre-existing esophageal abnormality.[8] Sixteen percent of these children presented with a foreign body on two or more occasions, all 16 of whom had a pre-existing esophageal abnormality.

**Table 6-1**
*Pediatric Foreign Bodies Ingested*
*(n = 122)*

| Type | Number | Percentage |
|---|---|---|
| Coins | 45 | 36% |
|    pennies | 33 | |
|    dimes | 3 | |
|    nickels | 6 | |
|    quarters | 3 | |
| Food | 41 | 34% |
| Toys | 11 | 9% |
| Buttons | 6 | 5% |
| Bones | 6 | 5% |
| Pins | 5 | 4% |
| Miscellaneous | 8 | 7% |

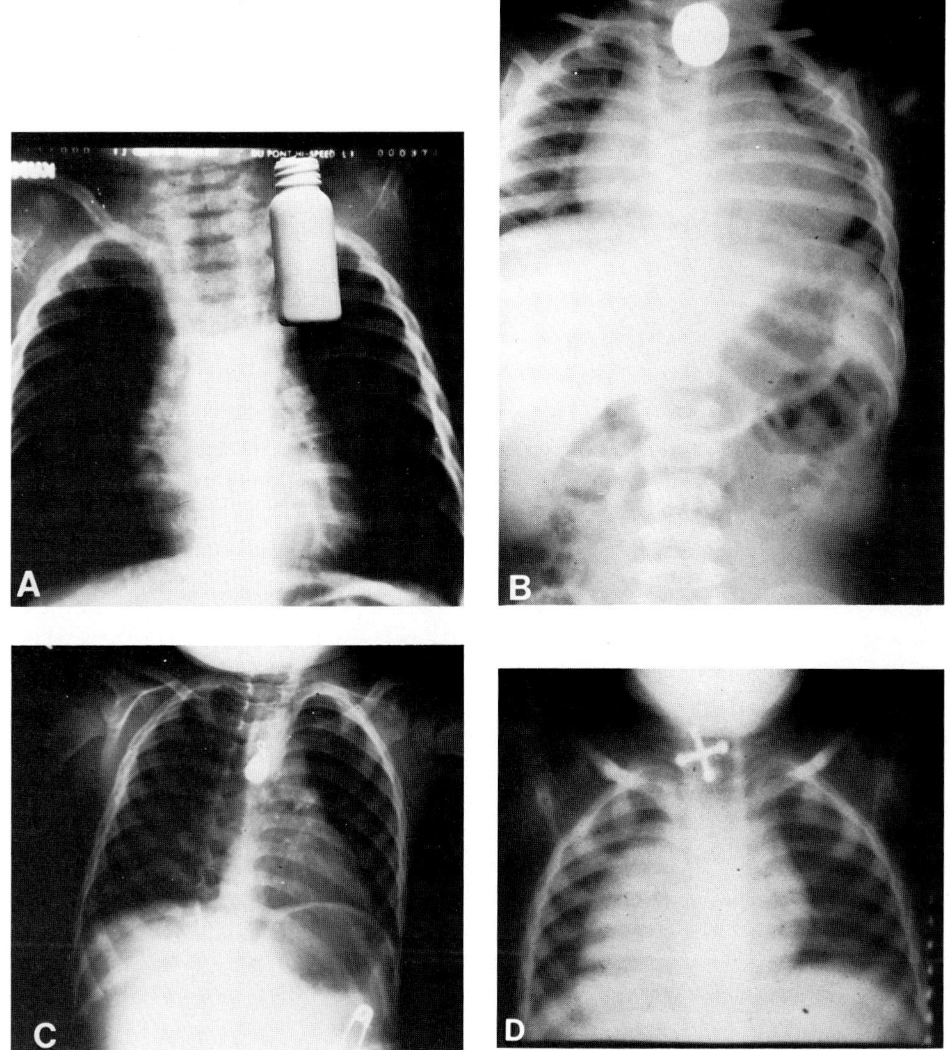

**Figure 6-1.** (A) This child presented in acute respiratory distress after the father attempted to retrieve a small bottle from the child's mouth. It was impacted into the child's esophagus. (By permission of Lucian L Leape, M.D.) (B) "Three coins in an esophagus": a typical configuration of a stack of coins. (C) This child avoided the hook and line but did swallow the sinker. He had an undiagnosed midesophageal stricture from ingestion of a clinitest tablet several months previously. (D) A jack in the esophagus.

The recent proliferation of miniaturized electronic devices powered by disk batteries has brought a new sense of urgency to the diagnosis and treatment of esophageal foreign bodies.[43] The National Poison Center Network estimated that 510–850 button battery ingestions occurred in 1980 alone. They accounted for 1.7 of every 10,000 poisonings reported in 1980.[28] In one of the largest reported series, consisting of 56 patients, ages ranged from 11 months to 90 years. Seventy-eight percent were less than five years of age. In this series, there were five serious complications; two of these resulted in death.[44] All of the deaths and two of the other serious complications were related to esophageal injury. The other serious complication occurred when the button battery became lodged in a Meckel's diverticulum.[54] The author's only case of button battery ingestion did not result in esophageal impaction; the battery was passed in the stool by 24 hours.

Fortunately, 90 percent of ingested foreign bodies in children pass through the gastrointestinal (GI) tract without incident. The ten percent that fail to pass most often become lodged in the esophagus and have the potential to cause serious morbidity and mortality.

## ANATOMY

The esophagus is a rather passive, nonadaptable organ, the peristaltic contractions of which are relatively weak.[32] This negative virtue, in addition to a number of anatomic narrowings, makes this organ more prone to impaction of foreign bodies than are other areas of the GI tract. The anatomic narrowings are in the cricopharyngeal area, the area of the aortic arch, the left main stem bronchus, and the region of the diaphragmatic hiatus.[46] In a series of 100 foreign bodies in children aged from seven months to 12 years, 74 percent of the foreign bodies were lodged in the cricopharyngeal region, 18 percent at the aortic arch, and 4 percent at the hiatus.[9] In the author's own series, 78 percent of the foreign bodies were lodged at the level of the cricopharyngeus and the remainder at the distal esophagus. Esophageal atresia patients with food impactions at the anastomotic site were included in the upper esophageal obstruction group. In adults, the relationship is the reverse as a general rule. The region of the esophagus just below the cricopharyngeus is the weakest peristaltic segment, which may account for the large number of foreign bodies in children that lodge in that area. The close relationship of heart, major vessels, trachea, and bronchi, and the lack of a serosal covering, make perforation of the esophagus by a foreign body much more serious than any other location in the GI tract. Unlike abdominal perforation, perforation in the mediastinum is poorly localized and infection spreads rapidly.

## PATHOPHYSIOLOGY

A vast majority of foreign bodies of the esophagus cause no pathophysiologic changes aside from mild obstruction to the usual flow of esophageal traffic. Foreign bodies can, however, cause significant pathophysiologic changes as a result of some or all of the following:

1.   physical characteristics
2.   chemical composition
3.   location in the esophagus
4.   duration of impaction
5.   abnormalities of the esophagus

These factors acting alone or in concert with one another can produce pathophysiologic changes that range from minor to major life-threatening complications.

Respiratory problems are not an uncommon complication of esophageal foreign body. They are either diagnosed acutely or, more often, much later (months to years in some cases). The acute cases result from a large object becoming lodged in the cricopharyngeal area, which compresses the membraneous portion of the trachea, resulting in acute airway compromise (Fig. 6-1).[20] This problem was appreciated by Dupuytren in earlier times when he vigorously kneaded a dying man's esophagus to break up a large piece of potato that threatened the man with asphyxia. This maneuver crushed the potato and allowed the victim to swallow it, thus relieving him of a life-threatening predicament.[13]

Delayed respiratory symptoms are usually secondary to erosion by a foreign body into the wall of the esophagus with resultant inflammation and edema formation. Figure 6-2 illustrates the edema formation that results from prolonged foreign body impaction. This 13-month-old child swallowed a large button three weeks prior to this radiograph. He presented with stridor and wheezing. His dietary pattern over this period of time was unchanged. Once relieved of the button, his symptoms rapidly subsided. In occasional cases, the foreign body will pass completely through the wall of the esophagus and form an abscess in the surrounding tissues. Foreign bodies have been reported to migrate into the lungs, heart, and major vessels.[39] The compression of

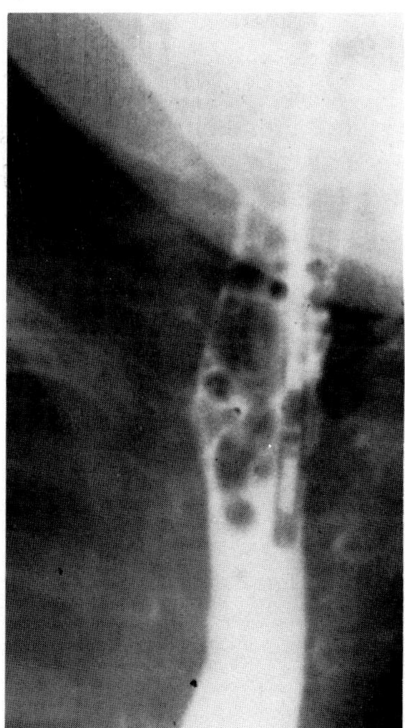
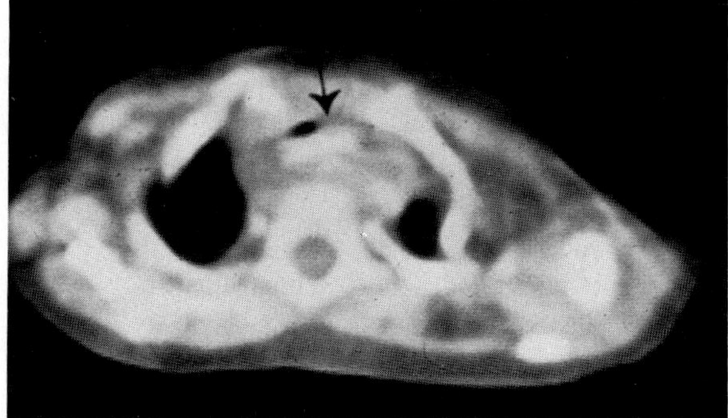

**Figure 6-2.** A thirteen-month-old male developed stridor, wheezing, and increased feeding difficulties over the three weeks prior to evaluation. His chest X-ray was negative. A barium swallow (A) did not demonstrate a foreign body. A CT scan (B) demonstrated a foreign body and soft tissue swelling which caused significant narrowing of the trachea. At endoscopy, a large button was retrieved. His stridor and wheezing gradually subsided during his uneventful recovery.

the membranous portion of the trachea by the inflammatory reaction, and/or abscess, causes compromise of the airway, which is manifested by wheezing, stridor, cyanosis, and, at times, persistent pneumonia.[4,22,36,38,47,50]

Exsanguinating hemorrhage is fortunately not a common problem in esophageal foreign body impaction, but it is nonetheless reported in larger series.[2,15,32,38,39] This catastrophic event arises when the esophagus is perforated by a sharp foreign body which subsequently erodes into a surrounding vessel, creating a fistula. Erosion and fistula formation have been reported to occur with smooth objects, such as coins.[32,39] Liquefaction necrosis secondary to ingestion of corrosives and enzymatic digestion (papain) have resulted in major-vessel esophageal fistulas and death from exsanguination.[48,50,54]

Mediastinal sepsis is a highly lethal complication if not detected and treated early.[39] The basic mechanism is perforation by a foreign body (or operator), followed by persistent leakage of esophageal content, resulting in a rapidly spreading cellulitis of the mediastinum. Because of the extensive communication of tissue planes of the neck with the mediastinum, a perforation anywhere in the cervical esophagus will eventually involve the mediastinum. The mortality rate is significantly lowered if a foreign body completely penetrates the esophagus and allows it to heal.[39]

Disk batteries pose a modern threat. Their smooth, round contour belies their true potential for harm. Most round, smooth objects less than 18 mm in diameter will pass through the esophagus without incident—witness the 17-mm dime, which is seldom impacted in a normal esophagus. The two reported deaths from disk battery ingestion were caused by batteries between 21 and 23 mm in diameter. The real danger, however, lies in the batteries' content, which readily leaks once in a fluid environment. These batteries usually contain some type of heavy metal (mercury, zinc, silver, or cadmium) and an alkali (potassium or sodium hydroxide).[28,31,51] The damage potential of button batteries arises from the corrosive effects of alkali. Electrical burns from the low-voltage current and mercury poisoning are a concern, but have not proven to be a significant problem as yet. Strong bases cause liquefaction necrosis which essentially soubilizes protein, saponifies lipids, and dehydrates cells. (See also Chapter 4.) Unlike the effects of acids, strong alkali effects are not rapidly neutralized but continue to act, in some cases, for days. Three phases of liquefaction necrosis have been characterized. The first phase is that of protein and lipid dissolution. The second phase is that of tissue slough and ulceration. The final phase is that of healing by scar formation and stricture.[6] This sequence of events is described, for the most part, in both cases of the two children who died from disk battery ingestion. They died some time after the removal of the battery and both were found at postmortem to have major liquefaction necrosis of the esophagus and surrounding vessels.[6,44] These batteries contain an eight-normal solution of potassium or sodium hydroxide, which has been shown to perforate the rabbit esophagus in less than 10 minutes.

The possibility of mercury poisoning from battery leakage has been of great concern, but to date this has not been reported. Mercury levels, in cases where the battery has been completely open, have not been significantly elevated. It is well known that the LD50 of mercuric chloride, which is readily absorbed, is less than 0.5 g. Most button batteries containing mercury have in the neighborhood of 21 g in the oxide form, which is poorly absorbed.[28,31,51] Because of the great potential for serious complications and possible death, esophageal foreign bodies should command the physician's full attention when the diagnosis is entertained.

## CLINICAL PRESENTATION

Most children harboring esophageal foreign bodies will present with a history of ingestion followed immediately by coughing, choking, drooling, poor feeding, dysphagia, or vomiting.[32,35,38] These acute symptoms, if not addressed early, can rapidly abate and the child will soon adapt to the foreign body by selecting foods which can be managed without symptoms.[17,35] Esophageal foreign bodies often present, however, in rather obscure ways.

In patients who present with acute obstructive airway symptoms, the possibility of an esophageal foreign body must be carefully considered.[51] Esophageal foreign bodies may present as chronic airway problems. Stridor, wheezing, cyanosis, and a persistent pneumonia are the most common signs in this setting.[4,19,22,36,38,47]

In the author's series, the duration of impaction was directly related to the likelihood of presenting with respiratory symptoms. After five days of impaction, 61 percent of patients presented with respiratory symptoms. After ten and twenty days of impaction, 83 percent and 90 percent, respectively, presented with respiratory symptoms as their primary complaint. In the author's series, five percent were under the age of six months. Seventh-one percent of this group had a foreign body in place for more than five days; 100 percent of this subgroup presented with predominantly respiratory symptoms. One must always consider esophageal foreign body when confronted with a child (especially a child under one year of age) in respiratory distress.

Acute upper GI bleeding may occasionally be the initial presentation of a patient with an esophageal foreign body. Such patients will often have a good history for foreign body ingestion that was never confirmed by X-ray or endoscopy, or they may have evidence of minor esophageal injury at endoscopy. These patients present with a sentinel hemorrhage that is self-limited or easily controlled. This placid beginning may be followed in hours or days by exsanguinating hemorrhage.[30,32] This complication is seen in roughly 30 percent of those who suffer esophageal perforation from a foreign body.[39]

Fever of unknown origin, failure to thrive, vocal cord paralysis associated with a mediastinal mass, torticollis, hemoptysis, pericardial effusion, and even sudden infant death have all been reported as the initial presentation in the case of esophageal foreign body.[3,38,48,50]

## DIAGNOSIS

A history of foreign body ingestion (usually obtained in over 50 percent of cases) accompanied by classic clinical presentation can be confirmed in most cases by a posterior-anterior (PA) and lateral chest X-ray and a good lateral neck film in the hyperextended position. This study will rapidly reveal any radio-opaque foreign body and will domonstrate the presence of mediastinal air. The hyperextended neck film will often align a relatively nonopaque foreign body (i.e., a pop top) so that it will present enough density to be visible on standard films.

In cases where the history and presentation are suggestive but the initial X-rays are negative, a barium swallow should be performed while the child is in the radiology suite. This examination can be aided by use of barium-soaked cotton if the foreign body is narrow and not detected on routine swallow.

Nonopaque foreign bodies that are embedded in the wall of the esophagus or that have migrated outside the esophageal lumen will not be demonstrated by barium swallow. These may be missed by endoscopy, as in two cases reported in children in which "pop tops" had migrated into the esophageal wall. They were readily visualized using computerized tomography (CT).[14,49] Children with atypical presentations (respiratory problems, esophageal bleeding, failure to thrive, fever of unknown origin, etc.), whose initial workup is negative, should undergo CT examination (Fig. 6-2).

## TREATMENT

The management of an esophageal foreign body is determined by the physical characteristics of the foreign body, the length of time it has been in place, the anatomy of the esophagus, the position of the foreign body relative to the esophagus, and at times the ingenuity of the surgeon.[21,29]

A smooth foreign body lodged in a normal esophagus for less than 72 hours can be very easily removed with a high degree of success using the Foley balloon catheter technique.[1,5,9,10,33] The basic requirements of this technique are a 16 or 18 French Foley catheter, a 10-cc syringe containing a few cubic centimeters of Hypaque (Winthrop), fluoroscopy with a tilting table, laryngoscope, Macgill forceps, suction, and good holding help. A fully-stocked resuscitation cart should be in the room. The child is placed in the lateral, steep, head-down position and the catheter passed orally beyond the foreign body. The balloon is then carefully inflated and gently but steadily withdrawn in a smooth motion all the way out of the mouth. The nasal route is discouraged because of the difficulty deflating the balloon which may hold the foreign body in the posterior pharynx where it can be aspirated or swallowed again.

Fluoroscopic guidance greatly enhances the safety and success rate of this procedure. The head down and lateral position utilizes gravity to help prevent aspiration of the object when it is pulled into the mouth. This method of extraction of smooth foreign bodies is simple and cost-effective and avoids the use of a general anesthetic. In the reported series, the success rate has been over 90 percent. No complications have been reported to date. This technique has been used in the author's institution for the last several years, likewise without complication. Its use has been reported in patients with nonopaque foreign bodies (mostly food) who have a history of esophageal stenosis due to peptic stricture or following repair of esophageal atresia. It was successful in 23 out of 25 cases with no complications.[33]

Food impactions, in particular meat impactions of the esophagus, have inspired novel approaches to removal. This particular problem is more common in the adult population than it is in children, but it not uncommon in children. Children with strictures from whatever cause, especially those with repaired esophageal atresia where poor motility adds to the problem, are at highest risk for food impactions. Papain, a trypsin-like enzyme obtained from the pawpaw tree, was advocated for treatment of this problem in 1945.[41] This method of removal of meat impaction in children is mentioned only to be condemned. In the 90 cases so treated which have been thus far reported, there has been a three percent mortality rate from esophageal perforation.[7,11,16,18] These patients died as a result of digestion and perforation of the esophagus. The use of papain prior to endoscopy makes this procedures more hazardous because of the partial digestion of the esophageal wall.

Another technique of removal of food foreign bodies involves the use of gas-forming agents. A mixture of 15 cc of tartic acid and 15 cc of sodium bicarbonate is instilled into the esophagus followed by a columnm of barium. The whole process is monitored by fluoroscopy. This technique has a reported 100-percent success rate in eight patients.[40]

Glucagon has been used for some time in radiographic procedures to facilitate examination of certain portions of the GI tract. A single dose of .25 to 0.5 mg, will give a nine–17-minute duration of action and a one-minute onset. One of the many actions of glucagon is the relaxation of smooth muscle. A 50-percent success rate has been reported in patients with food impactions of the esophagus.[7,16,18,37] The disimpaction may be aided by placing a barium column above the foreign body and then administering a glucagon bolus intravenously. If unsuccessful, a second try with a double dose of glucagon may be tried in 15–20 minutes. An unsuccessful trial of glucagon does not compromise a subsequent endoscopic procedure. The only contraindications to the use of glucagon are pheochromocytoma, insulinoma, and known hypersensitivity to the drug.

Disk battery ingestion constitutes a true emergency if the battery is demonstrated in the esophagus by plain roentgenogram[53] These batteries should be removed endoscopically, not only in order to rid the esophagus of the battery, but to also assess damage to the esophagus.[31] Some have advocated removal of disk batteries from the esophagus (if they have been in place for less than 24 hours) using the balloon method.[32] This is dangerous, as esophageal damage can occur early. The blind passage of a catheter into the injured esophagus and stretching as the balloon passes may prove very hazardous. Prompt endoscopic removal of all batteries which lodge in the esophagus is recommended.[28] If a battery has passed beyond the gastroesophagcal (GE) junction, it can safely be allowed to pass through the GI tract without operative intervention. The only reported complication of a disk battery that has passed beyond the esophagus was perforation of a Meckel's diverticulum.[54] This is indeed a rare occurrence. If the battery stays in one place longer than six–eight hours after passing through the esophagus, operative removal may be indicated. If any abdominal signs or symptoms develop, regardless of time, operative removal should be carried out.

Once the battery has been removed, the child should be treated with antibiotics while being observed in the hospital for several days. The corrosive effects of the battery alkali will often persist beyond the time of removal. A normal barium esophagram, which should be performed following removal, is no guarantee that catastrophic complications cannot follow.

Sharp foreign bodies, foreign bodies in patients with esophageal strictures, and foreign bodies that have been in place for more than 72 hours or an indeterminate length of time should be removed endoscopically under general anesthesia.

With the rapid proliferation of flexible endoscopists, there are those who advocate flexible endoscopy for foreign body removal. Most of these reports are small. Sufficient numbers have not accumulated to assess its safety; lower cost and increased safety are the claimed benefits.[45] In children, rigid endoscopy is more efficient and as cost-effective as flexible, since children require a general anesthetic for either modality. Most children with uncomplicated esophageal foreign bodies can be treated as outpatients. In the author's series, 36 percent were treated as outpatients. A majority of the remaining patients were overnight admissions.

All intraluminal penetrating foreign bodies should undergo contrast study to look for extravasation. If a leak is found, intravenous antibiotics should be started. The patient should be taken to the operating room soon thereafter for esophageal closure and thorough drainage.[26,52] These patients should have no oral intake and will therefore need intravenous hyperalimentation or a gastrostomy for nutritional management. Those who have a penetrating foreign body with no evidence of leakage should be started on antibiotics and observed in the hospital for several days.

If endoscopy cannot visualize a documented foreign body, a computerized tomographic (CT) scan should be done. Extraluminal or intramural foreign bodies that cannot be removed endoscopically will require a formal cervical or thoracic approach for removal. All patients with penetrating foreign bodies (with or without leakage) who experience hemoptysis or hematemesis should be considered for arteriography to rule out a vascular esophageal fistula.

## COMPLICATIONS

The potential for serious complications for esophageal foreign body rises with the duration of impaction.[12] Possible complications include erosion into major blood vessels, aspiration pneumonia, paraesophageal abscess, mediastinitis, airway obstruction, tracheoesophageal fistula, and esophageal stricture. Most of these potentially fatal complications result from erosion and perforation of the esophageal wall. The incidence of esophageal perforation by foreign body was one percent in two large series of 2902 and 2394 patients.

In the author's series of 122 patients, three (a 2.5 percent rate) documented perforations from foreign bodies occurred. One child suffered a perforation of the upper esophagus from a straight pin. He subsequently developed an abscess which was drained through a cervical incision. He responded to drainage and antibiotics. He died two weeks after discharge from asphyxia as a result of another foreign body aspiration. The second child swallowed a shard of glass that lacerated his upper esophagus. The perforation was demonstrated by esophagram. He was drained immediately and fed via gastrostomy for two weeks with an uneventful recovery. The last patient suffered perforation from a chicken bone. He showed no leakage on esophogram, but did have air evident in the soft tissue. He was treated with intravenous antibiotics and observed closely. His recovery was uneventful.

In an extensive review, a collected series of 321 cases of esophageal perforation secondary to foreign bodies found that of this total, 43 (13 percent) migrated extraluminally. Surprisingly, 25 of the objects were coins, with a 20-percent mortality rate reported in this subgroup. Several interesting facts emerged from this study. The male:female ratio was only slightly male predominant. The peak incidence was in the first ten years of life. Bones, pins, and coins were the most common perforating objects. The cervical esophagus was the most frequent site of injury, followed by the upper thoracic esophagus. The time interval from ingestion to diagnosis of perforation while the foreign body was intraluminal ranged from one hour to three years, with a mean of 24 days. Perforation and extraluminal migration of the foreign body required between one hour and seven years to occur, with a mean of 103 days. The overall mortality rate was 45 percent. When considered individually, the intraluminal foreign bodies had a mortality rate of 56 percent, as compared to a 14-percent mortality rate for the extraluminal foreign bodies. The antibiotic era improved the mortality by only a modest percentage, 13 percent and seven percent, respectively. There was no correlation between mortality and duration of impaction. In general, the more distal the perforation, the higher the mortality.

In this same series, vascular and suppurative complications carried the highest mortality. There were 112 vascular erosions: 101 involved the aorta, five the innominate, and six the carotid arteries. The mortality rate with a vascular fistula was 100 percent prior to 1940 and over 90 percent following that era. The principal reason for such a high mortality is delayed or missed diagnosis. The potential should always be entertained and arteriography quickly performed in any child with hemoptysis or hematemesis following removal of a penetrating foreign body.[2,32,39]

The suppurative complications carried a 66-percent mortality rate in the pre-antibiotic era and a 35-percent mortality rate after that time. Localized infections amenable to surgical drainage have a much better outlook.[34,38,39]

Tracheoesophageal fistula was found in six patients in Remsen's series. When these fistulas occur, they are often extensive and commonly require major reconstruction involving esophageal replacement and complicated repair of the trachea.[27,53]

As in any disease state, the treatment should not produce more morbidity than the disease. The overall perforation rate for rigid endoscopy is reported to be near 0.34 percent, with a reported mortality rate of 0.05 percent. Rigid endoscopy by experienced operators is the gold standard for treatment of esophageal foreign bodies.[17,42] The use of papain with its reported perforation and mortality rate of three percent is unacceptable.[11] Recent enthusiasm for flexible endoscopy by an ever-increasing number of endoscopists will have to be carefully monitored.[45] Use of the balloon catheter technique has numerous enthusiasts, with no serious complications reported thus far. This method should be limited to use in cases of smooth foreign bodies whose presence in the esophagus has been of short duration.

## PREVENTION

Public education to prevent foreign body ingestion is obviously the best treatment. In particular, the new threat that disk batteries pose should be countered by public education programs, warning labels, and efforts to develop a safer product.[53] The recent success in limiting the devastating injuries from drain cleaners from such an approach is apparent. It is to be hoped that similar efforts to inform the public regarding the dangers of the disk battery will help to reduce the incidence of ingestion and resultant injuries.

## REFERENCES


1. Aiken DW: Coins in the esophagus, a departure from conventional surgery. Military Med 130:182–183, 1965.
2. Barbary ASE: Oesophageal fistula caused by swallowed foreign bodies. J. Laryngol Otol 83:251–259, 1969.
3. Beal SM: Sudden infant death associated with an oesophageal problem. Med J. Aust 2:91, 1979.
4. Beer S, Avidan G, Viure E, et al: A foreign body in the oesophagus as a cause of respiratory distress. Pediatr Radiol 12:41–42, 1982.

5.  Bigler FC: The use of a foley catheter for removal of blunt foreign bodies from the esophagus. J. Thorac Cardiovasc Surg 51:759–760, 1966.
6.  Blatnik DS, Toohill RJ, Lehman RH: Fatal complication from an alkaline battery foreign body in the esophagus. Ann Otol 86:611–615, 1977.
7.  Bryant BG, Trout DJ: Treatment of esophageal food impaction—A new use for glucagon. Drug Intell Clin Pharm 16:407–409, 1982.
8.  Buchin PJ: Foreign bodies of the esophagus. N Y State J Med 81:1057–1059, 1981.
9.  Campbell JB, Foley C: A safe alternative to endoscopic removal of blunt esophageal foreign bodies. Arch Otolaryngol 109:323–325, 1983.
10.  Campbell JB, Quattromani FL, Foley LC: Foley catheter removal of blunt esophageal foreign bodies. Experience with 100 consecutive children. Pediatr Radiol 13:116–119, 1983.
11.  Cavo JW, Koops HJ, Gryboski RA: Use of enzymes for meat impactions in the esophagus. Laryngoscope 87:630–634, 1977.
12.  Clerf LH: Foreign bodies in the air and food passages. Surg Gynecol Obstet 70:328–339, 1940.
13.  Clerf LH: Historical aspects of foreign bodies in the air and food passages. S Med J 68:1449–1454, 1975.
14.  Crenshaw RT: "Pop Top" ingestion: A technique for localization. JAMA 237:1928–1929, 1977.
15.  Danis RK: Management of ingested foreign bodies in the esophagus in children. Missouri Med 77:27–28, 1980.
16.  Ferrucci JT, Long JA: Radiologic treatment of esophageal food impaction using intravenous glucagon. Radiology 125:25–28, 1977.
17.  Giordano A, Adams G, Boies L, et al: Current management of esophageal foreign bodies. Arch Otolaryngol 107:249–251, 1981.
18.  Glauser J, Lilja GP, Greenfeld B, et al: Intravenous glucagon in the management of esophageal food obstruction. JACEP 8:228–231, 1979.
19.  Goldsher M, Eliachar I, Joachims HZ: Paradoxical presentation in children of foreign bodies in trachea and oesophagus. The Practitioner 220:631–632, 1978.
20.  Handler, SD, Beaugard MR, Canalis RF, et al: Unsuspected esophageal foreign bodies in adults with upper airway obstruction. Chest 80:234–237, 1981.
21.  Himaldi GM, Fischer GJ: Magnetic removal of foreign bodies from the upper gastrointestinal tract. Radiology 123:226–227, 1977.
22.  Humphry A, Holland WG: Unsuspected esophageal foreign bodies. J Can Assoc Radiol 32:17–20, 1981.
23.  Jackson C: Peroral endoscopy and laryngeal surgery. Laryngoscope 27:583–584, 1917.
24.  Jackson C, Jackson CL: Diseases of the Air and Food Passages of Foreign Body Origin. Philadelphia: W B Saunders, 1936.
25.  Jackson CL: Foreign bodies in the esophagus. Am J Surg 93:308–312, 1957.
26.  Keszler P, Buzna E: Surgical and conservative management of esophageal perforation. Chest 80:158–162, 1981.
27.  Krespi YP, Grossman BG, Sisson GA: Repair of an intrathoracic tracheoesophageal fistula caused by an unsuspected esophageal foreign body. Am J Otolaryngol 3:339–343, 1982.
28.  Litovitz TL: Button battery ingestions. JAMA 249:2495–2500, 1983.
29.  Mack JW, Matthews JM, Takamoto RM: Swallowed endotracheal tube: A neonatal emergency case. Military Med 146:354–355, 1981.
30.  McCormack LR, Monroe LS: Esophageal perforation by swallowed foreign body causing arterial fistula with gastrointestinal hemorrhage. Gastrointest Endosc 23:157–158, 1977.
31.  Mofenson HC, Greensher J, Caraccio TR, et al: Ingestion of small flat disc batteries. Ann Emerg Med 12:88–90, 1983.

32. Nandi P, Ong GB: Foreign body in the oesophagus: Review of 2394 cases. Br J Surg 65:5–9, 1978.

33. Nixon GW: Foley catheter method of esophageal foreign body removal: Extension of applications. AJR 132:441–442, 1979.

34. Okafor BC: Lung abscess secondary to esophageal foreign body. Ann Otol 87:568–570, 1978.

35. O'Neill JA, Holcomb GW, Neblett WW: Management of tracheobronchial and esophageal foreign bodies in childhood. J Ped Surg 18:475–479, 1983.

36. Pasquariello PS, Kean H: Cyanosis of a foreign body in the esophagus. Clin Pediatr 14:223–225, 1975.

37. Pillari G, Bank S, Katzka I, et al: Meat bolus impaction of the lower esophagus associated with a paraesophageal hernia. Am J Gastroenterol 71:287–289, 1979.

38. Poncz M, Schwartz MW: Vocal cord paralysis and mediastinal mass. Clin Pediatr 17:196–198, 1978.

39. Remsen K, Biller HF, Lawson W, et al: Unusual presentations of penetrating foreign bodies of the upper aerodigestive tract. Ann Otol Rhinol (supplement 105) 92:32–44, 1983.

40. Rice BT, Spiegel PK, Dombrowski PJ: Acute esophageal food impaction treated by gas-forming agents. Radiology 146:299–301, 1983.

41. Richardson JR: A new treatment for esophageal obstruction due to meat impaction. Ann Otol Rhinol Laryngol 54:328–348, 1945.

42. Ritter FN: Questionable methods of foreign body treatment. Ann Otol 83:729–733, 1974.

43. Rumack BH, Rumack CM: Disk battery ingestion. JAMA 249:2509–2511, 1983.

44. Shabino CL, Feinberg AN: Esophageal perforation secondary to alkaline battery ingestion. JACEP 8:360–362, 1979.

45. Shaffer RD, Klug T: A comparative study of techniques for esophageal foreign body removal with special emphasis on meat bolus obstruction. Wis Med J 80:33–36, 1981.

46. Slovis CM, Tyler-Werman R, Solightly DP: Massive foreign object ingestion Ann Emerg Med 11:433–435, 1982.

47. Smith PC, Swischuk LE, Fagan CJ: An elusive and often unsuspected cause of stridor or pneumonia (the esophageal foreign body). Am J Radium Therapy Nucl Med 122:80–89, 1974.

48. So SY, Mok CK, Lam WK, et al: Haemoptysis due to unsuspected foreign body penetration of the oesophagus. Aust N Z J Med 12:533–535, 1982.

49. Spitz L, Hirsig J: Prolonged foreign body impaction in the oesophagus. Arch Dis Child 57:551–553, 1982.

50. Tauscher JW: Esophageal foreign body: An uncommon cause of stridor. Pediatrics 61:657–658, 1978.

51. Temple DM, McNeese MC: Hazards of battery ingestion. Pediatrics 71:100–103, 1983.

52. Turcot R, Gagnon RM, Joassin AM, et al: Anaerobic mediastinitis and septic shock secondary to esophageal perforation. Can J Surg 22:382–384, 1979.

53. Votteler RP, Nash JC, Rutledge JC: The hazard of ingested alkaline disk batteries in children. JAMA 249:2504–2506, 1983.

54. Willis GA, Ho WC: Perforation of Meckel's diverticulum by an alkaline hearing aid battery. CMAJ 126:497–498, 1982.

55. Arnold, E: The light of Asia. Roberts Bro, Boston 1891.

Max L. Ramenofsky

# 7

# Gastroesophageal Reflux: Clinical Manifestations and Diagnosis

The vast majority of newborn infants have an incompetent lower esophageal sphincter (LES) mechanism and with proper diagnostic maneuvers, gastroesophageal reflux (GER) can be demonstrated. It is known that, with growth and development, the LES becomes competent and that GER can no longer be demonstrated.[9,14] Competence of the gastroesophageal mechanism generally develops in the first year of life, as the child assumes an upright, walking position. The reason for the maturation of the LES is unclear. It has been suggested that the intra-abdominal esophagus lengthens and that the upright position adds the benefit of gravity to intragastric contents.* Identification of GER in a symptomatic toddler or older child is thought to be diagnostic of "pathologic" GER. It is difficult to differentiate from physiologic GER in the newborn and the infant. The purpose of this chapter is to describe the clinical manifestations of GER and to define the diagnostic modalities useful in its identification.

## CLINICAL MANIFESTATIONS

The symptoms produced by GER can best be divided into four general groups: vomiting, aspiration, esophagitis, and miscellaneous. In addition to these groups, there are a number of diseases in which GER is commonly present, which adds significantly to the overall morbidity of these entities. These conditions are listed in Table 7-1.

Pathologic reflux often results in more than one type of symptom. For example, a child may suffer from esophagitis and fail to thrive on that basis, but may also suffer from aspiration pneumonitis secondary to GER. In one series, the incidence of multiple symptoms from GER was 66 percent.[38]

---

* The presence of GER is not necessarily intrinsically damaging. Asymptomatic GER may be termed "physiologic reflux." Identification. . . .

Pediatric Esophageal Surgery
ISBN 0-8089-1776-5

**Table 7-1**
*Major Anomalies Associated with GER*

Neurologic
    mental retardation from any cause
    seizures
    Down's syndrome
    Cornelia-deLange syndrome
    microcephaly
    spastic quadriplegia
    Pierre-Robin syndrome
    Mobius syndrome
    hydrocephalus
Gastrointestinal
    esophageal atresia with or without TEF
    duodenal stenosis
    malrotation
    antral pylorospasm
    pyloric stenosis
    imperforate anus
    Hirschprung's Disease
    abdominal wall defects: omphalocele
    allergic enterocolitis
Cardiac
    ASD
    coarctation
    mitral stenosis
Respiratory/thoracic
    subglottic stenosis
    vocal cord paralysis
    cleft palate
    bronchial stenosis
    phrenic nerve palsy
    tracheomalacia
    pulmonary hypertension
    pectus excavatum
    asphyxiating thoracic dystrophy
    Klippel-Feil syndrome
    congenital diaphragmatic hernia of Bochdalek
Prematurity
Multiple anomalies

## Vomiting

The clinical presentations of GER are listed in Table 7-2. Most newborn infants vomit as a manifestation of their incompetent LES mechanism. Vomiting has been identified as the most common presentation in infants with GER.[2,25,43,66] The vomitus may be bile-stained or not.[58] It is usually effortless, but on occasion may be projectile. Vomiting as a manifestation of GER becomes significant when the loss of protein and calories results in failure to grow. GER has also been incriminated as one of the etiologies for rumination.[24,31]

**Table 7-2**
*Clinical Presentations of GER*

Vomiting
    failure to thrive
    rumination
Aspiration
    pneumonia—chronic and/or recurrent
    apnea
        laryngospasm
        reflex apnea
    bronchitis
    asthma
    URI—recurrent
    laryngitis
    otitis media
Esophagitis
    colic
    protein-losing enteropathy and finger clubbing
    gastrointestinal bleeding
    stricture
    Sandifer syndrome
    failure to thrive
Miscellaneous
    seizures
    hypotonia
    irritability
    cardiac arrhythmias

## Aspiration Syndromes

The aspiration syndromes form a constellation of disease processes which are the greatest threat to life from GER (Table 7-2).

Chronic and/or recurrent pneumonias are the second most common complication of GER,[2,38,58] although several reports have indicated that respiratory complications are the most common presentation.[4,36] The pneumonias are identifiable by the lack of consistent patterns in the same patient. Typically, the pneumonias are frequent and involve different pulmonary lobes with each attack. The identification of aspiration from GER is not often made, but, on occasion, tracheal aspirates will show fat-filled macrophages indicative of aspiration of fat-containing gastric contents.[67] Repeated episodes of aspiration will eventually lead to chronic fibrotic pulmonary changes.

The most difficult of the aspiration syndromes to document has been in infants with an "aborted sudden infant death".[1,5,26,28,32,35,36,42,46,53] Two mechanisms for apnea caused by GER have been suggested. Clinical and experimental proof exists for each mechanism.

GER causing reflux of gastric contents onto the larynx and down the trachea has been shown to result in severe, irreversible laryngospasm in piglets.[18] The laryngospasm can be abolished, however, by surgical transection of the superior laryngeal nerves or can be re-established by stimulation of the nerves. Rare reports have appeared which have documented death in infancy from aspiration of gastric contents.[27,47]

Clinically, this mechanism of the sudden infant death syndrome (SIDS) is correlated with certain epidemiologic aspects of SIDS. The age incidence in SIDS is from one to six months, which is similar to that of the GER/apnea group.[5,28,46] Most episodes of SIDS occur during sleep. Frequently, infants have been fed immediately prior to being put down for the night. There is a reported incidence of respiratory symptoms in the 48 hours preceding death in up to 45 percent of infants suffering SIDS. These symptoms could well have been secondary to minor degrees of aspiration.[1,35]

Laryngospasm has also been incriminated in an autopsy study.[5] Petechial hemorrhages were found in the lungs and on the thymus of infants succumbing to SIDS. This is thought to be evidence of vigorous respiratory efforts made against a closed glottis.

Further clinco-pathologic evidence for the laryngospasm hypothesis comes from the left ventricular $pO_2$ in autopsied infants. The $pO_2$ is lower in infants dying of SIDS than in those who die from other causes.[53] This evidence suggests that hypoxia preceded cardiac arrest.

Finally, changes have been identified in the larynxes of infants dying of SIDS which include fibrinoid necrosis of the larynx.[54,65] It has been postulated that the necrosis results from refluxed gastric acid or prolonged laryngospasm.

The second postulated mechanism for SIDS resulting from GER involves a reflex bradycardia mediated via receptor sites located above the esophagus.[42] This reflex, initiated by low pH fluid in the distal esophagus, has been termed a cardiac reflex, and has been shown to be independent of ventilation.

Clinically, this reflex has been demonstrated by simultaneous high and low esophageal pH measurements with heart rate and respiratory monitoring. The appearance of bradycardia in the presence of low, but not high, esophageal reflux seems to correspond to an experimental model.[26,42]

Stridor has also been incriminated as a symptom of GER. A clear temporal association has been depicted between episodes of GER and episodes of stridor by esophageal pH monitoring.[52] The disappearance of stridor has also been correlated with the clearance of refluxed acid from the esophagus. Other authors have also noted this association.[30,50] The mechanism of stridor in this situation has not been delineated, but, as with GER and apnea, the proposed mechanisms follow similar reasoning.

GER has been implicated as a cause of laryngitis.[16,52] There is evidence of laryngeal inflammation in such cases. The mechanism seems to be direct chemical damage to the larynx with secondary edema and inflammation. Parents of children suffering from laryngitis often report voice changes in the child as a precursor of full-blown laryngitis.

Chronic or recurrent bronchitis has been identified in children suffering from GER.[16] Reflux of gastric contents into the tracheobronchial tree has been shown both experimentally and clinically to result in bronchospasm.[16] Additionally, GER has been incriminated as a cause of asthma in childhood.[59]

Finally, an association has been noted between GER and frequent upper respiratory tract infections. This relationship has, however, not been adequately documented either clinically or experimentally.


## Esophagitis

A variety of clinical syndromes have been identified in children with GER/esophagitis.[3,7,12,33,34,44,49,51,55,63] In adults with esophagitis, a very common complaint is heartburn. In the infant who has reflux, crying is a very common complaint from the parents. Whether the crying is due to esophagitis or to some other cause has not been determined. When these children undergo esophagoscopy and biopsy, however, esophagitis is often identified.[12] Some authors have made the comment that one cause of infantile colic may be GER/esophagitis.

Failure to thrive has been identified in children with GER/esophagitis. Some have postulated that the inflammatory response to esophagitis may be of such a magnitude that growth is halted. An alternative explanation for the failure to thrive may be a protein-losing enteropathy secondary to the inflammatory changes in the esophagus.[33] Finger clubbing has been noted in children with GER/esophagitis who have a protein-losing enteropathy. These children were without evidence of chronic pulmonary or heart disease. The clubbing was reversed following successful therapy for GER.

Esophageal bleeding and stricture secondary to esophagitis is a well-known complication of GER.[7,34,51] Often, a young child will present with an anemia of unknown etiology. The finding of occult blood in the stool will often lead to the diagnosis of reflux esophagitis.

Stricture formation occurs primarily in the retarded child, again because of the lack of verbal ability. These children often present with dysphagia. A barium esophagram makes the diagnosis with ease. Patients in whom esophageal atresia has been repaired have a very high incidence of GER resulting in esophageal stricture.[3] The stricture most often occurs at the esophageal anastomotic suture line.

An association between hiatus hernia and contortions of the head and neck was first described in 1964.[44] This association has become known as the Sandifer syndrome. The abnormal head and neck posturing can take the form of opisthotonos or neural tics.[12,44,63] More recently, the term Sandifer's syndrome has been used to describe infants without hiatal hernia, but in who GER and esophagitis produce torticollis.[49,55]

Torticollis as a presenting sign of GER/esophagitis is not nearly as common as is torticollis from other causes. In the evaluation of the child with torticollis, the common etiologic factors (Table 7-3) must first be considered and evaluated.[33]

Benign muscular torticollis, which appears shortly after birth and which is associated with a characteristic benign muscular "tumor" of the sternocleidomastoid is generally easy to identify. Other forms of torticollis, such as those due to segmentation and fusion defects of the cervical spine, rotatory subluxation of the cervical spine after trauma or infection, and syndromes with C-1,2 instability (as in the bony dysplasias or Down's syndrome) can all result in torticollis. Radiographic evaluation of the cervical spine is generally sufficient for diagnosis. Torticollis can also result from intraspinal or posterior fossa tumors, acute inflammatory conditions of the neck such as tuberculosis,

**Table 7-3**
*Identifiable Causes of Torticollis*

Benign muscular torticollis
Intraspinal and posterior fossa tumors
C-1,2 dislocations, dysplasias, Down's syndrome
Cervical spine segmentation/fusion abnormalities
Neck inflammation, Tbc, rheumatoid arthritis
Extraocular muscle imbalance
Vestibular abnormalities
Gastroesophageal reflux

and abnormalities of the extraocular muscles or vestibular apparatus.[3,33,60] In all of these conditions, careful physical and radiologic examination will make the diagnosis.

After all other causes of torticollis have been ruled out, GER must be considered as a cause of the abnormality. The reason for the abnormal head and neck posturing has not been adequately determined. It has been suggested that the head is twisted in an attempt to empty the esophagus of refluxed gastric contents. The high frequency of the episodes of GER would then result in the head being held, more or less permanently, in a position which would open the LES to allow the esophagus to drain (Fig. 7-1). The constancy of the position may then result in more reflux, continued posturing, more reflux, and, hence, esophagitis.

In a small series of infants with the Sandifer syndrome, all had endoscopically and biopsy-proven esophagitis.[55] Medical therapy was unsuccessful. An antireflux operation was then performed, which resulted in prompt disappearance of the torticollis in each case. Reflux torticollis should be adequately treated before the child reaches the age of one year, because of calcification of the cranium, which will maintain the abnormally shaped head even after the torticollis is corrected (Fig. 7-2).[64]

## Miscellaneous

The final group of presenting signs cannot be grouped as easily as can those previously described. This miscellaneous group consists of such entities as seizures, hypotonia, and irritability. The pathophysiology of these entities has not been eluci-

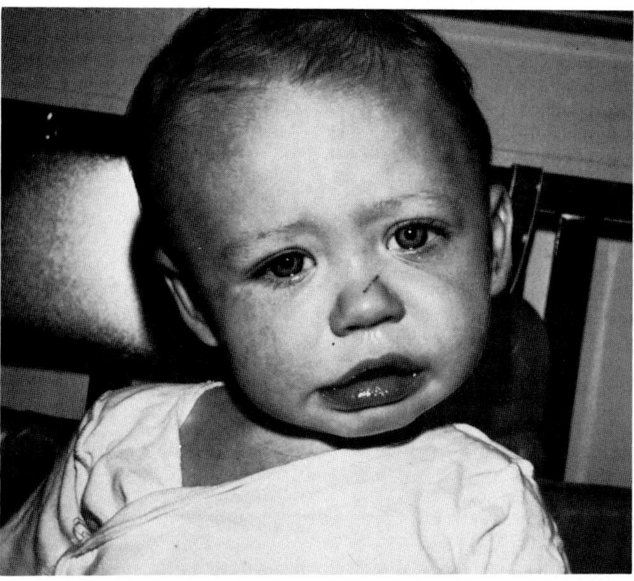

**Figure 7-1.** Torticollis in an infant with GER/esophagitis (Sandifer's syndrome). The only identifiable cause of the torticollis was GER which did not respond to medical therapy for GER. From: Ramenofsky ML, Buyse M, Goldberg MJ: Gastroesophageal reflux and torticollis. J Bone Joint Surg 60-A:1140–1141, 1978. With permission.

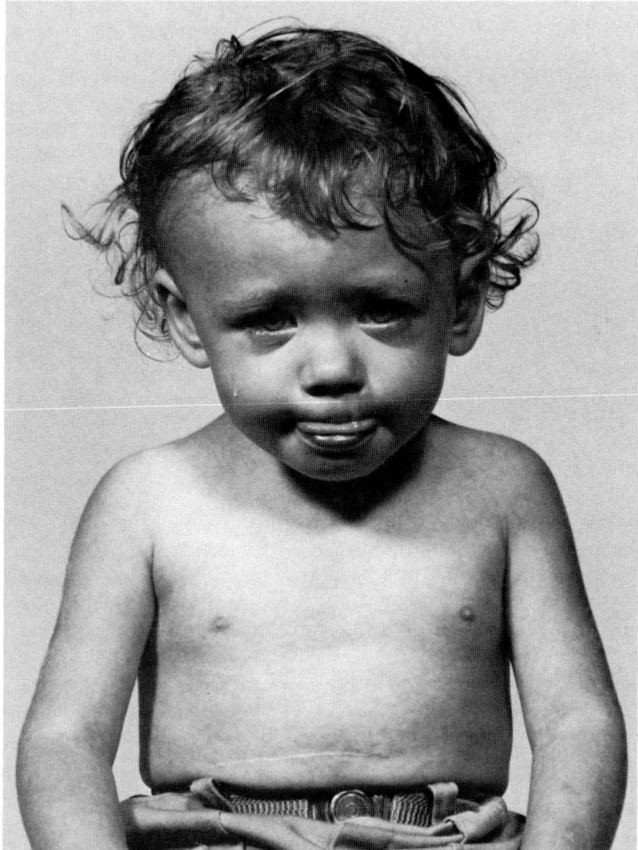

**Figure 7-2.** Postoperative photograph of the patient pictured in Figure 7-1. The operation was performed at 13 months of age. The esophagitis responded rapidly to the antireflux procedure. Although the head straightened immediately after the operation, facial asymmetry and a very slight head tilt remained. From: Ramenofsky ML, Buyse M, Goldberg MJ: Gastroesophageal reflux and torticollis. J Bone Joint Surg 60-A:1140–1141, 1978. With permission.

dated satisfactorily, but theoretical explanations exist. Seizure activity secondary to GER may be a result of hypoxia but may also be a reflex as yet undelineated. Similarly, hypotonia could result from seizure activity. Irritability could be a manifestation of esophagitis, but, in some instances, irritability may persist after adequate treatment of GER.

Much of the evidence for these various manifestations being the result of GER is indirect. For example, it has been difficult to prove that GER can cause aborted SIDS unless an episode of reflux can be temporally related to the "dying spell". The proof, however indirect, rests in a number of series of infants with aborted SIDS and GER who have been treated either medically or surgically.[26,32,46] No further episodes of apnea were identified in these groups of patients after successful therapy.

## DIAGNOSIS

A variety of diagnostic modalities have been utilized for the diagnosis of GER (Table 7-4). Some, such as the barium esophagram, have been used primarily to establish the diagnosis.[17,48] Others, such as extended esophageal pH monitoring, have been used both for diagnosis and to identify the severity of the disease process.[10,37,38,39,56,57,61] Still other modalities, such as esophageal manometry, do not identify GER per se, but offer indirect evidence of its presence and can potentially identify those patients requiring surgical therapy.[11,13,19,20,21,22,62] The purpose of this section is to describe the various diagnostic modalities available, to briefly describe the application of those modalities, and to compare the efficacy of each.

### Barium Esophagram

The time-honored method of making the diagnosis of GER is by the barium esophagram. In 1977, a technique for the performance of the barium swallow in infants and children was described; this technique has become the standard technique for radiographic diagnosis.[17,48] During the barium study, the infant must be kept warm and comfortable. Crying and fussing are discouraged by an experienced pediatric radiological nurse. The volume of the barium meal should be the same volume as the infant is usually fed. Deglutition and peristalsis are studied from the right lateral view if the patient will drink the barium. Should the infant fail to drink the barium, a soft rubber tube is placed transorally into the stomach, the appropriate volume of barium is infused, and the tube is removed. The infant is then positioned comfortably on a well-padded X-ray table in the supine position. Without using external abdominal pressure, reflux is sought. The infant is turned to the prone position and, again, the presence of reflux is evaluated. The water siphon test, allowing the infant to take small sips of water after the barium, is on occasion utilized. Thirty minutes after all the barium has been ingested, an overhead antero-posterior radiograph is taken for delayed reflux.

By means of this technique, GER is classified according to the height reached by the refluxing barium column and other factors (Table 7-5). Six grades of GER have been described. Grade I is reflux into the distal esophagus below the level of the carina (Fig. 7-3). Grade II is defined as reflux into the proximal thoracic esophagus, but below the level of the clavicles (Fig. 7-4). Grade III is reflux into the cervical esophagus (Fig. 7-5). Grade IV is continuous reflux to the neck with a widely patulous gastroesophageal junction (Fig. 7-6). Grade V GER is the aspiration of barium into the tracheobronchial tree (Fig. 7-7). Grade D is the delayed reflux seen on the film taken 30 minutes after completion of the study (Fig. 7-8).

**Table 7-4**
*Modalities Used in the
Diagnosis of GER*

Barium esophagram
intraesophageal pH probe
Gastroesophageal scintiscan
Esophagogastric manometry
Esophagoscopy
Esophageal biopsy

**Table 7-5**
*Barium Esophagram*
*Grading of GER*

| Grade | Height of Barium Column |
| --- | --- |
| 1 | Distal esophagus |
| 2 | Proximal thoracic esophagus |
| 3 | Cervical esophagus |
| 4 | Continuous GER |
| 5 | Aspiration barium |
| D | GER on 30 min X-ray |

From: McCauley RG, Darling DB, Leonidas JC: Gastroesphageal reflux in infants and children: A useful classification and reliable physiologic technique for its demonstration. Am J Roentgenol 130:47–50, 1979. With permission.

Although this technique generally does not identify the severity of the reflux, it does provide a standard means of identifying the presence of reflux. The correlation of GER with severity can be made in two situations using the barium esophagram: aspiration of refluxed gastric content (Grade V GER) and the presence of severe esophagitis and/or stricture. A study done well allows evaluation of the swallowing mechanism and esophageal peristalsis.

It must be noted that the barium esophagram provides information on the presence of GER only during the time of the study, not on that GER which occurs throughout the day. Still, in trained hands this method is an extremely sensitive test for the presence of GER.

## Esophageal pH Monitoring

The most accurate method for diagnosing GER and for identifying its temporal relationships to feeding and other physiologic events is the intraesophageal pH probe.[10,37,38,39,56,57,61] A variety of probes are available which are small enough to be easily used in the newborn infant. Appropriate monitoring systems make possible the simultaneous recording of esophageal pH, respiration, and heart rate. A system has been developed in Europe which monitors the lower esophageal sphincter pressure (LES) simultaneously with esophageal pH, respiration, and heart rate.

The esophageal pH probe is passed into the esophagus, transnasally, positioned in either the distal or proximal esophagus, and attached to a pH meter. The intraesophageal pH level is continuously recorded on a physiologic recorder for whatever length of time the physician deems appropriate (Fig. 7-9). The recording times have been as short as three hours and as long as 24 hours.[37,39,56,57]

Normal esophageal pH is between 5.5 and 7.0. An episode of reflux is considered to be a fall in pH below 4.0. An example of a simultaneous monitoring of esophageal pH, respiration, and heart rate is seen in Figure 7-10. Four episodes of GER occurred in a 20 minute period. During these episodes, neither changes in respiration nor heart rate were identified.

Another use of the esophageal pH probe is to determine the best position in which to medically treat an infant with GER. In one study, it was determined that the prone position was the most efficacious.[56] This study pointed out, however, that some in-

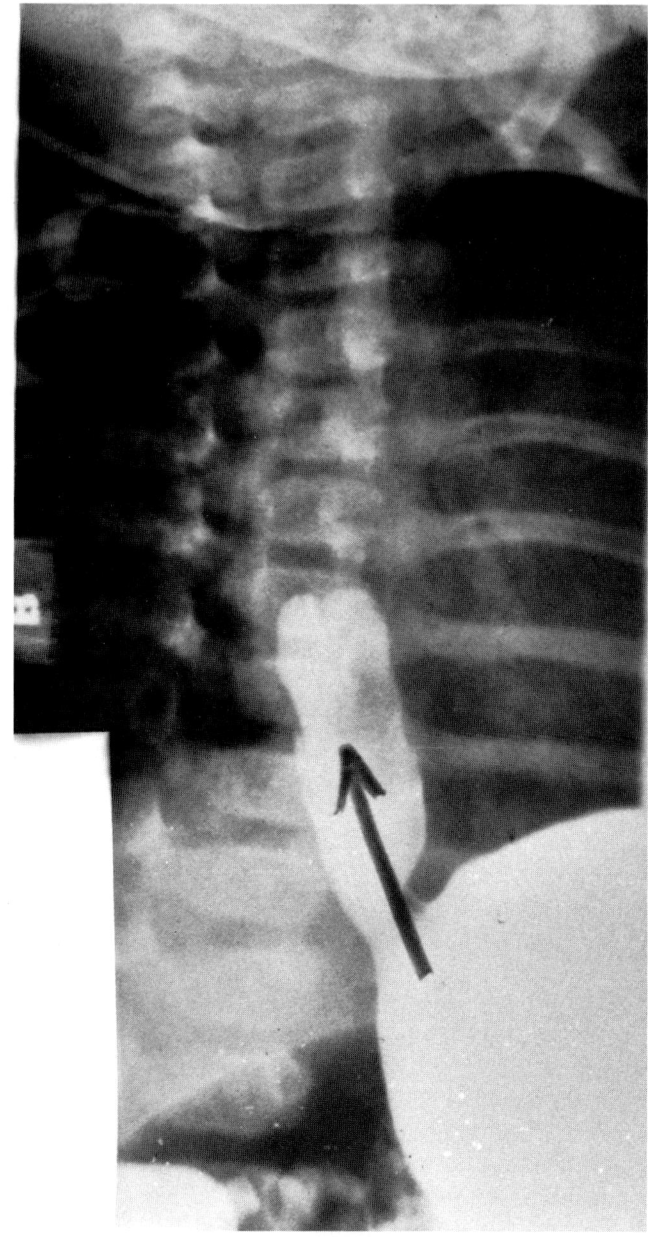

**Figure 7-3.** Grade 1 GER as demonstrated by barium esophagram. The height reached by the refluxing barium column remains below the level of the carina.

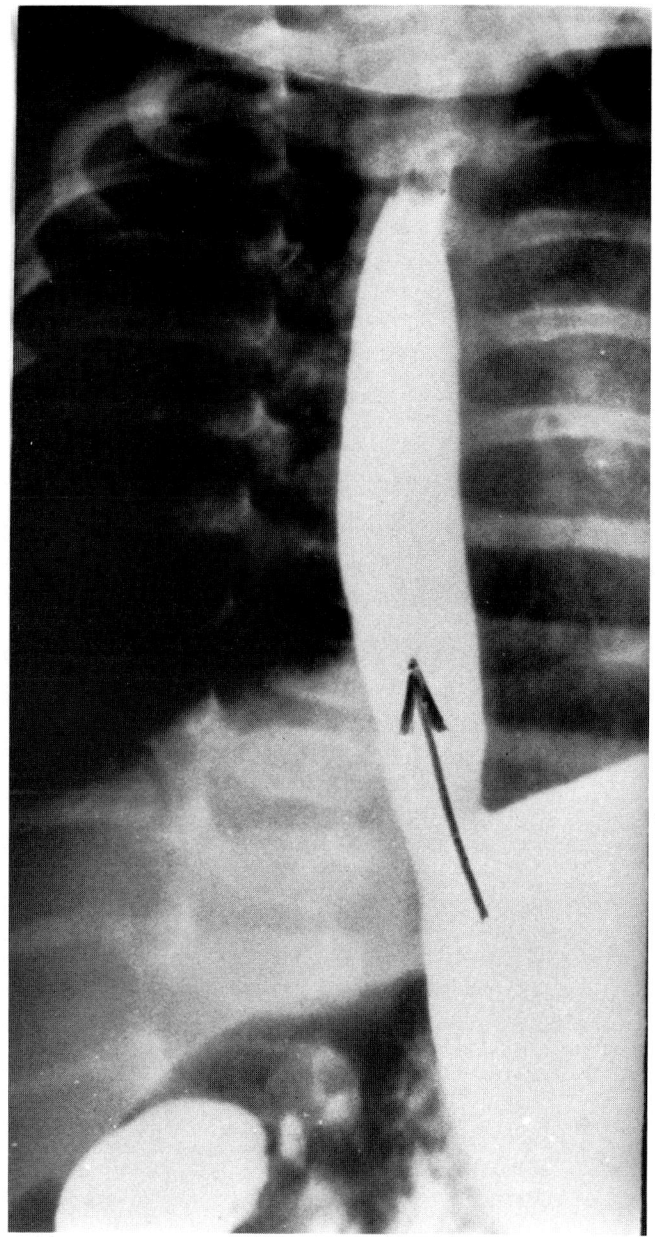

**Figure 7-4.** Grade 2 GER as demonstrated by barium esophagram. The height reached by the refluxing barium column is the proximal thoracic esophagus, but below the level of the clavicles.

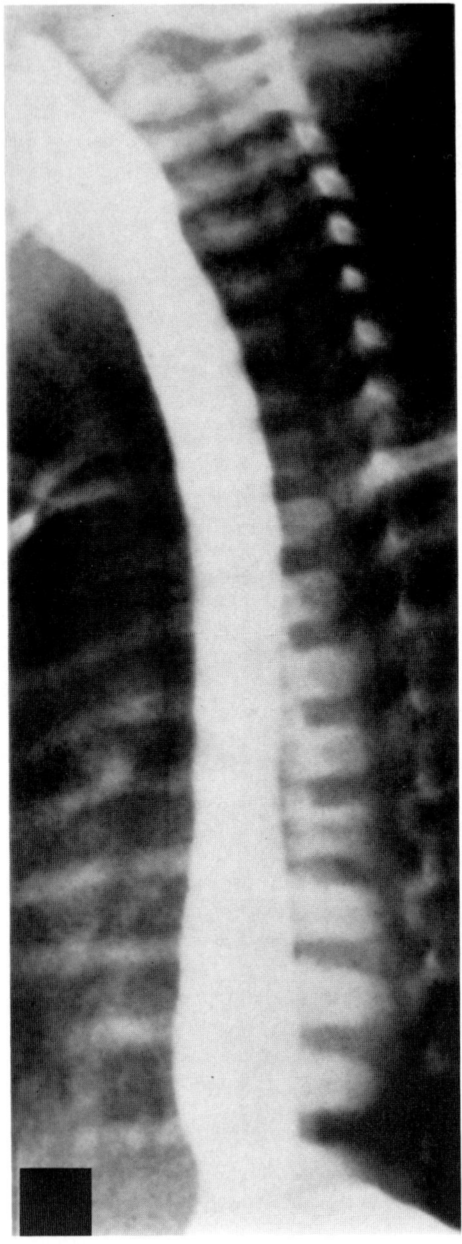

**Figure 7-5.** Grade 3 GER as demonstrated by barium esopha-gram. The height reached by the refluxing barium column is above the clavicles into the cervical esophagus.

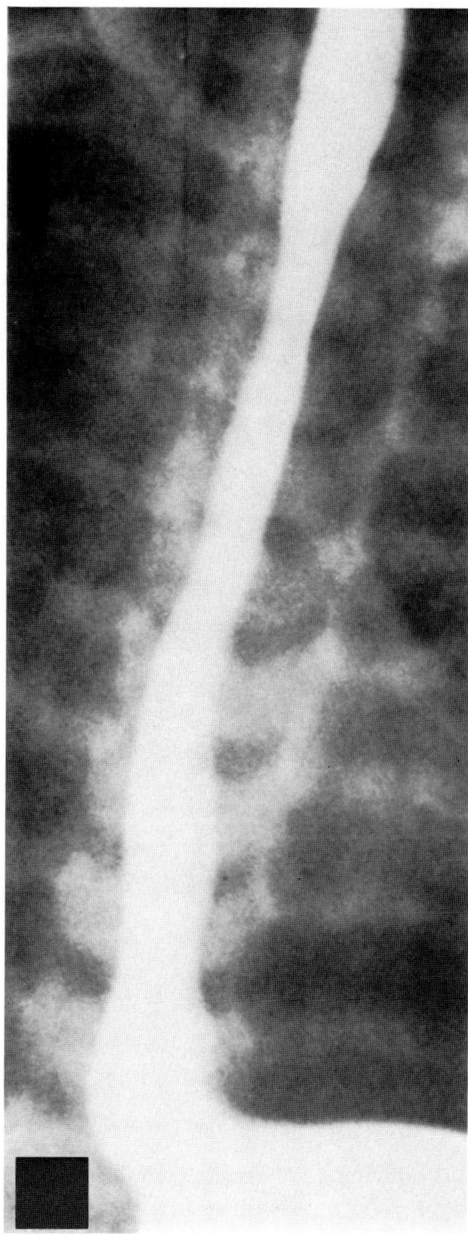

**Figure 7-6.** Grade 4 GER as demonstrated by barium esopha-gram. The height reached by the refluxing barium column is the same as for Grade 3, but the reflux is continuous and the gastro-esophageal junction is widely patulous.

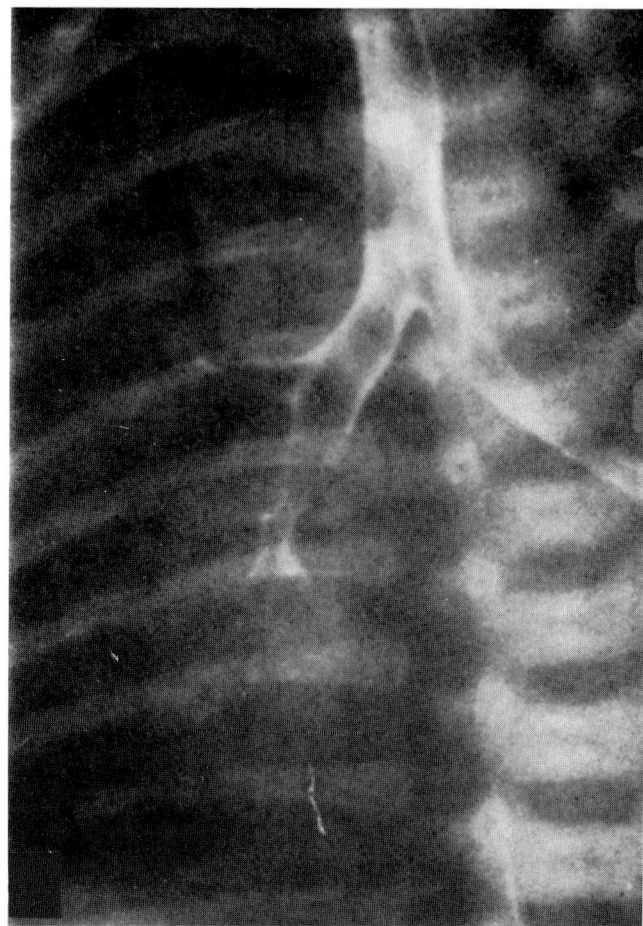

**Figure 7-7.** Grade 5 GER as demonstrated by barium esophagram. The refluxed barium has been aspirated into the tracheobronchial tree.

fants are best managed in a chalasia chair, whereas others are best managed supine. The esophageal pH probe was able to identify which position was optimal for the individual.

To determine the significance of GER a very complex scoring system was developed.[38,39] Thirty-six children younger than 12 years were evaluated by esophageal pH monitoring. Twenty-four served as asymptomatic controls and the remaining 14 patients all had symptoms of GER. Extended esophageal pH monitoring (18–24 hours) was utilized in all patients. Reflux was defined as a fall in distal esophageal pH to less than 4.0 for at least 15 seconds. The number of reflux episodes, the number each 12 hours, the duration of the longest single reflux episode, and the percentage of time the esophageal pH was less than 4.0 were measured while the child was awake, asleep, upright, and supine. The result was a 16 pH-data set combination in each post-cibal interval. The asymptomatic patients had low pH scores, 39.0 plus or minus 8.8, whereas symptomatic patients had uniformly high scores, 221.0 plus or minus 153.5. It was suggested that by the use of subscores, certain patients with esophagitis, peptic

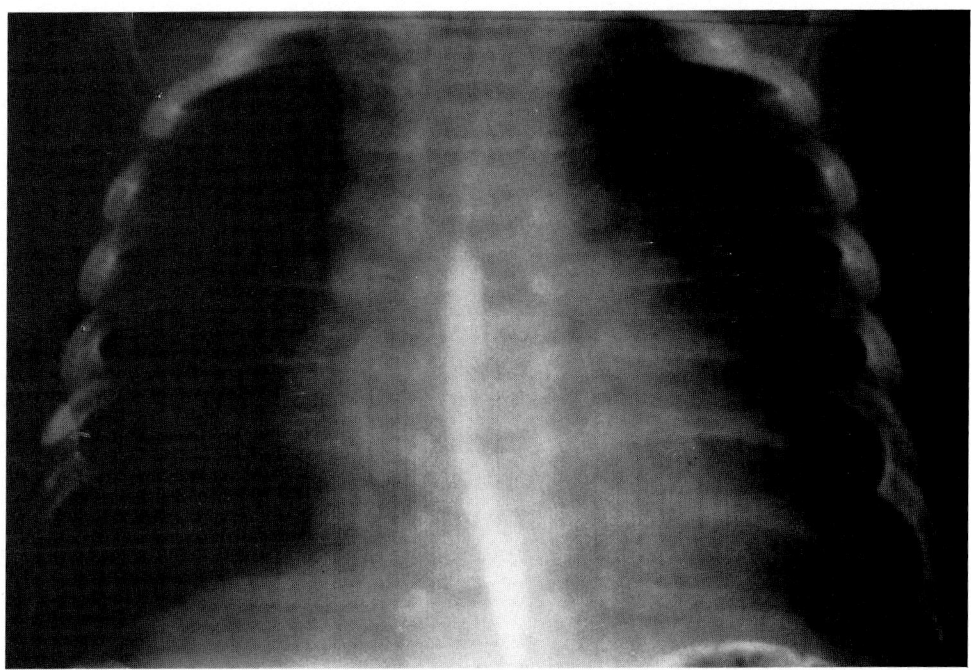

**Figure 7-8.** Grade D or *delayed GER* is identified 30 minutes after the completion of the barium esophagram by an antero-posterior radiograph.

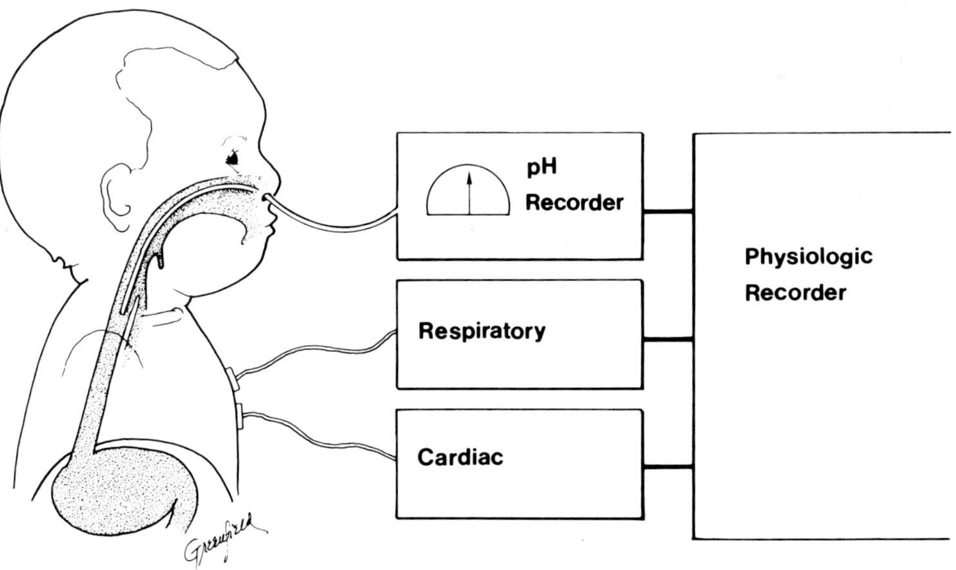


**Figure 7-9.** An example of simultaneous intraesophageal pH, heart rate, and respiratory monitoring and recording.

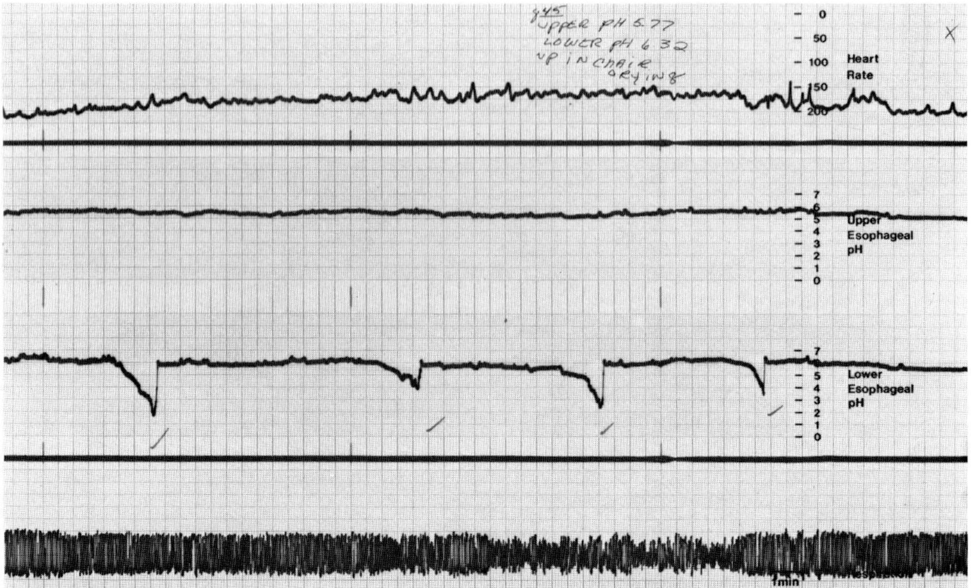


**Figure 7-10.**   Simultaneous upper and lower esophageal pH, heart rate, and respiratory monitoring. In this example, four episodes of pathologic GER occurred in a 20-minute period. No
upper esophageal reflux was identified during this recording.

strictures, and respiratory complications could be separated from the general group of
children with physiologic GER.

A related study identified the presence of GER and classified reflux into one of
four patterns.[38] Based upon the pattern of GER which the patient demonstrated, it
was possible to predict which patient had a greater likelihood of spontaneously recov-
ering from GER and which would require surgical intervention.

The majority of infants had GER which was considered to be physiologic and
which disappeared in time as the LES matured (Fig. 7-11). Type I GER was described
as continuous, type II as discontinuous, and type III as mixed (Fig. 7-11). There were
93 patients evaluated, all less than two years of age, all of whom had symptoms of
GER. Fifty-six percent of these children had the type I pattern 35 percent had type II,
and nine percent had type III.

Large hiatus hernias were found in 19 percent of patients with the type I pattern.
Fifty-two percent of this group eventually required antireflux surgery. Fourteen percent of these patients having respiratory symptoms or growth retardation were not
controlled by the surgical procedure. Their symptoms were subsequently related to
other major disorders. Forty-eight percent of patients in this group received medical
therapy alone. Sixty-five percent of these resolved their symptoms spontaneously by
ten months of age. Two-thirds of the medically treated patients who were restudied,
however, revealed a persistence of the type I pattern despite the fact that they were
asymptomatic. Thirty-five percent of the children who were medically treated experienced persistence of their GER symptoms.

Hiatus hernia was absent in patients with the type II pattern. Antral pylorospasm
was, however, present in 24 percent. Five patients in this group required surgical

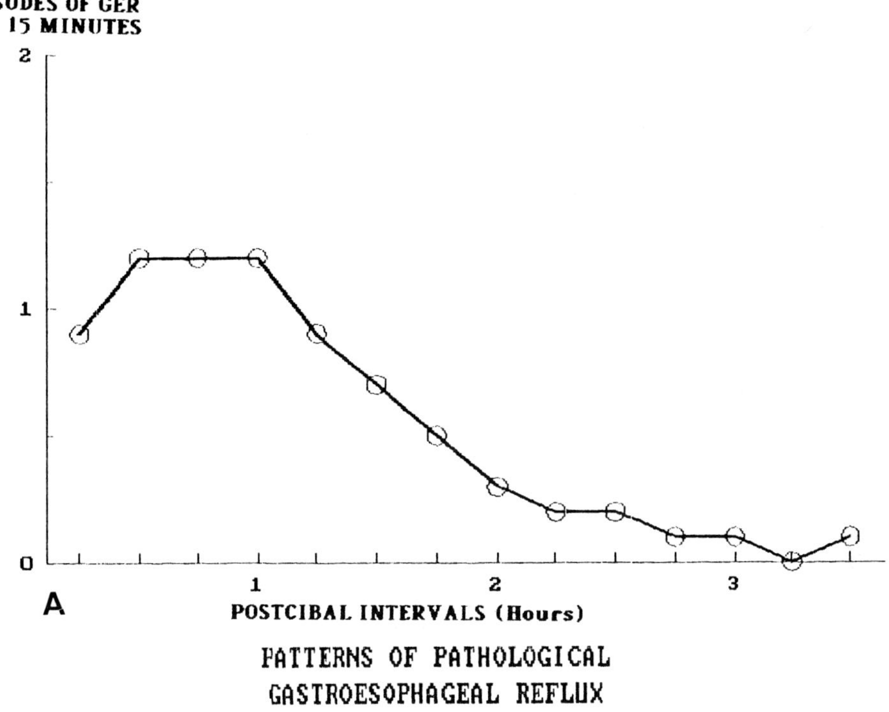



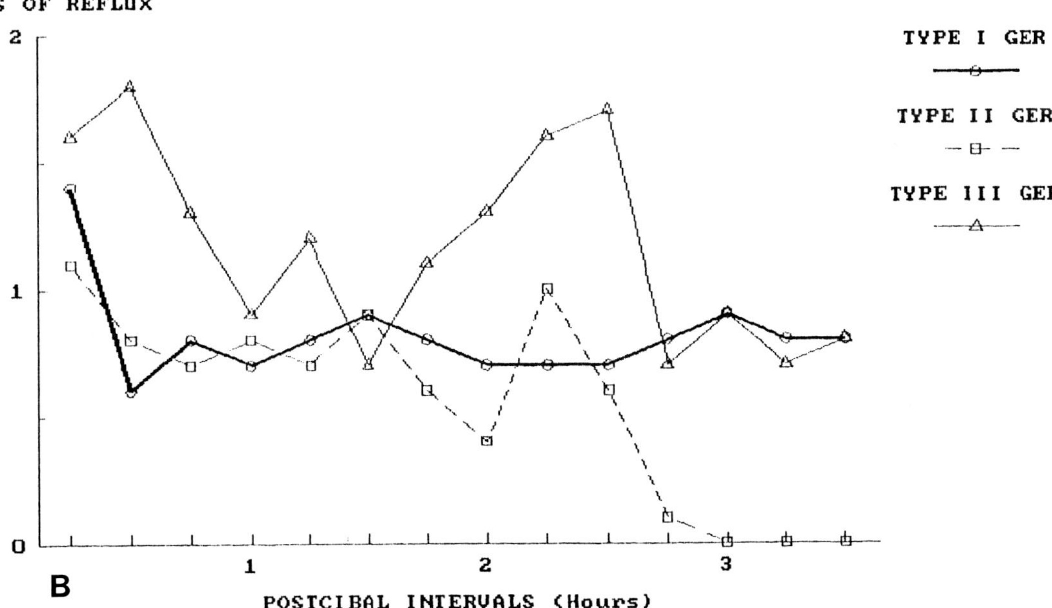

**Figure 7-11.** (A) Esophageal pH monitoring pattern in infants without symptoms of GER. Note the frequency of GER in the one-hour post-cibal interval, followed by a rapid decrease in the number of episodes of GER. From: Froggatt P: Sudden death in babies: Epidemiology. Am J Cardiol 22:457, 1968. With permission. (B) Patterns of pathological GER. From: Jolley SG, Johnson DG, Herbst JJ, et al: The significance of gastroesophageal reflux patterns in children. J Pediatr Surg 16:859–865, 1981. With permission.

therapy, but this therapy did not control the respiratory or growth retardation manifestations in two of the five. The persistence of symptoms in this group was subsequently related to other major associated disorders rather than to the GER per se, a finding similar to that in type I patients who were not helped by surgical therapy. Two-thirds of the patients in this group were treated with medical therapy alone. Slightly over 75 percent of these had spontaneous resolution of the reflux symptoms. In the other 25 percent, the abnormal reflux pattern and the symptoms persisted. There was, however, no asymptomatic patient who had a persistent abnormal reflux pattern. When spontaneous resolution occurred, it did so by ten months of age when both the frequency and duration of the abnormal reflux returned to the normal range.

In the type III pattern, an occasional patient with a hiatus hernia was found. Three required surgical therapy for control of symptoms, and, in one of these, symptoms were unrelieved. Symptoms resolved spontaneously in one-third of this group during medical therapy, but, of these, only one patient (13 percent) hàd a normal esophageal pH study on follow-up. The reflux pattern changed, however, from a type III to a type I pattern in all patients with persistent reflux. This transition from type III to I, as well as the spontaneous resolution of GER, occurred by ten months of age.

The patterns described by Jolley et al. appear to be useful in clarifying the mechanisms and prognosis in children with GER. The type I children appear to have an abnormality of the gastroesophageal junction, evidenced by the high proportion of hiatal hernia and low-normal LES pressures. The persistence of the type I pattern may offer prognostic information regarding peptic esophageal strictures in the older child. Additionally, the low frequency of spontaneous resolution in this group mandates close long-term follow-up.

The mechanism of GER in those children with type II patterns seemed to be related to delayed gastric emptying. This has been confirmed on upper gastrointestinal (UGI) series and on gastroesophageal scintiscan. Spasm of the antrum or pylorus was accompanied by an elevation of the LES pressure and nonspecific watery diarrhea.[50] Children with the type II pattern infrequently required antireflux surgery due to the high rate of spontaneous resolution of the GER.

The patients with the type III pattern behaved as did those with the type I, based on the clinical course followed by these children. The evidence for this mixed type is the presence of an occasional hiatus hernia, delayed gastric emptying, and conversion to a type I pattern by age ten months.[40]

## Gastroesophageal Scintiscanning

One of the criticisms of the standard barium esophagram has been that it provides information on the presence of GER only at the time that the examination is being performed. Gastroesophageal scintiscanning using technetium (Tc 99m) sulfur colloid was developed in order to obviate this perceived disadvantage of barium examination.[18,15,23,41] The sulfur colloid form was considered to be adequate because of its lack of absorption in the GI tract and also because the scanning of the patient could be performed repeatedly without increasing the exposure to radiation. Another theoretical advantage of this method is the ability to identify aspiration of the the radio-labeled sulfur colloid secondary to GER on the delayed scan, thus identifying those patients at risk of developing aspiration pneumonia. The addition of milk to the radio-labeled sulfur colloid makes it more likely that the infant will drink the mixture and also has the advantage of increasing the gastric volume to that which the patient usually takes at each feeding.

The scintiscan provides graphic evidence of the presence of GER or of its absence (Fig. 7-12). The value of being able to re-scan the patient after the initial ingestion with no added radiation is obvious.

The value of the scintiscan has been assessed in both the pediatric and adult populations. In adults, there appears to be a 90-percent correlation of positive gastro-esophageal scintiscans to symptoms of GER.[23] The accuracy of scintiscan is not, how-ever, as high in the pediatric population. One study reported an 80-percent positive correlation with symptoms,[15] whereas another study was able to identify only a 57 percent positive correlation.[2] Without providing anatomic detail of the barium esophagram, one group reported that the scintiscan was twice as accurate as the barium examination for the identification of GER.[41] In another study, scintigraphy was compared to the barium esophagram; both were judged to be equally efficient in diagnosing the presence of GER.[8]

An increase in the accuracy and specificity of scintigraphy can be provided by computer enhancement. Figure 7-13 A demonstrates a GE scintiscan in which there is no perceptible gamma radiation in the lung fields. Figure 7-13 B provides graphic evidence of the presence of aspirated radionuclide into the lung after computer en-hancement.

Information on gastric emptying obtainable by scintiscan also helps in assessment of GER. After the child ingests the radio-labeled milk, the length of time needed to empty the stomach can be quantitated by using the gamma camera and a dedicated computer (Fig. 7-13). The stomach of the child without GER empties by 44 percent or more in one hour. Stomachs of children with GER will empty only five–21 percent in the same period of time.

## Esophagogastric Manometry

The LES and its relationship to GER has long been debated. Although the LES is not an anatomically identifiable sphincter, a region of increased resting pressure has been found in the lower esophagus which provides a positive pressure zone between the stomach and the esophagus. Development and maintenance of this high-pressure zone has been related to muscular, neural, and hormonal mechanisms. Although each has a role, muscular mechanisms either by themselves or initiated by neurotransmitters appear to have the greatest importance in the maintenance of competence. Acetylcho-line plays a significant role in this respect. Intestinal hormones play a role in esophago-gastric continence, but their exact mechanism of action has yet to be determined.

Muscular factors such as an acute gastroesophageal angle, compression of the lower esophagus by the sling and by diaphragmatic fibers, the pinchcock mechanism of the diaphragm, and the location of the LES below the diaphragm all contribute to esophagogastric (EG) competence. In the neonate, the gastroesophageal angle has not been established and the LES has been shown to lie at or above the diaphragm.[29] These two anatomicical factors are significant when the frequency of GER in the neonate and infant are considered.

Esophagogastric manometry has been used to diagnose children with GER, to identify the best position for medical therapy[13,22] and even to identify which children are most likely to benefit from surgical correction of reflux.[21]

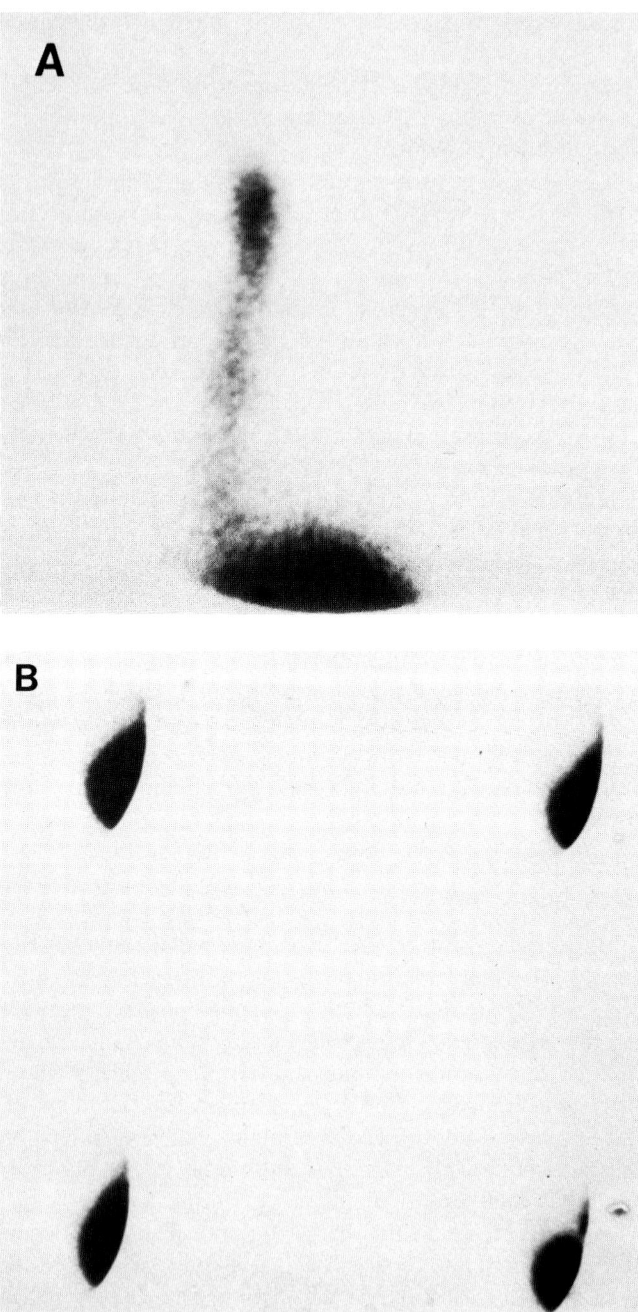

Figure 7-12. (A) Gastroesophageal scintiscan demonstrating GER 40 minutes after ingestion of the radionuclide. (B) Gastro-esophageal scintiscan without evidence of GER. (Courtesy of Myron L. Lecklitner, M.D., Department of Radiology, University of South Alabama College of Medicine.)

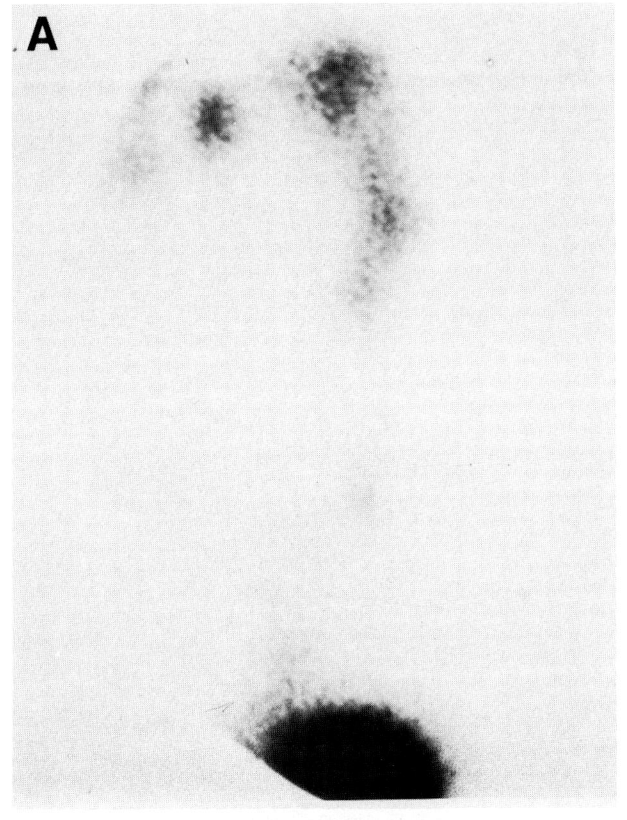

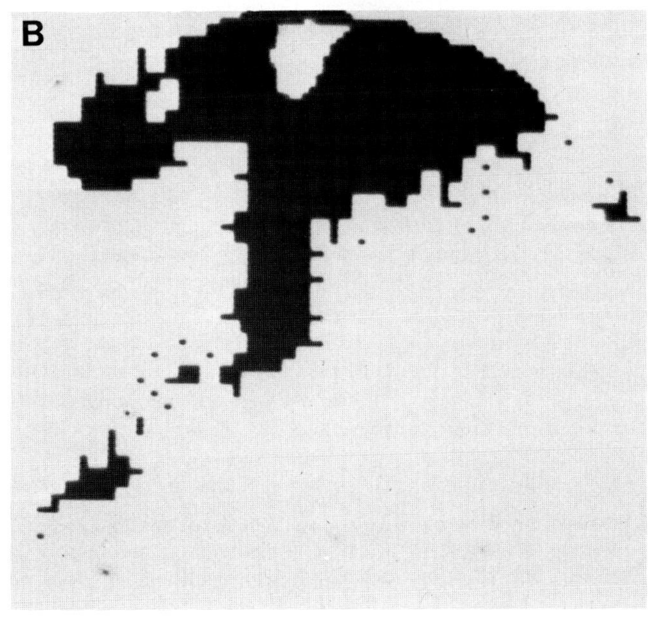

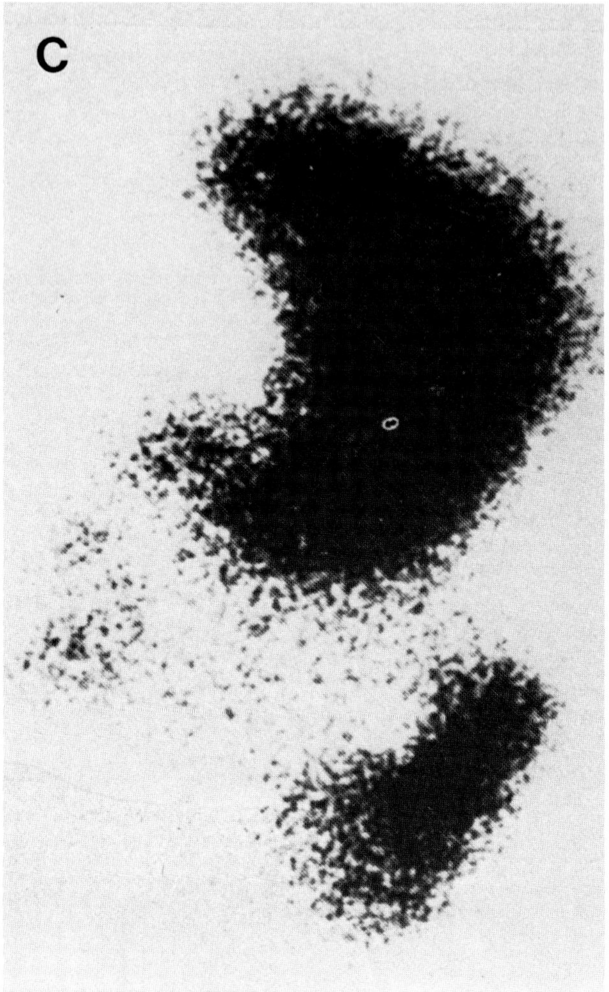



**Figure 7-13.**   Gastroesophageal scintiscan without evidence of aspiration. (B) A scintiscan of the patient in Figure 7-13A, but with the addition of computer enhancement. Note the presence of radionuclide in the upper lung fields. (Courtesy of Myron L. Lecklitner, M.D., Department of Radiology, University of South Alabama College of Medicine.) (C) Gastroesophageal scintiscan one hour after ingestion of radionuclide meal. Computer analysis indicated that 20 percent of the ingested material had exited the stomach at one hour.

There is good correlation between GER symptoms and a decreased lower esophageal sphincter pressure (LESP) in adults,[6,11,19] but little similar data are available for the pediatric age group. Two techniques for manometric evaluation have been used. One technique is that of the non-perfused catheter. Studies using a non-perfused catheter technique have reported decreased LESP in infants with GER.[29,62] The non-perfused system for LESP measurements is quite inaccurate and not comparable to those data derived from multiple-lumen perfused catheters.

The now-accepted method of EG manometry utilizes a perfusion catheter assembly with four continuously perfused tubes of different lengths. This assembly is passed transorally, positioned in the stomach, and withdrawn into the esophagus while transducer pressure measurements are recorded.[21] In addition to measurements of the intragastric, LES, and intrathoracic esophageal pressures, a pneumatic collar placed around the neck of the patient identifies swallowing. This technique allows for simultaneous pressure measurement at various levels and, in addition, allows for measurement of peristaltic activity in the esophagus. Unfortunately, infants and children undergoing EG manometry almost always require sedation in order for this test to be performed.[13,21,22,66]

Normal values for LESP have been difficult to establish in infants and children. One study indicated that an LESP of greater than 15 mmHg is present in children without GER.[2] In another series of 70 infants (less than one year of age) without symptoms of GER, the resting LESP was 21.5 mmHg.[20] These "normal" values have been compared to a series of 15 infants and children with symptomatic GER.[21] These patients experienced vomiting, recurrent pulmonary infections, esophagitis, esophageal stricture, and failure to thrive. EG manometry revealed that the nine children who eventually responded to medical therapy for GER had significantly higher LESP (19.6 mmHg; range: 15.0–25.0 mmHg), than did those requiring surgical therapy (12.7 mmHg; range: 11.3–15.0 mmHg). Although the difference between the means in these groups was significant (p less than 0.001), the overlap at the lower range of the medical responders and the upper range of the surgical responders makes the test relatively insensitive as a selector for either surgical or medical therapy.

An evaluation of 30 infants and children with signs and symptoms of GER whose symptoms included vomiting, recurrent pneumonia, hematemesis, iron deficiency anemia, persistent radiographic pulmonary abnormalities, melena, and nocturnal coughing and wheezing has been reported.[2] These patients were compared to 15 randomly selected controls in whom GER could not be demonstrated by any means. The mean LESP for the control group was 29.0 plus or minus five mmHg, with a range of 14–56 mmHg. The mean LESP for the reflux group was 18.0 plus or minus four mmHg, with a range of four–48 mmHg. The conclusion from this study was that a normal LESP does not exclude GER, although a low LESP is frequently associated with GER, and a very low LESP is often associated with esophagitis.

It has been documented that children with the most severe clinical manifestations of GER have LESP well below the normal range.[22] Another study documented that positional therapy had no effect on the LESP.[8] The latter group postulated that if positional therapy were successful, it was due to the effect of gravity on the gastric pool rather than through an increase in the LES pressure.

Two studies have commented on the presence or absence of a hiatus hernia and its effect on GER.[11,21] Neither found the presence of a hiatus hernia to be a factor contributing to LES dysfunction.

Although EG manometrics can be performed in infants and children in a safe and reproducible manner, the sedation which is often required may invalidate the measurements due to lessening of LESP by the sedative. Normal LESP does not necessarily rule out the presence of GER. Low LESP is often associated with GER and a *very* low pressure is frequently associated with esophagitis. Manometry may help to identify which infants and children will respond to medical therapy.

**Table 7-6**
*Endoscopic Grading of
GER/Esophagitis*[45]

| Grade | Findings |
|---|---|
| 0 | Slight erythema/edema |
| 1 | Definite erythema/edema |
| 2 | Mucosal friability |
| 3 | Bleeding/slough mucosa |
| 4 | Ulceration mucosa |

## Esophagoscopy

Esophagoscopy is useful in determining the presence of esophagitis but will not diagnose GER in the absence of esophagitis. Esophagoscopy by itself is not, however, necessarily sufficient to make the diagnosis of esophagitis.[45] In severe cases of esophagitis, the findings of bleeding, ulceration, and stricture are quite evident endoscopically. In patients with milder forms of esophagitis, the mucosal turnover rate is rapid and the typical inflamed area may not be seen. Biopsy at the time of esophagoscopy is therefore necessary in all cases except the most severe forms of esophagitis.

**Table 7-7**
*Histological Grading in Patients with GER/Esophagitis*[45]

| Grade | Degree | Inflammation Cell Type | Basal Cell Layer |
|---|---|---|---|
| 0 | 0-6 cells/HPF in epithelium. Rare cells in lamina propria. | Lymphocytes in epithelium. Lymphocytes, monocytes, and plasma cells in lamina propria. | 3 or fewer cell layers. |
| $\frac{1}{2}$ | Single small focus $>6$ cells/HPF in basal Also small inflitration in lamina propria. | Same. | Same. |
| 1 | Mild inflammation, infiltration in clusters in epithelium and lamina propria. | Same. | $>3$ cells layers thick, but $<\frac{1}{3}$ of total thickness. |
| 2 | Moderate inflammation, infiltration in epithelium and lamina propria $>$ Grade 1. | Same with or without eosinophils. | Between $\frac{1}{3}$ and $\frac{2}{3}$ the thickness of epithelium. |
| 3 | Severe inflammation, infiltration of full epithelium. | Same with or without eosinophils and neutrophils. | $>\frac{2}{3}$ the thickness of epithelium. |
| 4 | Ulceration. | Same. | Same. |

[45] From: Leape LL, Bhan I, Ramenofsky ML: Esophagyeal biopsy in the diagnosis of reflux esophagitis. J Pediatr Surg 16:379–384, 1981. With permission.

In the pediatric patient older than one year, both rigid and flexible endoscopes may be used. Flexible instruments which are appropriate for use in a neonate or infant do not have an operating channel for the biopsy forceps. The Storz rigid esophagoscope with quartz rod telescopic magnification and a fiberoptic light source is frequently used. Most often, general anesthesia is required, particularly in the very young patient. Biopsies should be taken from the distal esophagus and from the most commonly dependent portion of the esophageal wall. Cup or suction biopsies should be taken under direct vision.

Endoscopic and histologic grading is helpful in determining the degree of esophagitis (Tables 7-6 and 7-7).[45] Five grades of esophagitis have been identified endoscopically. Grade 0 is normal or with very slight erythema or edema, whereas Grade 4 involves ulceration. Endoscopic findings correlate poorly with biopsy results, except with the more advanced grades (Grades 3 and 4), in which biopsy is not really necessary.

Histologic grading is based on the degree of inflammation present and on the amount of basal cell hyperplasia (Table 7-7).[45] Six grades have been defined. The mildest degree of inflammation (Grade 0) involves a minimal increase in infiltration of lymphocytes in the mucosa and lamina propria and a normal basal cell layer. The most severe degree of inflammation (Grade 4) reveals ulceration in addition to infiltration of

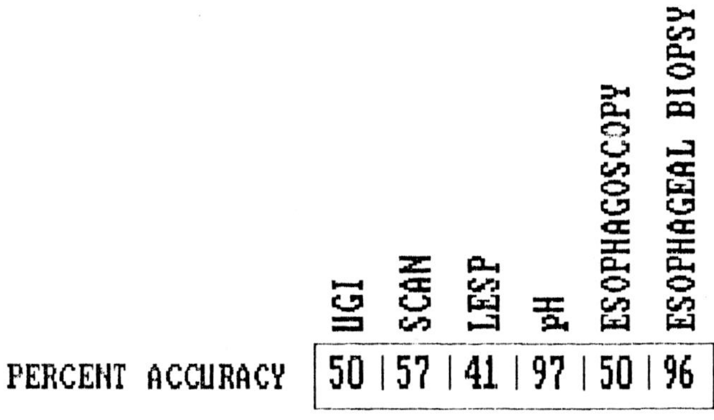


Figure 7-14.   This table indicates the overall accuracy rates of individual diagnostic tests for the presence of GER.

lymphocytes, eosinophils, and neutrophils. The basal cell layer increases to more than two-thirds of the thickness of the epithelium.

## Comparative Accuracy of Diagnostic Modalities

Figures 7-14 and 7-15 indicate the accuracy of individual diagnostic tests and the comparative accuracy of diagnostic tests in patients who are known to have GER. The standard against which all other diagnostic modalities are measured is the barium esophagram. Some believe that this examination is only 50-percent accurate,[2] while others believe that it rivals the sensitivity of the pH probe.[17,48]. The most accurate diagnostic examination is the intraesophageal pH probe. Most studies report an accuracy rate of between 92 and 100 percent. Esophagoscopy to determine the presence of esophagitis is accurate 50 percent of the time, although the addition of esophageal biopsy to the esophagoscopic procedure increases the accuracy to 96 percent (Figs. 7-14 and 7-15). The next most accurate diagnostic method is the scintiscan with computer enhancement, accurate 57 percent of the time. Esophagogastric manometry of

**COMPARATIVE ACCURACY**

**OF**

**DIAGNOSTIC MODALITIES FOR GER**

| | UGI + (15) | SCAN + (17) | LO LESP (12) | NI LESP (17) | PH (29) |
|---|---|---|---|---|---|
| UGI% + | | 65 | 42 | 59 | 52 |
| SCAN% + | 73 | | 58 | 59 | 55 |
| LO LESP% + | 33 | 29 | | | 41 |
| NI LESP% + | 67 | 54 | | | 59 |
| pH% + | 100 | 100 | 92 | 100 | |

**Figure 7-15.** This table compares the accuracy of individual diagnostic modalities for GER to other common modes of diagnosis. (2) Numbers in the chart are the percentage of positive tests for the indicated diagnostic modality. In 15 patients in whom the barium esophagogram was positive, 100 percent had a positive pH probe evaluation. Twenty-nine patients with a positive pH probe had a positive barium esophagogram, 52 percent of the time.

LESP measurement is the least accurate method currently employed (41 percent accurate), but may in time prove useful in identifying which infants and children will respond to medical therapy and which ones will require surgical intervention. At present, manometrics do not identify GER with any degree of reliability.

A heightened awareness of GER in infants and children, greater knowledge of the clinical manifestations and complications of GER, and more accurate diagnostic techniques, now make the recognition of the presence of GER possible with considerable accuracy.

## REFERENCES


1. Adelson L: Specific studies of infant victims of sudden death. In Wedgwood RJ, Benditt EP (Eds.): Sudden Death In Infants. US Dept. of Health, Education and Welfare, pp. 11–40, 1965.
2. Arasu TS, Wyllie R, Fitzgerald JF, et al: Gastroesophageal reflux in infants and children: Comparative accuracy of diagnostic methods. J Pediatr 96:798–803, 1980.
3. Ashcraft KW, Goodwin C, Amoury RA: Early recognition and aggressive treatment of gastroesophageal reflux following repair of esophageal atresia. J Pediatr Surg 12:317, 1977.
4. Ashcraft KW, Holder TM, Amoury RA: Treatment of gastroesophageal reflux in children by Thal fundoplication. J Thorac Cardiovasc Surg 82:706–712, 1981.
5. Beckwith JB: The Sudden infant death syndrome. Curr Problems Ped 3(8):3–37, 1973.
6. Benz LJ, Hootkin LA, Marguilies S, et al: A comparison of clinical measurements of gastroesophageal reflux. Gastroenterology 62:1, 1972.
7. Berlatzky Y, Cohen OM, Freund HR, et al: Surgical treatment of gastroesophageal reflux with esophageal stricture in infancy and childhood. Am J Surg 143:205–208, 1982.
8. Blumhagen JD, Rudd TG, Christie DL: Gastroesophageal reflux in children: Radionuclide gastroesophagography. Am J Roentgenol 135:1001–1004, 1980.
9. Boix OJ, Carrals J: Maturation of the lower esophageal esophagus. J Pediatr Surg 11:749, 1976.
10. Boix-Ochoa J, Lafuente JM, Gil-Vernet JM: Twenty-four hour pH monitoring in gastroesophageal reflux. J Pediatr Surg 15:74–78, 1980.
11. Bombeck CT, Battle WS, Nyhus LM: Preoperative manometry in the choice of operations for gastroesophageal reflux. Am J Surg 125:99, 1973.
12. Bray PF, Herbst JJ, Johnson DG, et al: Childhood gastroesophageal reflux: Neurologic and psychiatric syndromes mimicked. JAMA 237:1342–1345, 1977.
13. Byrne WJ, Euler AR, Campbell M: Body position and esophageal sphincter pressure in infants. Am J Dis Child 136:523–525, 1982.
14. Carre I: The natural history of the partial thoracic stomach (hiatal hernia) in children. Arch Dis Child 34:344, 1959.
15. Christie D, Rudd TG: Radionuclide test for gastroesophageal reflux in children. Pediatr Res 12:432, 1978.
16. Danus O, Carlos C, Larrain A, et al: Esophageal reflux, an unrecognized cause of recurrent obstructive bronchitis in children. J Pediatr 89:220–224, 1976.
17. Darling DB: Hiatal hernia and gastroesophageal reflux in infancy and childhood: Analysis of the radiologic findings. Am J Roentgenol Radium Ther Nuclear Med 123:724–736, 1975.
18. Downing SE, Lee JC: Laryngeal chemosensitivity: A possible mechanism for sudden infant death. Pediatrics 55:640, 1975.
19. Ellis FH, Garabedian M, Gregg JA: Fundoplication for gastroesophageal reflux: A comparison of preoperative manometric findings. Chest 62:142, 1972.

20. Espinoza J, Heitman P: The gastroesophageal sphincter in the first year of life. Clin Res 5:773, 1971.
21. Euler AR, Ament ME: Value of esophageal manometric studies in the gastroesophageal reflux in infancy. Pediatrics 59:58–61, 1977.
22. Euler AR, Ament ME: Decreased lower esophageal sphincter pressure in children with symptoms of gastroesophageal reflux. Am J Dis Child 132:528–529, 1978.
23. Fisher RS, Malmud LS, Roberts GS, et al: Gastroesophageal reflux (GE) scintiscanning to detect and quantitate GE reflux. Gastroenterology 70:301, 1976.
24. Fleisher DR: Infant rumination syndrome. Am J Dis Child 133:266–269, 1979.
25. Fonkalsrud EW, Ament ME, Byrne WJ, et al: Gastroesophageal fundoplication for the management of reflux in infants and children. J Thorac Cardiovasc Surg 76:655–664, 1978.
26. Fontan JP, Heldt GP, Heyman MB, et al: Esophageal spasm associated with apnea and bradycardia in an infant. Pediatrics 73:52–55, 1984.
27. Forshall I: The cardio-esophageal syndrome in childhood. Arch Dis Child 30:40, 1955.
28. Froggatt P: Sudden death in babies: Epidemiology. Am J Cardiol 22:457, 1968.
29. Gryboski JD, Tayer WR, Spiro HM: Esophageal motility in infants and children. Pediatrics 31:382, 1963.
30. Henry RL, Mellis CM: Resolution of inspiratory stridor after fundoplication: Case report. Aust Paediatr J 18:126, 1982.
31. Herbst J, Friednland GW, Zboralske FF: Hiatal hernia and "rumination" in infants and children. J Pediatr 78:261–265, 1971.
32. Herbst JJ, Book LS, Bray PF: Gastroesophageal reflux in the "near miss" sudden infant death syndrome. J Pediatr 92:73–75, 1978.
33. Herbst JJ, Johnson DG, Oliveros MA: Gastroesophageal reflux with protein-losing enteropathy and finger clubbing. Am J Dis Child 130:1256, 1976.
34. Hicks LM, Christie DL, Hall DG, et al: Surgical treatment of esophageal stricture secondary to gastroesophageal reflux. J Pediatr Surg 15:863–868, 1980.
35. Houstek J: Sudden infant death syndrome in Czechoslovakia. In Bergma AB, Beckwith JB, Ray CG (Eds.): Sudden Death Syndrome. Seattle: University of Washington Press pp. 55–63, 1970.
36. Johnson DG, Jolley SG, Herbst JJ, et al: Surgical selection of infants with gastroesophageal reflux.
37. Jolley SG, Herbst JJ, Johnson DG, et al: Patterns of postcibal gastroesophageal reflux in symptomatic infants. Am J Surg 138:946–950, 1979.
38. Jolley SG, Johnson DG, Herbst JJ, et al: The significance of gastroesophageal reflux patterns in children. J Pediatr Surg 16:859–865, 1981.
39. Jolley SG, Johnson DG, Herbst JJ: An assessment of gastroesophageal reflux in children by extended pH monitoring of the distal esophagus. Surgery 84:16–24, 1978.
40. Jolley SG, Johnson DG, Roberts CC, et al: Patterns of gastroesophageal reflux in children following repair of esophageal atresia and distal tracheoesophageal fistula. J Pediatr Surg 15:857–862, 1980.
41. Jona JZ, Sty JR, Glickich M: Simplified radioisotope technique for assessing gastroesophageal reflux in children. J Pediatr Surg 16:114–117, 1981.
42. Kenigsberg K, Griswold PG, Buckley BJ, et al: Cardiac effects of esophageal stimulation: Possible relationship between gastroesophageal reflux (GER) and sudden infant death syndrome (SIDS). J Pediatr Surg 18:542–545, 1983.
43. Kim SH, Hendren WH, Donahoe PK: Gastroesophageal reflux and hiatus hernia in children: Experience with 70 cases. J Pediatr Surg 15:443–451, 1980.
44. Kinsbourne M: Hiatus hernia with contortions of the neck. Lancet 1:1058–1061, 1964.
45. Leape LL, Bhan I, Ramenofsky ML: Esophagyeal biopsy in the diagnosis of reflux esophagitis. J Pediatr Surg 16:379–384, 1981.

46. Leape LL, Holder TM, Franklin JD, et al: Respiratory arrest in infants secondary to gastroesophageal reflux. Pediatrics 60:924–928, 1977.

47. Lilly JR, Randolph JG: Hiatal hernia and gastroesophageal reflux in children. Pediatrics 43:527, 1969.

48. McCauley RG, Darling DB, Leonidas JC: Gastroesophageal reflux in infants and children: A useful classification and reliable physiologic tecnnique for its demonstration. Am J Roentgenol 130:47–50, 1979.

49. Murphy WJ, Gellis SS: Torticollis with hiatus hernia in infancy. Sandifer Syndrome. Am J Dis Child 131:564–565, 1977.

50. Nielson DW, Heldt GP: Gastroesophageal reflux and stridor in infancy. Pediatr Res 16:358A, 1982.

51. O'Neill JA, Betts J, Ziegler MM, et al: Surgical management of reflux strictures of the esophagus in childhood. Ann Surg 196(4), 453–460, 1982.

52. Orenstein SR, Orenstein DM, Whitington PF: Gastroesophageal reflux causing stridor. Chest 843:126, 1982.

53. Patrick JR; Cardiac or respiratory death. In Bergma AB, Beckwith JB, Ray CG (Eds.): Sudden Infant Death Syndrome. Seattle: University of Washington Press, p. 131, 1970.

54. Pinkham JR, Beckwith JB: Vocal cord lesions in the sudden infant death syndrome. In Berham AB, Beckwith JB, Ray CC (Eds.): Sudden Infant Death Syndrome. Seattle; University of Washington Press, pp. 104–107, 1970.

55. Ramenofsky ML, Buyse M, Goldberg MJ: Gastroesophageal reflux and torticollis. J Bone Joint Surg 60-A:1140–1141, 1978.

56. Ramenofsky ML, Leape LL: Continuous upper esophageal pH monitoring in infants and children with gastroesophageal reflux, pneumonia, and apneic spells. J Pediatr Surg 16:374–378, 1981.

57. Reyes HM, Ostrovsky E, Radhakrishnan J: Diagnostic accuracy of a 3-hr continuous intraluminal pH monitoring of the lower esophagus in the evaluation of gastroesophageal reflux in infancy. J Pediatr Surg 17:625–631, 1982.

58. Rhode H, Cywes S, Davies RQ: The phreno-pyloric syndrome in symptomatic gastro-esophageal reflux. J Pediatr Surg 17:152–157, 1982.

59. Shapiro GG, Christie DL: Gastroesophageal reflux in steroid dependent asthmatic youths. Pediatrics 63:207–212, 1979.

60. Snyder CH: Paroxysmal torticollis in infancy. A possible form of labyrinthitis. Am J Dis Child 117:458–460, 1969.

61. Sondheimer JM: Continuous monitoring of distal esophageal pH: A diagnostic test for gastroesophageal reflux in infants. J Pediatr 96: 804–807, 1980.

62. Strawczynski J, Beck JT, McKenna RD, et al: The behavior of the lower esophageal sphincter in infants and its relationship to gastroesophageal regurgitation. J Pediatr 64:17, 1964.

63. Sutcliffe J: Torsional spasms and abnormal postures in children with hiatus hernia: Sandi-fer syndrome. In Kaufman HJ (Ed.): Gastrointestinal Tract. New York: Karger, pp. 190–197, 1969.

64. Tachdjian M: Pediatric Orthopedics. Philadelphia: W.B. Saunders Company, 1972.

65. Valdes-Dapena M: Sudden infant death syndrome and necrosis of the larynx. J Forensic Sci Soc 3:503, 1958.

66. Weissbluth M: Gastroesophageal reflux. Clin Pediatr 20:7–14, 1981

67. Williams HE, Freeman M: Inhalation pneumonia: The significance of fat filled macro-phages in tracheal secretions. Aust Paediatr J 9:286–288, 1973.

John J. Herbst

# 8

# Medical Treatment of Gastroesophageal Reflux

Gastroesophageal reflux (GER) occurs normally in all individuals, especially in the postprandial period, and is severe enough to cause significant problems in one of every 300–1000 children.[9] In older patients, reflux symptoms occur at least occasionally in seven–36% of individuals.[32] Perhaps because of the frequency of the problem and the fact that symptoms are often bothersome but not life-threatening, gastroesophageal reflex is often ignored or self-treated. In the past, antacids were the major form of therapy used and they were used mainly for symptomatic relief of heartburn. In recent years, improved knowledge of the pathophysiology of reflux has stimulated the use of several methods of therapy; many of these therapies have been subjected to clinical trials that demonstrate their usefulness.

The primary problem in gastroesophageal reflux is the frequent movement of irritating, acidic gastric contents into the esophagus. The material may be expelled into the mouth and cause vomiting and malnutrition, or it may be aspirated and cause respiratory symptoms. The presence of acid contents in the esophagus can cause esophagitis, pain (heartburn), chronic blood loss, hematemesis, or even stricture formation.[25] Many patients with gastroesophageal reflux and esophagitis have altered esophageal motility and are less efficient than normal in clearing acid contents from the esophagus.[5] Perfusion of the distal esophagus of cats with dilute acid has been shown to decrease lower esophageal sphincter pressure.[16] Studies of adults and children have shown that patients with esophagitis have decreased tone in the lower esophageal sphincter, a factor which predisposes to further reflux.[24,40] Conversely, when esophagitis is treated by medical or surgical means, the improvement in esophagitis is associated with improvement in esophageal motility, increased lower esophageal sphincter pressure, and decreased gastroesophageal reflux. Recent studies by Dodds and coworkers have shown that reflux occurs not only across a chronically lax sphincter, but also during spontaneous relaxations in sphincter pressure, and during times of elevated abdominal pressure, such as during coughing.[15] Another factor contributing to the prevalence of GER is that approximately two-thirds of children and adults with reflux

Pediatric Esophageal Surgery
ISBN 0-8089-1776-5

will have delayed gastric emptying.[26,28] The resulting increase in gastric contents will encourage gastroesophageal reflux. Thus, individuals often have a combination of several meachnisms that predispose them to gastroesophageal reflux.

Medical treatment of gastroesophageal reflux takes many forms because of the many mechanisms predisposing to reflux. Some therapies seek to prevent reflux of gastric contents into the esophagus. This may be done by keeping meal volumes small, by using position and gravity to minimize reflux, by keeping stomach contents very viscous with the use of thickened formula, or by stimulating lower esophageal sphincter tone. Efforts to increase gastric emptying, thereby decreasing the volume of material available for reflux, will also minimize reflux. Avoidance of drugs or foods that encourage reflux by altering sphincter pressure or delaying gastric emptying is also important.

Another major therapeutic approach involves the use of methods that will make the refluxed material less irritating to the esophagus than they might ordinarily be. This is usually accomplished by altering the pH. Antacid therapy will not prevent reflux, but it is the most prevalent method for treating heartburn. It is also thought that reducing esophageal inflammation will improve esophageal motor function. The various methods of achieving these goals are discussed below. Some patients may require very little or no therapy; others with very severe symptoms may require use of all modes of therapy.

## GENERAL CARE

General medical care is important in the overall treatment of patients with reflux, since they often have other medical problems. They may be anemic or iron deficient from chronic blood loss. They may have delayed development and failure to thrive because of malnutrition due to vomiting, or anorexia due to stricture or severe esophagitis. Other patients will have problems which are often complicated by gastroesophageal reflux.[25] Patients with cerebral palsy or trisomy 21 often suffer from gastroesophageal reflux.[7,41] Almost two-thirds of patients with repaired esophageal atresia will have significant reflux.[35] Patients with scleroderma or dermatomyositis may have poor esophageal motility with subsequent poor clearance of noxious gastric contents from the esophagus. Patients with chronic cough or asthma have wide changes in abdominal pressure which encourages gastroesophageal reflux.[10] In some patients with pulmonary disease, the reflux induced by wide swings in abdominal pressure can result in aspiration which compounds the seriousness of the pulmonary disorder. Optimal management of these associated problems can minimize factors that may increase reflux. Management of relux can also minimize aggravation of other medical problems, e.g., coughing and wheezing in patients with reactive airway disease caused by aspiration of refluxed gastric contents.

## FEEDING PRACTICES

Alterations in the type and amount of feeding are among the simplest therapeutic efforts, yet these measures are often very effective. Small, frequent meals, careful burping, and gentle handling of the child after feeding are simple maneuvers which are elementary principles of care for the child suffering from GER. These measures are especially important when one considers that approximately two-thirds of patients with reflux experience delayed gastric emptying.[26,28] In the older patient, it is wise to avoid snacks just prior to going to bed, since the recumbent position favors reflux. It is assumed that a stomach less distended with air or food will be less likely to expel its contents into the esophagus. If other methods of therapy do not control reflux, one might consider the ultimate approach to providing freqeunt small feedings, i.e., constant nasogastric feeding. Realizing that gastroesophageal reflux is a self-limited disease in most infants, Ferry and associates employed a short-term trial of constant nasogastric feeding in children not responding to conventional therapy for gastroesophageal reflux and growth failure.[20] There was a favorable response in approximately half of the infants. If they did not show weight gain in the first week, they were unlikely to improve with longer periods of nasogastric feeding. The author's group has increased growth velocity and improved lower esophageal sphincter function in some very premature infants with gastroesophageal reflux by using constant nasojejunal feedings. Thickening of formula, usually with cereal, is recommended in infants on the assumption that thick, viscous feedings are less likely to "slosh" up into the esophagus. Thickening feedings also increases the caloric density of the food so that the volume of feedings can be reduced. It has been recommended that enough cereal be used so that a spoon will stand upright when placed in a bottle of the thickened formula. The use of thickened feedings was vigorously advanced by Carre as a supplementary measure in the treatment of GER, but has not been subjected to a controlled study.[9] It is the author's experience that this measure is useful, but occasional patients experience increased vomiting when fed the thickened feedings.

It is possible that the increased caloric density of thickened feedings may delay gastric emptying. Attention to the type of feeding can be important. Very fatty meals may predispose to reflux and it is especially important to keep this in mind when treating older patients with fatty-food intolerance. Substances such as chocolate, alcohol, tobacco, and peppermint oil decrease lower esophageal sphincter pressure and should be avoided.[36] Some patients have food intolerances that may cause vomiting or may exacerbate gastroesophageal reflux. Milk allergy or intolerance is relatively common, and it may exacerbate vomiting caused by reflux or may even be the primary problem. This possibility should be considered if the patient is not responding to routine treatment.

How caustic the refluxed material is to the esophageal epithelium depends on many factors, including the acidity of the material and the presence of peptic enzymes and bile salts. Except for a temporary buffering of gastric pH by food, these factors are altered very little by feeding practices. Some substances, such as aspirin, tea, and alcohol, can increase the esophageal permeability to hydrogen ions and contribute to the severity of esophagitis.[38,39] These agents also stimulate gastric acid production, which further damages esophageal epithelium. Tart fluids, especially citrus juices, may elicit pain in patients with esophagitis and their avoidance is often helpful in controlling symptoms.


## POSITIONAL THERAPY

One of the simplest and most frequently used modes of therapy is positional therapy. This method uses gravity to pool stomach contents in the dependent portions of the stomach, away from the gastroesophageal junction. Even if symptoms are not noticed, continuation of therapy at night is important, since nighttime reflux is very important in causing esophagitis. One reason that nighttime positional therapy is so vital is that salivation is decreased at night. Although the buffering capacity of saliva is minor, it is an important mechanism in washing the last traces of gastric acid from esophageal mucosa.[22] In adults and older children, positional therapy is usually accomplished by raising the head of the bed approximately eight inches. Elevating the head of the bed further will usually cause the patient to slide down. Elevating the head of the mattress or propping the patient with pillows is not nearly as effective as is raising the head of the bed. Once the head of the bed is elevated, no further patient compliance is required. Avoidance of silk or similar cloth for pajamas can minimize the tendency to slide down the inclined mattress. This therapy is especially useful for those patients who are primarily nighttime refluxers as described by Demeester and coworkers.[14]

In infants who are usually recumbent and sleep for many hours a day, positional treatment should be continued throughout the day. Carre first emphasized that the sitting position must be at an angle of at least 60°.[8] In older studies, special chairs or even partial body casts were often fashioned to help maintain the position. This was pursued to such an extreme that flattening of the occiput from constant positioning was noted as a frequent occurrence.

In infants, muscular tone is poor, especially in truncal muscles; infants often slump when placed in infant seats, causing increased abdominal pressure which can induce reflux episodes, particularly when the stomach is full. Placing the child prone on a flat surface at a 30° angle prevents this increased abdominal pressure.[23] Another reason that placing the child prone with the head elevated 30°may be superior to having the child propped in an infant seat is that the esophagus enters the stomach in the most dorsal portion of the abdomen. When lying prone, the fundic pool of food is moved away from the lower esophageal sphincter, thereby decreasing the tendency to reflux into the esophagus. (Fig. 8-1)

Meyers and coworkers studied the effect of position on reflux in over 70 patients with gastroesophageal reflux who had a mean age of 11.6 months.[31] Using prolonged esophageal pH monitoring during supine, prone, and sitting positions, they showed that the percentage of time spent in reflux was least in the 30° head-elevated, prone position. The upright position was better than the supine position, and the prone position (both 30° head elevated and horizontal) was associated with less reflux than the supine position. Orenstein and Whitington have also documented the superiority of the 30° head elevated, prone position.[33] Blumenthal and Lealman have shown that low-birth-weight infants have less reflux in the prone position than when placed on the right or left side.[4] Orenstein et al. have shown that in infants less than six months of age, positioning a child upright in an infant seat may be associated with more reflux than simply placing the infant in a horizontal prone position.[34] They also speculated that the poor truncal muscle strength in these very young children contributed to increased abdominal pressure which can induce reflux.

The author's group has found that the best way to maintain the head elevated, prone position is to place the child on a padded board with the head elevated 30°. Placing rolled towels on either side of the child and wrapping both the board and child with a sheet (or cloth secured with velcro) keeps the child from rolling off the board, yet allows easy access for routine child care. The child can be kept from slipping down by having the child straddle a padded post, or by inserting the child into a harness

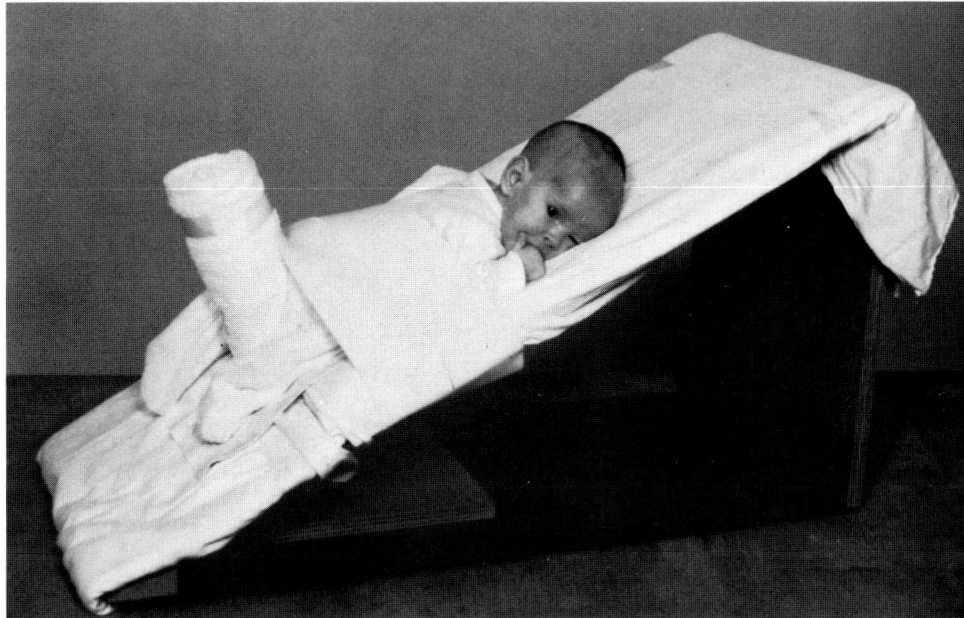

**Figure 8-1.**   Infant in 30° head elevated, prone position. Note the wide cloth wrapped around patient and board to help maintain position.

resembling a large pair of shorts that is anchored to the board. In most cases, such treatment will decrease the amount of relux in symptomatic infants so that the percentage of time spent in reflux is similar to that of normal patients.[31] It has been found that the 30° head elevated, prone position can be easily maintained around the clock until the child is approximately one year of age. Beyond this age, increased mobility and desire not to be restrained makes such intensive positional therapy impractical.

Positional treatment is effective in both the awake and the asleep child, but is so by different mechanisms. In both cases, the end result is a decrease in the percentage of time that esophageal pH is less than four. When a symptomatic patient is awake, the decrease in reflux during positional therapy is due to a decreased frequency of reflux episodes; the mean of duration of episodes remains unchanged. Conversely, while asleep, the number of episodes is not affected, but mean duration of reflux episodes is shortened.[31]

The use of tight abdominal clothing, belts, or girdles should be avoided during positional therapy since increased abdominal pressure will negate all the effects of gravity gained in positioning the patient.


## DRUG TREATMENT

The use of drugs to prevent gastroesophageal reflux has been receiving increased attention over the last few years. There are several drugs that are useful in treating gastroesophageal reflux; conversely, there are also some drugs that predispose to gastroesophageal reflux and should be avoided if possible.

Secretin, Isuprel (Breon), atropine, and alcohol will depress tone in the lower esophageal sphincter and thereby predispose to reflux.[36] Atropine also tends to suppress secondary stripping waves in the esophagus, thereby compromising an important protective mechanism. Tetracyclines on occasion may be the cause of severe esophagitis, especially if the capsule disintegrates in the esophagus. Many of the reported cases of esophagitis occurred in patients with a history of pyrosis.[11] A number of drugs may cause nausea alters vagal tone and decreases lower esophageal sphincter pressure and results in an increased likelihood of reflux. Theophylline is often used in patients who have reactive airway disease, but it will stimulate gastric acidity and depress smooth muscle tone of the gastrointestinal (GI) tract, actions which favor reflux. A frequent side effect of theophylline is nausea, which also lowers sphincter pressure and encourages reflux.[43] In patients treated with theophylline for reactive airway disease, pulmonary problems may be worsened by aspiration of gastric contents that are refluxed due to the effects of theophylline.

Drug therapy may also be directed at rendering the refluxed gastric contents less noxious to esophageal mucosa by increasing the gastric pH. The results of trials of antacids in adults are mixed. Extensive clinical experience indicates that use of antacids can relieve the pain of heartburn and in many studies, the amount of antacids needed to give relief of symptoms was as a measure a measure of the effectiveness of other therapy.[2,29] Some studies did not show a significant improvement of esophagitis, either at endoscopy or microscopically, even though heartburn was improved, but Thanik et al. were able to show improvement in symptoms and severity of esophagitis by using large doses of antacids in adults.[45] Recently Cucchiara and coworkers were able to show clinical improvement and healing of esophagitis in 13 of 15 patients aged two–42 months with gastroesophageal reflux using positional therapy and large doses of antacids.[12] They used a liquid preparation of magnesium and aluminium hydroxide (Maalox—Rorer) at a dosage of 700 meq/1.73m$^2$/day, given one and three hours after meals and at bedtime. It is important that full therapeutic doses of antacids be given, just as in ulcer therapy. The volume of each dose will vary with the buffering capacity of the antacids, but a dose of approximately 10 ml/m$^2$ of the concentrated therapeutic antacids should be given one and three hours after each meal and at bedtime. Additional doses may be taken to relieve hearburn. Liquids are the most potent antacids. If tablets are used, they must be thoroughly chewed; this prolonged, tiresome effort usually offsets the convenience of the easy portability of tablets except for occasional use.

Antacid therapy may be combined with alginic acid (Gaviscon—Marion). This agent concentrates the antacid in a foam that coats the esophagus and floats on top of the gastric fluid, so that, with reflux, this foam is the first material expelled into the esophagus. Double-blind studies in adults and children have shown the mixture to be effective.[1,46]

Another class of drugs that can alter gastric contents is the hydrogen receptor antagonists, cimetidine and the more recently introduced ranitidine (Zantac®). A number of studies on the effect of the hydrogen receptor antagonists on reflux esophagitis in adults have been performed.[2,12,29] Most have demonstrated relief of symptoms, especially heartburn. Some studies have been able to document an improvement in histologic or endoscopic changes of esophagitis, while other studies failed to show objective improvement in esophagitis.

Cucchiara and coworkers compared the effects of antacids and cimetidine in combination with positional therapy on esophagitis caused by gastroesophageal reflux in children.[12] Using a dosage of 20 mg/dg/day of cimetidine, they showed healing of esophagitis at endoscopy in seven of 14 patients after 12 weeks and showed some improvement in an additional six patients. These results are almost identical with those of another 15 patients treated with large doses of antacids. Cimetidine was as effective as large doses of antacids in the treatment of esophagitis, and was not associated with significant side effects. In contrast, two of the antacid-treated children developed diarrhea and dropped out of the study.

Neither rantidine nor cimetidine have been approved for use in children. Ranitidine can be taken twice a day and in adults seems to have fewer side effects than does cimetidine. Cimetidine has the disadvantage of being administered four times a day, but the childhood experience with this drug is much greater than with ranitidine, and a liquid preparation is available.

It would appear that large and frequent doses of oral antacids and the hydrogen receptor antagonists are both effective therapy of reflux-induced esophagitis. The clinician must consider the convenience and possible side effects of cimetidine and ranitidine against the complications of large doses of oral antacids. These include diarrhea and possible development of bezoars in very small infants.

Another approach to drug therapy is to use agents that increase lower esophageal sphincter pressure and hasten gastric emptying, which is prolonged in two-thirds of patients with reflux. Bethanechol is a cholinergic drug that stimulates motor activity in the upper intestinal tract. Studies in adults and children indicate that bethanechol increases esophageal transit and acid clearance and also increases lower esophageal sphincter pressure.[17,18,19] Three separate studies have documented the therapeutic effect of bethanechol in children with gastroesophageal reflux.[17,42,44] The usual recommended dosage is nine mg/m$^2$/day divided into three doses given 30 minutes before meals. If no improvement is noted, the dosage is increased four times a day and each dose is cautiously increased to as much as double the initial dose as long as there are no side effects. The drugs come in tablets and an injectable form. Diluting the injectable form to one mg/ml provides a convenient oral dosage form for infants and toddlers. Side effects are infrequent, but include sweating, flushing, abdominal cramps, and diarrhea. In patients with reactive airway disease, an asthmatic attack may be stimulated and this would be a contraindication for use of this drug. The author's group has not hesitated to use the drug in patients with recurrent aspiration pneumonia or apnea if there is no evidence of reactive airway disease.

Metoclopramide increases motor activity in the upper intestinal tract without stimulating gastric, biliary, or pancreatic secretions. It increases gastric emptying and increases lower esophageal sphincter pressure. It has been used extensively in adults. There are several abstracts describing its effectiveness in children.[3,6,30,37] The drug has been shown to reduce the frequency of reflux episodes and the duration of reflux. The usual dosage is 0.1 mg/kg/dose, given prior to meals and at bedtime. Metoclopramide is a dopamine antagonist and can produce sedation and extrapyramidal reactions. These are rare if the above dosage is used, but are common if large amounts which can cross the blood-brain barrier are administered. In larger dosages (one mg/kg/dose) metoclopramide is used as a central antinauseant. Extrapyramidal reactions are common in children at this dosage, but can be treated with diphenlhydramine. One advantage of metoclopramide over bethanechol is that is will not stimulate an asthmatic attack.

Domperidone is a peripheral dopamine antagonist available in Europe, but not approved for use in this country.[13] It also hastens gastric emptying and stimulates esophageal contractions. In an abstract, Grill et al. demonstrated that, in infants with gastroesophageal reflux, this drug increased gastric emptying, increased peristaltic waves in the esophagus, decreased postprandial reflux time, and improved symptoms.[21]

In some patients with severe esophagitis, there may be severe pain on deglutition, so that even swallowing of saliva is very painful. This is thought to be related to diffuse esophageal spasm. Nitroglycerine has been shown to decrease lower esophageal sphincter pressure and decrease amplitude and duration of esophageal contractions in patients with esophageal spasm.[27] Careful use of sublingual nitroglycerine can help provide transient symptomatic relief in patients with severe reflux esophagitis and dysphagia caused by esophageal spasm. It should always be used in conjunction with aggressive antacid therapy of gastroesophageal reflux and esophagitis.

## CLINICAL APPROACH

From these different modes of medical therapy which have been shown to be effective, the clinician must choose the optimal therapy for the individual. A rational approach to the use of the various modes of therapy will be suggested in the following paragraphs.

If an infant has some regurgitation and vomiting, but is otherwise well with no evidence of other problems that could cause vomiting, it is reasonable to institute positional therapy. It is usually unnecessary to study all of these very mild cases with barium if they respond promptly. Therapy could consist of frequent feeding, careful burping of the child, and positioning in the prone rather than supine position (preferably with the head elevated 30°). If symptoms are more bothersome and the diagnosis of reflux has been confirmed, it would be reasonable to institute either bethanechol or metoclopramide therapy 30 minutes prior to feeding three times a day and at bedtime. Which of the drugs is chosen is somewhat arbitrary. They should be used in full dosage. If no improvement is noted in two–three weeks, or if there are side effects, the physician may wish to try the alternate drug. Both drugs should not be given at the same time. If the patient has reactive airway disease, bethanechol should not be used, but the author has not hesitated to use the drug if the patient has recurrent aspiration pneumonia, coughing, or apnea without other evidence of bronchospasm.

No firm guidelines can be given concerning the use of antacids and hydrogen receptor antagonists. If there is evidence of esophagitis, such as iron deficiency, heartburn, friability of mucosa at esophagoscopy, or an infiltration of eosinophils or polymorphonuclear leukocytes into the epithelium on biopsy, vigorous therapy to raise the pH of gastric contents should be employed. It has been noticed that many infants who have gastroesophageal reflux are very irritable or feed poorly because of severe esophagitis. With effective antacid therapy, the healing of the esophagitis is accompanied by an improvement in eating and temperament.

Use of antacids is effective in treating GER, but they must be given multiple times throughout the day; the total volume is quite large. For most preparations, the single dose for a 12 kg child will be between ten and 20 ml. Some patients may develop diarrhea, and compliance may be a real problem in older children. The hydrogen receptor antagonists cimetidine and ranitidine are not approved for use in children under 16, although there are numerous reports of their safe use in children. Cimetidine is favored for use in the very young, since there is an oral liquid preparation available and compliance may be better than for regimens involving vanitidine.

Once a full range of vigorous therapy is instituted, one should persist in treatment for at least six weeks. Past experience has shown that, sometimes, easily detectable improvement may not be noted for several weeks. In patients under 15–18 months, persistence with intensive medical therapy is indicated, since development of functional competence of the lower esophageal sphincter mechanism can be expected with time. A rapid spontaneous improvement often occurs at eight–ten months of age. If failure to thrive is the major problem and the patient is responding slowly to treatment, a trial of continuous nasogastric feeding is reasonable. In very small, premature infants, one may want to institute a cautious trial of continuous transpyloric feeding.

In contrast to the developing infant, patients over 18–24 months, can be expected to respond in a manner similar to that of adults. There is unlikely to be rapid spontaneous improvement in lower esophageal sphincter function with time. Gastroesophageal reflux in older children and adults tends to be a chronic problem. If there is no satisfactory improvement in four–six weeks of intensive medical therapy, a surgical procedure could be contemplated.

Patients who have severe, life-threatening complications, such as repeated episodes of coughing, choking, apnea, or severe bradycardia that do not respond promptly, may reasonably be considered for early surgical correction of gastroesophageal reflux.

In children with esophageal stricture, medical therapy usually will be only an interim measure. Until there is cessation of reflux, it is highly unlikely that the esophagitis will heal and stricture formation will continue or recur.

Except in patients with esophageal strictures, it is difficult to identify those patients who will ultimately fail medical therapy. As is particularly true of children less than 15 months of age, most patients will respond to medical therapy. In the experience of the author's group, even in groups of patients with severe esophagitis, over half will respond to intensive medical groups of management.


## SUMMARY

Medical therapy of gastroesophageal reflux will be effective in most patients experiencing GER and only a few will require surgical correction. Unlike the situation in adults, where reflux is likely to be present for decades, most patients under two years will experience a complete cure of the reflux problem. The challenge to the physician is to choose from the several modes of therapy discussed that mode which is most likely to benefit the individual while causing the least inconvenience and side effects.


## REFERENCES


1. Barnardo DE, Lancaster-Smith M, Strickland ID, et al: A double-blind controlled trial of Gaviscon in patients with symptomatic gastro-oesophageal reflux. Curr Med Res Opin 3:388–391, 1975.
2. Behar J, Brand DL, Brown FC, et al: Cimetidine in the treatment of symptomatic gastroesophageal reflux. Gastroenterology 74:441–448, 1978.

3.  Behar J, Ramsby G: Gastric emptying and antral motility in reflux esophagitis. Gastroenterology 74:253–256, 1978.

4.  Blumenthal I, Lealman GT: Effect of posture on gastroesophageal reflux in newborns. Arch Dis Child 57:555, 1982.

5.  Booth DJ, Kemmerer WT, Skinner DB: Acid clearing from the distal esophagus. Arch Sug 96:731–734, 1968.

6.  Byrne WJ, Marino LR: Metoclopramide increases lower esophageal sphincter pressure (LESP) and reduces the number of episodes and duration of relux in infants with gastroesophageal reflux (GER). Pediatr Res 18:191A, 1984.

7.  Cadman D, Richards J, Feldman, W: Gastroesophageal reflux in severely retarded children. Dev Med Child Neurol 20:95–98, 1978.

8.  Carre IJ: Postural treatment of children with a partial thoracic stomach ("hiatus hernia"). Arch Dis Child 35:569, 1960.

9.  Carre IJ: Disorders of the oro-pharynx and esophagus. In Anderson CM, Burke V, Anderson CM, et al. (Eds.): Pediatric Gastroenterology. Oxford: Blackwell Scientific Publications, pp. 33–79, 1975.

10. Christi DL, O'Grady LR, Mack DV: Incompetent lower esophageal sphincter and gastroesophageal reflux in recurrent acute pulmonary disease of infancy and childhood. J Pediatr 93:23–27, 1978.

11. Crowson TD, Head LH, Ferrante WA: Esophageal ulcers associated with tetracycline therapy. JAMA 235:2747, 1976.

12. Cucchiara S, Staiano A, Romaniello G, et al: Antacids and cimetidine treatment for gastro-oesophageal reflux and peptic oesophagitis. Arch Dis Child 59:842–847, 1984.

13. Deloore I, Van Ravensteyn H, Ameryckx L: Domperidone drops in the symptomatic treatment of chornic paediatric vomiting and regurgitation. A comparison with metoclopramide. Postgrad Med J (supplement 1) 55:40–42, 1979.

14. Demeester TR, Johnson LF, Joseph GJ, et al: Patterns of gastroesophageal reflux in health and disease. Ann Surg 184:459–470, 1976.

15. Dodds WJ, Dent J, Hogan WJ, et al: Mechanisms of gastroesophageal reflux in patients with reflux esophagitis. N Engl J Med 307:1547–1552, 1982.

16. Eastwood GL, Castell DO, Higgs RH: Experimental esophagitis in cats impairs lower esophageal sphincter pressure. Gastroenterology 69:146–153, 1975.

17. Euler AR: Use of bethanechol for the treatment of gastroesophageal reflux. J Pediatr 96:321–324, 1980.

18. Farrell RL, Roling GT, Castell DO: Stimulation of the incompetent lower esophageal sphincter. A possible advance in therapy of heartburn. Amer J Dig Dis 18:646–650, 1973.

19. Farrell RL, Roling GT, Castell DO: Cholinergic therapy of chronic heartburn. Ann Intern Med 80:573–576, 1974.

20. Ferry GD, Selby M, Peitro TJ: Clinical response to short-term nasogastric feeding in infants with gastroesophageal reflux and growth failure. J Pediatr Gastroenterol Nutr 2:57–61, 1983.

21. Grill BB, Hillemeier AC, McCallum RW, et al: Efficacy of domperidone in the treatment of gastroesophageal reflux in infancy. Gastroenterology 84:1175, 1983.

22. Helm JF, Dodds WJ, Pelc LR, et al: Effect of esophageal emptying and saliva on clearance of acid from the esophagus. N Engl J Med 310:284–287, 1984.

23. Herbst JJ: Medical progress; Gastroesophageal reflux. J Pediatr Vol. 98, No. 6:859–870, 1981.

24. Herbst JJ, Book LS, Johnson DG, et al: The lower esophageal sphincter in gastroesophageal reflux in children. J Clin Gastroenterol 1:119–123, 1979.

25. Herbst JJ, Meyers WF: Gastroesophageal reflux in children. Adv Pediatr 28:159–186, 1981.

26. Hillemeier AC, Lange R, McCallum R, et al: Delayed gastric emptying in infants with gastroesophageal reflux. J. Pediatr 98:190–193, 1981.

27. Kekendall JW, Mellow MH: Effect of sublingual nitroglycerin and long-acting nitrate preparations on esophageal motility. Gastroenterology 79:703–706, 1980.

28. McCallum RW, Berkowitz DM, Lerner E: Gastric emptying in patients with gastroesophageal reflux. Gastroenterology 80:285–291, 1981.

29. McCallum RW, Eshelman F, Nardi R, et al: A double-blind multicenter trial to compare the efficacy of ranitidine (R) and placebo (P) in the short-term treatment of chronic gastroesophageal reflux disease (GER). Gastroenterology 86:1179, 1984.

30. McCallum RW, Fink SM, Lerner E, et al: Effects of metoclopramide and bethanechol on delayed gastric emptying present in gastroesophageal reflux patients. Gastroenterology 84:1573–1577, 1983.

31. Meyers WF, Herbst JJ: Effectiveness of positioning therapy for gastroesophageal reflux. Pediatrics 69:768–772, 1982.

32. Nebel OT, Fornes MF, Castell DO: Symptomatic gastroesophageal reflux: Incidence and precipitation factors. Amer J Dig Dis 21:953–956, 1976.

33. Orenstein SR, Whitington PF: Positioning for prevention of infant gastroesophageal reflux. J Pediatr 103:534–537, 1983.

34. Orenstein SR, Whitington PF, Orenstein DM: The infant seat as treatment for gastroesophageal reflux. N Engl J Med 309:760–763, 1983.

35. Parker AF, Christie DL, Cahill JL: Incidence and significance of gastroesophageal reflux following repair of esophageal atresia and tracheoesophageal fistula and the need for antireflux procedures. J Pediatry Surg 14:5–8, 1979.

36. Pope CE II: Physiology. Gastronintestinal Disease. In Sleisenger MH, Fordtran JS (Eds.): Gastrointestinal Disease (2nd ed.). Philadelphia: W.B. Saunders Company, pp. 504–512, 1978.

37. Rozen P, Hallak A, Gelfond M, et al: A comparison of the lower esophageal sphincter response of reflux patients to metoclopramide or domperidone. Gastroenterology 86:1225, 1984.

38. Safaie-Shirazi S, Brubacher M: Effect of cold and hot tea on mucosal permeability of esophageal mucosa. Gastroenterology (abst) 70:932, 1976.

39. Safaie-Shirazi S, Zike WL, Brubacher M, et al: Effect of aspirin, alcohol, and pepsin on mucosal permeability of esophageal mucosa. Surg Forum 25:335–337, 1974.

40. Scheurer U, Halter F: Lower esophageal sphincter in reflux esophagitis. Scand J Gastroenterol 11:629–634, 1976.

41. Sodheimer JM, Morris BA: Gastroesophageal reflux among severely retarded children. J Pediatr 94:710–714, 1979.

42. Sondheimer JM, Mintz HL, Michaels M: Bethanechol treatment of gastroesophageal reflux in infants: Effect on continuous esophageal pH records. J Pediatr 104:128–131, 1984.

43. Stein MR, Weber RW, Tower TG: The effect of theophylline on the lower esophageal sphincter pressure (LESP), abstracted. J Allergy Clin Immunol 61:136, 1978.

44. Strickland AD, Chang JHT: Results of treatment of gastroesophageal reflux with bethanechol. J Pediatr 103:311–315, 1983.

45. Thanik KD, Chey WY, Shah AN, et al: Reflux esophagitis: Effect of oral bethanechol on symptoms and endoscopic findings. Ann Int Med 93:805–808, 1980.

46. Weldon AP, Robinson MJ: Trial of Gaviscon in the treatment of gastro-oesophageal reflux of infancy. Aust Paediatr J 8:279–281, 1972.

Dale G. Johnson

# 9

# The Nissen Fundoplication

Nissen's own description concerning the development of his fundoplication operation for control of gastroesophageal reflux implies that he borrowed the idea from the Japanese

> The first successful operation of this kind outside Japan was performed in 1937 on a man with a perforating ulcer of the cardia. To reinforce the sutures connecting the esophageal stump and the stomach, the latter was mobilized and the distal segment of the esophagus implanted in it in much the same manner as the rubber tube in Witzel's gastrostomy . . . . Sixteen years later, we were able to re-examine the patient. In contrast to our usual experience following esophagogastrostomy, there was no history of gastric reflux.[10]

Nissen subsequently applied this technique specifically for the control of reflux and reported two cases in 1956.[9] His later description in English amplifies the details of those first operations.

> From an abdominal incision, the distal part of the esophagus was mobilized and drawn down 6 cm. into the abdominal cavity; the fundus ventriculi was then wrapped round the latter and the folds fixed with sutures. This procedure was termed fundoplication . . . . When it was found that the favorable clinical and radiological results were maintained, we adopted this procedure in combination with gastropexy in those cases of sliding hiatal hernia which involved severe reflux manifestations. As a rule, these were small hernias.[10]

Nissen had previously been working with paraesophageal and hiatal hernias, and he had been treating these disorders with an anterior gastropexy. His description continued.

> A method does exist which enables one to restore the angle of His and to correct the hernia by simultaneous abdominal invagination of the hernial sac . . . . This method is a

Pediatric Esophageal Surgery
ISBN 0-8089-1776-5

type of gastropexy in which the stomach is fixed to the anterior abdominal wall under traction.

This operation was first performed by us in 1946 as an emergency measure. The patient was a 66-year-old man in very poor general condition, with a history of a large incarcerated paraesophageal hiatal hernia of several days' standing. In view of the critical situation, we contented ourselves with extracting the hernial contents (four-fifths of the stomach) from the hernial sac and, to prevent renewed incarceration, fastening the fundus under traction to the anterior wall of the abdomen. Soon after this, we were obliged to perform a similar operation on a 70-year-old patient. Both patients remained symptom-free, despite the fact that the hernial orifice was not constricted nor the hernial sac removed.[10]

Two years after Nissen's first report of fundoplication for reflux, Adler et al. advocated the same procedure based upon animal experiments, finding it superior to other mechanical methods for combating reflux disorders.[1] In 1959, Nissen and Rossetti summarized their results with fundoplication plus gastropexy in 96 cases, reporting a "clinical and radiological healing rate" of 88 percent (85/96 patients) over an observation period ranging from three months to 3.5 years. Seven cases showed "relapse of the hernia", but the patients remained "symptom free," so control of symptoms was recorded as 96 percent (92/96 patients).[11]

In 1960, Nissen published a paper discussing the connection between reflux esophagitis and hiatal hernia in the light of his own experience. He emphasized that "[r]elief from gastroesophageal reflux should constitute the primary objective of surgical intervention."[8]

Nissen's first English-language description of his operation with his clinical experience was published in 1961 under the title "Gastropexy and 'Fundoplication' in Surgical Treatment of Hiatal Hernia", from which paper the above quotations have been taken.[10] At that time, he reported 122 cases of fundoplication, "partly as the only procedure, partly in combination with gastropexy". Nissen's experience evolved in such a manner as to suggest that he considered the gastropexy important for control of herniation into the chest, with the fundoplication being added for specific control of reflux.


## OBJECTIVES IN FUNDOPLICATION

Control of intractable gastroesophageal reflux remains the sole indication for fundoplication today, as it was when Nissen first described it. The controversies which have arisen over alternative operations have developed not because Nissen's operation has proven ineffective. Rather, the search for different procedures continues because the side effects from complete control of reflux have, in the hands of many surgeons, proven to be troublesome and almost unacceptable in frequency.

Ideally, a properly constructed antireflux operation should allow normal swallowing, produce no troublesome alteration of esophageal, gastric, or intestinal motility, and permit release of gas from the stomach by belching, even while eliminating any reflux of acid or gastric content. Comprehensive postoperative studies with objective testing for reflux in adults following the Nissen fundoplication, the Belsey Mark IV operation, or the Hill posterior gastropexy have demonstrated superior control of reflux with Nissen's procedure.[3] Similar studies comparing different operations by objective testing have not been published for children. Until proven otherwise, the

Nissen fundoplication must still be considered the best procedure for elimination of gastroesophageal reflux.

It also seems clear, however, that both potential and actual complications are probably highest with the complete fundoplication. Modifications of the Nissen operation are still being developed and evaluated for the purpose of decreasing the troublesome side effects of gas bloat, varying degrees of dysphagia, and postoperative vagal dysfunction. Technical simplification and better reproducibility are also desirable modifications for an operation that has produced good results only with experience and a compulsive attention to detail. These goals must be achieved without serious compromise of the excellent control of reflux which is the main justification for any of the antireflux procedures.

## THE NORMAL BARRIER TO REFLUX

The physiologic control of reflux in the normal and asymptomatic person depends upon multiple factors, some of which probably are not even known. Closing pressure of the abdominal segment of the lower esophageal sphincter is due to the intrinsic muscle tone, intra-abdominal pressure, a closing suction effect from the negative intra-thoracic influence,[4] and a mucosal sealing pressure.[13] In addition, the quality of peristalsis clearly affects esophageal emptying and the rate of esophageal clearance when reflux does occur. Also, the acute angle of insertion between the esophagus and stomach, the angle of His, has been assumed to be an important component of the antireflux mechanism since before the time of Nissen, but there are few recent objective data either to prove or disprove this point.

This angle of insertion, however, is one of the things the surgeon can alter, and most of the operations for reflux have been designed to do so. Other factors under the surgeon's control involve the ability to lengthen the intra-abdominal segment of esophagus and to fix it in that position, the ability to increase resistance at the gastroesophageal junction by sutures which restrict lower esophageal expansion, and the ability to construct various types and degrees of valve mechanisms at the gastroesophageal (GE) junction. There is no surgical technique for increasing the intrinsic tone in the lower esophageal sphincter, but studies with in vitro sphincter models have revealed that lengthening the abdominal segment increases the suction and mucosal sealing effects.[12] The same authors have also documented, from experimental models and from analysis of manometric data in adult patients, that "[t]he resistance to reflux provided by a sphincter is a function of its pressure distributed over the abdominal length (of the esophagus)." And, "[a]s the abdominal length is shortened, the pressure needs to be increased exponentially to maintain competence. However, with a sphincter in the abdomen less than 1 cm in length, competence cannot be achieved by pressure increases."[12]

## MODIFICATIONS SINCE NISSEN

Nissen used the fundoplication to control reflux, and the anterior gastropexy to maintain the stomach (and the wrapped intra-abdominal segment of esophagus) within the abdominal for control of the hiatal (or paraesophageal) hernia. His patients were adults, and the patients described in the early papers had large hernias. As early as

1964, Bettex and Stillhart stated that "[i]t is superfluous to fasten the stomach, cardia, or cuff in the abdominal cavity."[2] They were reporting experience in 20 infants and children operated upon for complications of reflux, and they also said, as did Nissen, that surgical narrowing of the hiatus was not necessary.

What today is called a Nissen operation may deviate widely from Nissen's original procedure. Most surgeons do not perform supplemental gastropexy routinely, and most do narrow the esophageal hiatus by suturing. The length of the intra-abdominal esophagus and the length of the fundoplication seem to vary with the individual surgeon, making comparisons for success rates and complications difficult. Additional variables include the alignment of the wrap (with or without twisting as the fundoplication is constructed); the technique of suturing the wrap; the position of the wrap in relation to the GE junction; the extent of mobilization of the greater and lesser curvatures; the treatment of the vagus nerves (within or outside the wrap); the size of intraesophageal bougie during fundoplication and the tightness of the wrap around the esophagus; construction of the wrap from anterior, posterior, or both walls of the fundus; the use of supplemental pyloromyotomy or pyloroplasty; supplemental gastrostomy; and so on. Each variation or combination has its advocates—or at least practitioners—and this diversity of techniques and beliefs about what constitutes a Nissen antireflux operation has confused the interpretation of results. How much this matters is still uncertain.

This author believes, however, that most of the complications and side effects attributed to complete fundoplication can be ascribed to technical errors and lack of precision in performing the technical aspects of the operation. This position is supported by the studies of Joelsson, DeMeester, Skinner, et al., who also suggest that not only the details of the fundoplication but also the decision regarding whether or not to perform a fundoplication in addition to esophageal lengthening should be tailored to the patient and the particular aberration in function.[6] Important details in the fundoplication procedure, according to this author's own bias, are presented below.

## TECHNICAL ASPECTS OF FUNDOPLICATION IN CHILDREN

The Nissen fundoplication can be performed either transabdominally or transthoracically, but the author's group favors the abdominal approach in the majority of patients. Transthoracic or thoracoc-abdominal approaches are reserved for patients with strictures or significant esophageal shortening, or for complex reoperations for reflux.

The best exposure can be obtained by an incision which takes into account the patient's size and body contour. For infants and small children, and for anyone with a relatively flat or transverse costal arch, a transverse incision across both rectus muscles with a one-cm extension into the obliques on each side will provide superior access. Older children with a high costal arch are usually best approached through a vertical midline incision from xyphoid to umbilicus.

The esophageal hiatus is approached by first laying a gauze pack over the splenic flexure of the colon and the small bowel below it. A malleable retractor is than placed over the pack, with the tip positioned just below the hilum of the spleen. The first assistant then retracts in a downward direction.

The surgeon should then lay a second gauze pack over the body of the stomach for subsequent downward retraction with the left hand.

The leading edge of the left lobe of the liver should be grasped between the thumb and fingers of the surgeon's left hand for traction outward and to the right to expose the left triangular ligament of the liver.

Two blades of a self-retaining, table-attached Thompson retractor, or one Richardson retractor in the hands of a second assistant, should be placed beneath the left costal arch for an upward and cephalad retraction.

The left triangular ligament should be incised under tension and in a bloodless plane over to the right side of the esophagus, but measurably short of a large left hepatic vein which may come into view. The lateral segment of the left lobe of the liver can then be folded under to the right and covered with a third gauze pad.

The esophageal attachment of the phrenoesophageal ligament can be visualized clearly if the surgeon will retract the stomach downward with the left hand while the first assistant lifts the diaphragmatic muscle anteriorly with a long atraumatic forceps. The attachment to the esophagus will then appear as loose areolar tissue, which can be cut with dissecting scissors in an avascular plane. Bleeding during this separation of the phrenoesophageal ligament from the esophagus means that the surgeon is in the wrong plane and is cutting either esophagus or diaphragm. The left vagus nerve, on the right anterior aspect of the esophagus at the hiatus, should be clearly visualized and protected from injury (Fig. 9-1).

Encirclement of the esophagus for placement of a one-quarter-inch rubber drain to provide downward traction must be performed cautiously to avoid injury to the posterior wall of the esophagus. A large rubber bougie should be maintained within the lower esophagus to aid the dissection and to prevent excessive narrowing during the subsequent crural suturing and the construction of the fundoplication. For infants, a minimum size of 26–28 French is used, with 36–38 French used for a five-year-old. Appropriate sizes are chosen forages in between.

The structures at the hiatus are too small in infants and children to permit the usual blunt dissection with the surgeon's index finger posterior to the esophagus. Rather, the dissection can be performed carefully and precisely with a long-nosed, right-angled clamp. The nose of the clamp should be placed parallel to the esophagus and pointing in a cephalad direction into the mediastinum. With downward pressure on the clamp to place the tips parallel but posterior to the esophagus, the jaws of the clamp can be opened and closed several times on each side of the esophagus to dissect the posterior wall free from the mediastinal areolar tissue. In the presence of extensive esophagitis, this dissection will be particularly sticky and dangerous. It is very important to have the stomach retracted downward with the surgeon's left hand and to dissect in the mediastinum well above the GE junction during this maneuver. Once the posterior esophagus has been freed from the mediastinal tissue, the nose of the right-angled clamp, introduced from the right side and with the jaws still parallel but posterior to the plane of the esophagus can be rotated downward and to the left, behind the esophagus in the mediastinum. The Penrose rubber drain can then be safely drawn behind the esophagus for downward traction.

Division of the short gastric vessels is the next step in mobilization of the fundus. In the infant, the spleen may hug the greater curvature closely with no apparent length to the uppermost short gastric vessels. Exposure can be obtained safely and systematically by first incising the anterior leaf of the gastrosplenic ligament between the

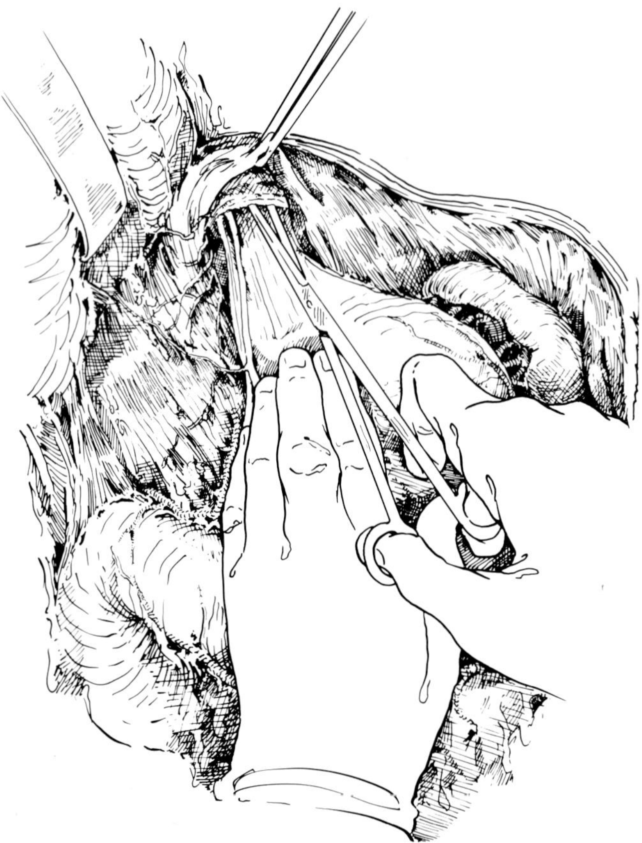

**Figure 9-1.**  The phrenoesophageal attachments can be divided bloodlessly if the hiatal muscle edge is tented upward by the assitant's forceps while the surgeon places downward traction on the stomach with the left hand.

esophagus and the uppermost splenic vessel. The posterior leaf of the ligament should not be penetrated because the adrenal and, inferiorly, the pancreas lie in this deeper plane. A right-angled clamp, in infants, or the surgeon's left index finger, in older children, can then be passed between the leaves of the gastrosplenic ligament and behind the short gastric vessels to expose and place these vessels on gentle tension (Fig. 9-2). The splenic side of each vessel is ligated and the gastric side suture-ligated as a precaution against slippage of the ligature with subsequent gastric distention. Sufficient short gastric vessels are divided to provide mobilization of about five cm of upper fundus for subsequent wrap around the esophagus. Areolar tissue is dissected from the posterior aspect of the stomach up to the hiatal crus in order to prevent kinking or restriction of the fundus as it is later rotated behind the esophagus. The left gastric vessels will come into view from this posterior approach and should not be disturbed. This is also the place in the operation where the posterior right vagus nerve must be identified in order to preserve it from injury. Both vagus nerves are usually included with the esophagus inside the Penrose drain and, later, within the fundoplication.

In order to complete exposure of the right side of the left crus of the diaphragm,

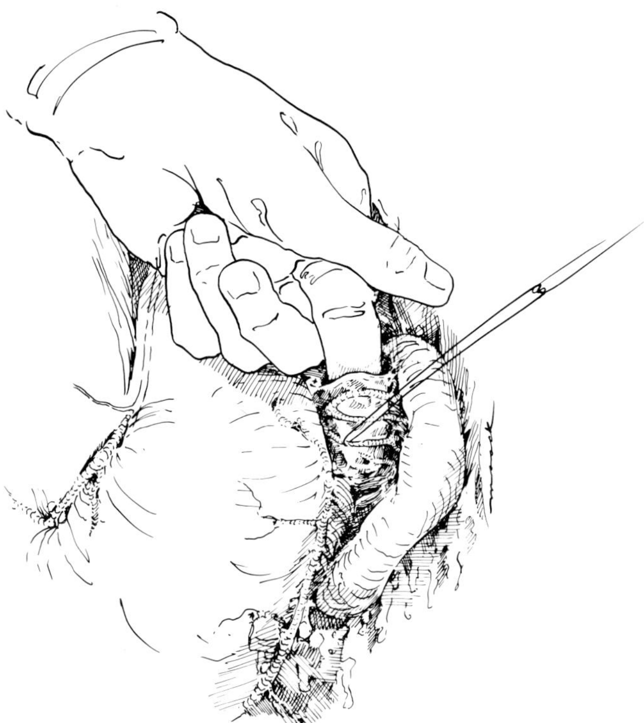

**Figure 9-2.** The short gastric vessels can be easily exposed and divided by incising the anterior leaf of the gastrosplenic ligament and placing a right-angled clamp or the surgeon's left index finger behind the vessels.

the gastrohepatic ligament is entered through its avascular midportion, with the esophagus retracted to the left. The ligament is then incised to a point just below the GE junction where the hepatic branch of the left vagus nerve angles upward through the ligament toward the liver. Ordinarily, this hepatic branch is preserved and the fundoplication is performed above it, although sometimes it is necessary to divide the hepatic branch to obtain sufficient room for the wrap. Care is taken not to injure the left anterior vagus trunk, or the nerve of Lartarjet which continues from it along the lesser curvature. A plexus of lymphatics runs between the liver and the posterior abdomen just above the hepatic branch of the vagus. These lymphatics must be clamped and ligated to obtain sufficient exposure of the right leaf of the left crus and also to provide sufficient room for the fundoplication between the diaphragm and the downwardly displaced GE junction (Fig. 9-3).

The esophageal hiatus is then narrowed by suturing the two sides of the left crus behind the esophagus. Some have suggested that this is unnecessary, but the experience of having the fundoplication slip into the chest when these sutures have cut through will convince the surgeon otherwise. To prevent such recurrent herniation, it is important to preserve the peritoneum on the surface of the crural muscle and to tie the sutures loosely to minimize cutting through the muscle. A bougie of appropriate size remains in the lumen of the esophagus while the hiatus is narrowed, and sufficient additional room is left between the esophagus-with-bougie and the hiatal margin to

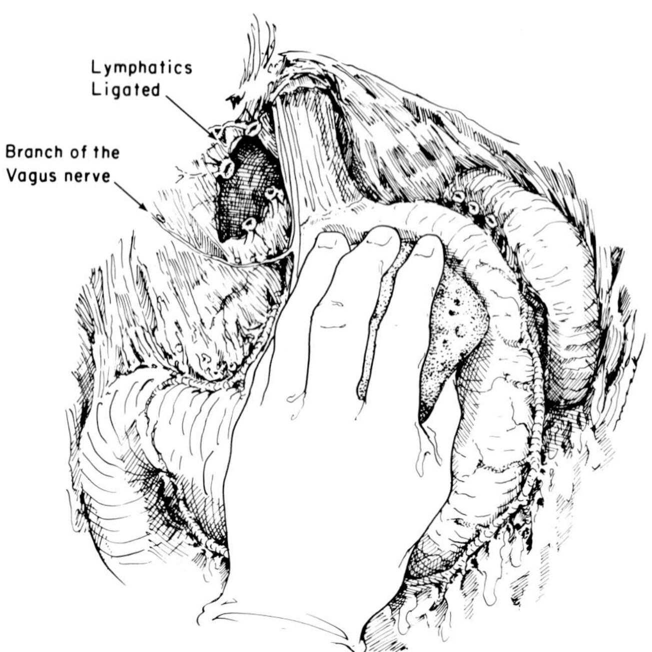


**Figure 9-3.** The hepatic branch of the left vagus nerve extends into the gastrohepatic ligament just below the gastroesophageal junction. The portion of the ligament cephalad to the nerve is rich with lymphatics, and these should be ligated to expose the right side of the diaphragmatic crus. The hepatic branch serves as a convenient marker for the lowermost portion of the fundoplication and can usually be preserved.

allow passage of a #12 Hegar dilator. Recently, at the suggestion of Dr. Tom DeMeester, who has experienced similar problems with fundal herniation in adults, the author's group has reinforced the crural sutures with small teflon patches on either side in order to minimize the cutting through of the stiches. The author prefers to place these crural stitches from the left side with the esophagus retracted to the right. Exposure is obtained by passing a long, flat instrument to the left of the esophagus and to the right of the two crural limbs. Two mattress sutures with teflon reinforcement usually suffice (Fig. 9-4).

Construction of the fundoplication is organized first by measuring the appropriate length of fundus along the greater curvature and then placing traction sutures, prior to rotation of the fundus behind the stomach, to obtain proper alignment and placement of the wrap. For infants and small children, two traction sutures are placed at the GE junction anteriorly, near the lesser curvature, for downward pull on the esophagus. The Penrose drain around the esophagus is bulky and interferes with alignment of the wrap in small patients, so this is removed. A third traction suture is placed in the posterior wall of the fundus a measured distance below the GE junction and at least the width of the esophagus posterior to the greater curvature. With the sutures at the GE junction held on downward traction, the suture in the posterior wall is passed behind the esophagus to bring its point of fixation in the stomach to the right of and two cm above the GE junction. This aligns the invaginated portion of the greater

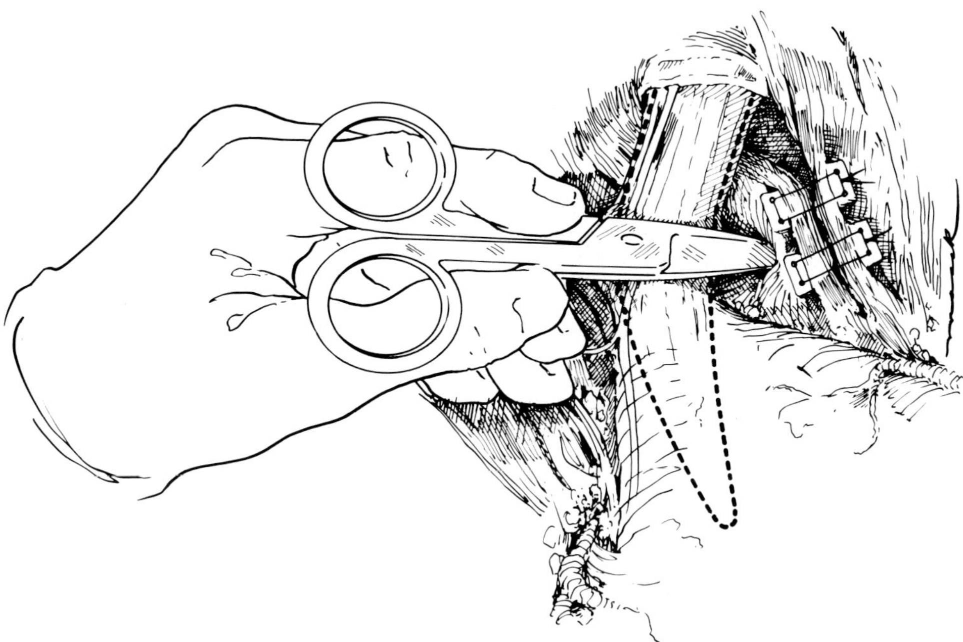

**Figure 9-4.**   Good exposure for both sides of the diaphragmatic crura can be obtained by using a flat instrument or a pair of straight scissors placed to the right of the right crus for retraction of the esophagus to the right. The muscle is thin and friable in small infants. Reinforcing teflon patches are currently being used to lessen the chance of fundal herniation due to stitches tearing through the crura.

curvature parallel to the left side of the esophagus without twisting and insures a loose wrap if the subsequent sutures are properly placed (Fig. 9-5).

The fundoplication is then completed by starting the suture line in the anterior stomach wall at the level of the GE junction, passing the suture through the muscular wall of the esophagus just above the junction, and catching the posterior wall of the stomach again as it has been rotated from behind the esophagus. Four–five sutures are used for this first layer, progressing in a cephalad direction. The wrap is currently constructed no longer than 1.5 cm in infants and two cm in older children, although formerly wraps have been constructed as long as three cm. The longer the wrap and the tighter the wrap, the higher the incidence of unpleasant side effects. Two cm is now the maximum length used by the author's group. The wrap should also be very loose around the esophagus while it contains a large bougie. Currently, a double layer of sutures is favored to secure the wrap. The author's group has had experience with subsequent disruption of a single suture line with recurrence of reflux. Reinforcement of mattress sutures by small teflon patches has also been tried, as suggested by DeMeester, but the double row of sutures seems tidier.

Two or three additional sutures are usually placed between the upper portion of the wrap on either side of the esophagus and the hiatus or the adjacent diaphragm. It is hoped that these additional sutures will provide insurance against subsequent slippage or unraveling of the fundoplication.

Supplemental anterior or posterior gastropexy, in the author's practice, is reserved for those cases where esophagitis has caused shortening and the fundoplication does

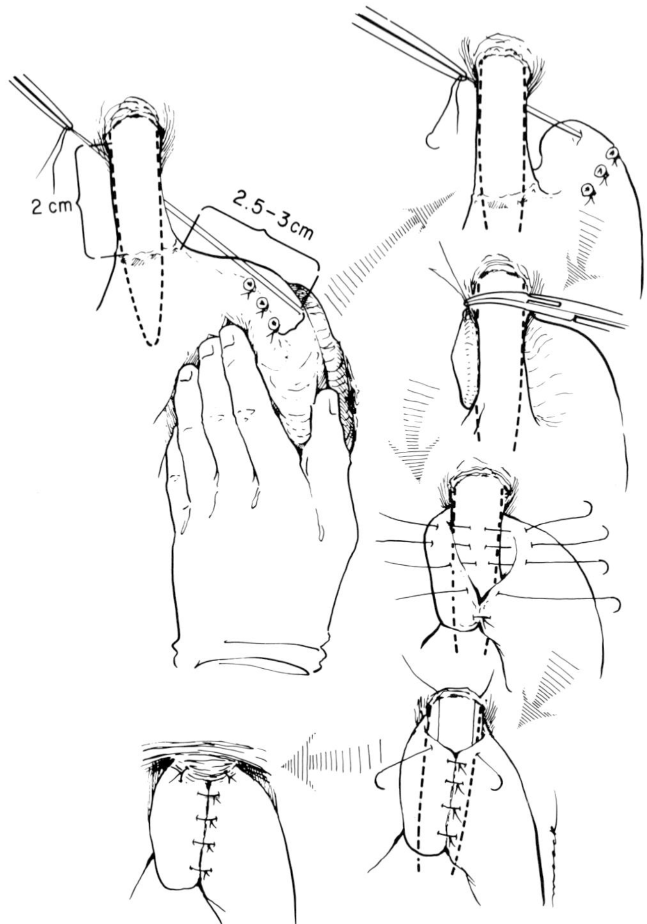



**Figure 9-5.** Suture alignment of the wrap during fundoplication minimizes rotational twisting and contributes to a loose
and functional result. Two temporary sutures placed anteriorly
at the gastroesophageal junction for downward traction, not
shown here, are also useful. The wrap must be constructed
loosely over a large intraluminal bougie. A double row of sutures provides additional security against subsequent disruption. Sutures between the diaphragmatic hiatus and the top of
the wrap lessen the chance of downward slippage.

not sit loosely against the diaphragm without tension. If it has been possible to
mobilize three–five cm of esophagus below the diaphragm and to wrap the lower two
cm without tension, no gastropexy is performed.

Anterior gastropexy, when utilized, involves the placement or four–five sutures
inferior to the wrap between the lesser curvature and the anterior abdominal wall.
Slight tension is created to maintain the intra-abdominal segment of esophagus and the
wrap below the hiatus. In small infants, the left lobe of the liver is relatively larger
than it is in later life, and this makes the construction of an anterior gastropexy
difficult without awkward rotation of the left lobe.

Posterior gastropexy in the author's experience usually involves the anchoring of the lowermost sutures of the fundoplication, or the traction sutures in the GE junction, to the lowermost suture or teflon patch used for narrowing the hiatus; supplemental gastropexy has been used in only a small minority of cases. The author's group has experienced a bothersome incidence of radiographic (though usually asymptomatic) partial slippage of the fundoplication through the hiatus at late follow-up, however, and perhaps the gastropexy should be added more liberally.

Gastrostomy is usually not a part of the antireflux operation in the author's experience. Neurologically damaged children who have swallowing disorders, and some small infants with failure to thrive, may have gastrostomy for those specific reasons, but gastrostomy is not routinely necessary, in the opinion of the author's group, if the wrap is made loose and short.

## EXTENDED APPLICATIONS OF COMPLETE FUNDOPLICATION

Severe esophagitis with significant longitudinal shortening of the esophagus may make intra-abdominal fundoplication impossible. Surgeons handle this problem in a variety of ways, but modified Nissen fundoplications have been constructed intrathoracically, as a complete fundoplication around a Collis gastroplasty, and as a complete wrap around a Thal gastric patch. The indications and details of these procedures are beyond the scope of this discussion, but it is worth noting here that these extended procedures are available as options because the valve mechanism of the complete fundoplication does function even when displaced into the negative-pressure environment above the diaphragm. It is critical, however, that the hiatus be enlarged and that the edges of the hiatus be sewn to the stomach without tension if the fundoplication is to be left partially in the mediastinum. This will prevent hourglass deformity of the stomach by pinching at the hiatus, a situation reported by several authors to cause serious problems.

## COMMON TECHNICAL ERRORS IN FUNDOPLICATION

### A Too-tight Wrap

The intraluminal bougie should be large (28 for infants; 38 for children), and the wrap should be loose (allowing passage of a 12–14 Hegar dilator between esophagus with bougie and the wrap).

### Insufficient Abdominal Esophagus

Inadequate mobilization of the esophagus causes tension on the wrap and leads to disruption and recurrence of reflux. Three–five cm of esophagus should be mobilized for a two-cm wrap.

### A Twisted Wrap

Failure to align the fundus properly before passing it around the esophagus may lead to uncontrolled increases in lower esophageal pressure and increased incidence of unwanted side effects such as gas bloat and dysphagia.

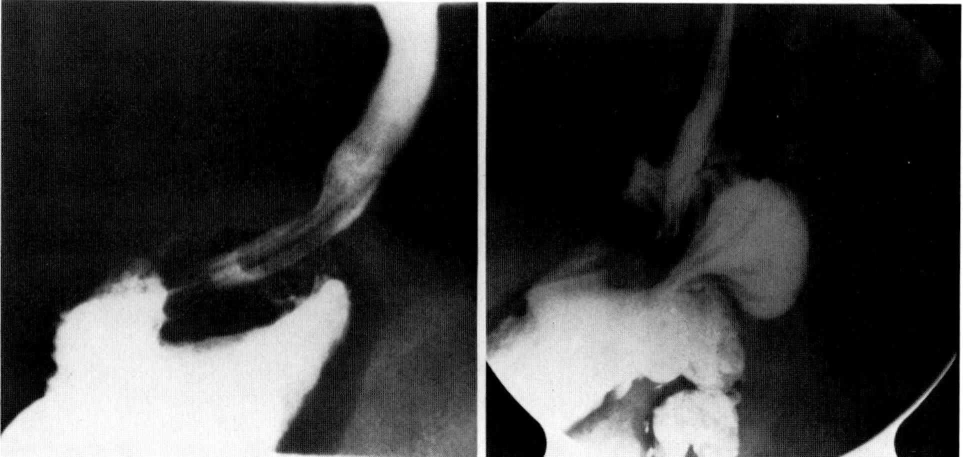

**Figure 9-6.**   Fundoplication in a seven-month-old infant with active esophagitis was functionally and anatomically satisfactory at follow-up one month after operation (left), and symptoms were completely relieved. Return of pinching pain and substernal burning two years later prompted the repeat study (right), which demonstrated herniation through the hiatus, partial disruption of the wrap, and recurrent reflux.

## Wrapping of the Stomach

Wrapping of the stomach rather than the lower esophagus will fail to control reflux and often will cause dysphagia.

## Inadequate Hiatal Closure

Inadequate hiatal closure leads commonly to partial slippage of the fundus into the mediastinum. This slippage may result in hourglass deformity with pain, partial breakdown, and sometimes recurrent reflux, if the hiatus has not been surgically enlarged (Fig. 9-6).

## Errors Causing Vagal Injury

Vagal injury can be caused by initial hiatal and esophageal dissection, tight wrapping, or actual suture entrapment of the vagus.

## POSTOPERATIVE SIDE EFFECTS

Unpleasant side effects or complications of a tight fundoplication include gas bloat, inability to vomit, dysphagia, and early satiety. Within the first week after operation, most patients have several or all of these symptoms, at least in mild degree. If the wrap is short and constructed loosely, however, the dysphagia and the gas bloat are minimal within one–three weeks. Inability to vomit usually persists, with occasional exception, as long as the wrap is intact, and the early satiety may persist for several weeks until the stomach accommodates or the patient develops the ability to burp. Abdominal meteorism with increased amounts of flatus following fundoplication

**Table 9-1**
*Control of Reflux and Control of Main Symptoms*
*with Nissen Fundoplication*

|  | None | Partial | Complete |
|---|---|---|---|
| GER relief |  |  |  |
| <3 weeks | .2% (3/155) | 2.6% (4/155) | 95% (148/155) |
| >3 weeks | 5.7% (9/158) | 9.5% (15/158) | 85% (134/158) |
| Main symptom relief |  |  |  |
| <3 weeks | .3% (4/141) | 18% (26/141) | 79% (111/141) |
| >3 weeks | 8.5% (13/153) | 24% (37/153) | 67% (103/153) |

may be noticed by mothers of one-third of the pediatric patients, although good quantitation of the incidence, severity, or the duration of this side effect is not available. The infants who are air swallowers obviously experience greater discomfort from gas bloat, early satiety, and flatus following fundoplication than do non-air swallowers.

Results and complications associated with individual modifications of the Nissen fundoplication operation in children have been reported recently.[7,14,15] It is difficult to make comparisons, however, because follow-up criteria were not defined, objective testing was minimal, and the rigor of the clinical evaluation was not specified. Reported success in controlling reflux symptoms ranged from 88 to 96 percent.

The author's own series in Salt Lake City includes 216 complete fundoplications

**Table 9-2**
*Principal Reason for Operation—Nissen Fundoplication*

| Symptom | No. of Patients | Average Age |
|---|---|---|
| Vomiting | 60 | 38 months |
| Failure to thrive | 28 | 12 months |
| Respiratory symptoms |  |  |
| recurrent pneumonia | 52 | 24 months |
| apnea | 41 | 6 months |
| stridor/cough | 3 | 33 months |
| asthma | 2 | 101 months |
| Esophagitis |  |  |
| irritability | 4 | 14 months |
| pain | 8 | 84 months |
| dysphagia | 2 | 32 months |
| hematemesis | 1 | 360 months |
|  | (severely retarded— weight 40 kg) |  |
| stricture | 8 | 82 months |
| Sandifer's syndrome | 1 | 56 months |
| anemia | 2 | 112 months |
| Neuropsychiatric indications | 1 | 36 months |
| Other | 3 | 18 months |
| Total | 216 |  |

**Table 9-3**
*Complications of Complete Fundoplication*

|                                                      | Early | Late | Total | Percentage |
|------------------------------------------------------|-------|------|-------|------------|
| Postoperative herniation of fundoplication through hiatus (any degree) | 5 | 18 | 23 | 10.6% |
| Wound infection                                      | 12    | 1    | 13    | 6.0%       |
| Postoperative pneumonia                              | 5     | 2    | 7     | 3.0%       |
| Intestinal obstruction                               | 4     | 5    | 9     | 4.0%       |
| Dysphagia, severe                                    | 1     | 0    | 1     | 0.5%       |
| Systemic sepsis                                      | 1     | 0    | 1     | 0.5%       |
| Wound disruption                                     | 3     | 0    | 3     | 1.4%       |
| Esophageal leak                                      | 2     | 0    | 2     | 1.6%       |
| Disruption of repair                                 | 7     | 8    | 15    | 6.9%       |
| Death, related                                       | 0     | 0    | 0     | 0%         |
| Death, unrelated                                     | 3     | 3    | 6     | 2.8%       |
| Other                                                | 3     | 4    | 7     | 3.2%       |

performed or closely supervised by three pediatric surgeons. Reflux symptoms have been controlled in 95 percent of these patients, but this required two operations in 18 patients because of partial disruption of the initial wrap. Control of the main symptom which prompted operation was achieved in 91 percent of the cases (Table 9-1). Reasons for operation in these children are presented in Table 9-2. Operative complications are listed in Table 9-3. Functional side effects are tabulated in Table 9-4.

**Table 9-4**
*Functional Side Effects of Complete Fundoplication*

|               | None | Mild | Moderate | Severe |
|---------------|------|------|----------|--------|
| Gas bloat     |      |      |          |        |
| <3 weeks      |      |      |          |        |
| >3 weeks      | 72% (73/101) | 17% (17/101) | 10% (10/101) | 1% (1/101) |
| Dysphagia     |      |      |          |        |
| <3 weeks      | 65% (50/77) | 22% (17/77) | 9% (7/77) | 4% (3/77) |
| >3 weeks      | 73% (70/96) | 15% (14/96) | 9% (9/96) | 3% (3/96) |
| Diarrhea      |      |      |          |        |
| <3 weeks      | 72% (59/82) | 12% (10/82) | 15% (12/82) | 1% (1/82) |
| >3 weeks      | 58% (37/64) | 25% (16/64) | 16% (10/64) | 1% (1/64) |

|               | No | Yes |
|---------------|----|-----|
| Slow eater    |    |     |
| <3 weeks      | 76% (47/62) | 24% (15/62) |
| >3 weeks      | 64% (49/77) | 0% (0/77) |
| Able to burp  |    |     |
| <3 weeks      | 63% (30/48) | 38% (18/48) |
| >3 weeks      | 50% (29/58) | 50% (29/58) |
| Able to vomit |    |     |
| <3 weeks      | 94% (78/83) | 6% (5/83) |
| >3 weeks      | 80% (78/98) | 20% (20/98) |

Long-term follow-up has been reported for 25 of these patients who returned four–nine years after antireflux surgery for overnight hospitalization and re-study.[5] Testing involved a structured interview by a nonsurgeon (pediatric gastroenterologist), physical examination, extended esophageal pH monitoring, and, in selected patients, a barium esophagram. The results are interesting. The preoperative symptoms of vomiting, recurrent pneumonia, esophagitis, hematemesis, and apnea were controlled in all 25 patients. Several minor problems were identified, however. Roughly one-third of the children had mild symptoms of gas bloat, inability to vomit, slow eating habits, and choking on solids. These problems were reported, however, independent of each other, and the symptoms of gas bloat were not necessarily in the same patients who were unable to vomit. More interesting is the fact that the Boerema anterior gastropexy without fundoplication was used in early patients in this series. Seventeen of the 25 patients studied had the anterior gastropexy, and only seven had the Nissen fundoplication. The postoperative symptoms, particularly gas bloat, were not found to correlate more strongly with either the Nissen or the Boerema procedures. Parental satisfaction with the long-term results of the surgery was unanimous. Nineteen were very happy with the surgical repair; six were happy with the surgery and would have it done again, but they expressed minor concerns over residual gas bloat symptoms.

## SUMMARY

The term "Nissen fundoplication" is generic for a variety of antireflux operations which involve complete wrapping of the gastric fundus around the lower esophagus. This procedure is both praised for providing the most complete possible control of reflux and criticized for producing the most frequent and the most troublesome side effects. The numerous modifications by way of addition and subtraction from the original operation make the term "Nissen" inappropriate for most current antireflux procedures.

Preserving effective reflux control while minimizing the side effects of treatment is the motivation behind the proliferation of modified operations. Simplification of a demanding technical procedure is also desirable, because it is likely that many of the undesirable side effects and complications of fundoplication are in fact the result of technical or judgment errors in the performance of the operation. Standardization of the procedure would be desirable for the sake of reproducibility and comparison of results. Unfortunately, there is still no real agreement upon precisely which details of the operation should be standardized. Because the reported experience of the author's group represents a pooling of cases from three surgeons, all of whom perform the procedure differently, and because the author's own experience has evolved, as did Nissen's, from simple anterior gastropexy through a variety of additions and subtractions to the fundoplication, the results, at present, do not make a compelling argument for the author's biases.

It is particularly interesting that the long-term follow-up study by the author's group included both Boerema anterior gastropexy patients with no wrap and Nissen fundoplication patients with a complete wrap. The side effects of gas bloat, inability to vomit, early satiety, meteorism, and diarrhea were found in comparable frequencies for both operations, thus challenging the dogma that these problems are all attributable to a wrap which is too complete and too tight. A prospective clinical study with standardization of surgical procedures and of the follow-up methodology would greatly clarify the complications and their etiologies. The present clinical evidence from both pediatric and adult patients, plus the laboratory evidence, still favors the complete fundoplication as the standard for reflux control. It remains a significant challenge for clinical surgeons to minimize the associated symptoms and complications.

## REFERENCES


1. Adler RH, Firme CN, Lanigan JM: A valve mechanism to prevent gastro-esophageal reflux and esophagitis. Surgery 44:63–76, 1958.
2. Bettex M, Stillhart H: Operation for hiatus hernia and cardioesophageal chalasia by fundoplication after Nissen. Surgery 55:451–454, 1964.
3. DeMeester TR, Johnson LF, Kent AH: Evaluation of current operations for the prevention of gastroesophageal reflux. Ann Surg 180:511–525, 1974.
4. DeMeester TR, Wernly JA, Bryant GH, et al: Clinical and in vitro determinants of gastroesophageal competence: A study of the principles of antireflux surgery. Am J Surg 137:39–46, 1979.
5. Harnsberger JK, Corey JJ, Johnson DG, et al: Long-term followup of surgery for gastro-esophageal reflux in infants and children. J Pediatr 102:505–508, 1983.
6. Joelsson BE, DeMeester TR, Skinner DB, et al: The role of the esophageal body in the antireflux mechanism. Surgery 92:417–424, 1982.
7. Leape LL, Ramenofsky ML: Surgical treatment of gastroesophageal reflux in children. Results of Nissen's fundoplication in 100 children. Am J Dis Child 134:935–938, 1980.
8. Nissen R: Beziehungen zwischen Hiatushernien und Refluxosophagitis. MMW 102:1472–1474, 1960.
9. Nissen R: Eine einfache Operation zur Beeinflussung der Refluxosophagitis. Schweiz Med Wochenschr 86:590–592, 1956.
10. Nissen R: Gastropexy and "fundoplication" in surgical treatment of hiatal hernia. Am J Digest Dis 6:954–961, 1961.
11. Nissen R, Rossetti M: Die Behandlung von Hiatushernien und Refluxosophagitis mit Gastropexie und Fundoplicatio. Stuttgart: Thieme, 1959.
12. O'Sullivan GC, DeMeester TR, Joelsson BE, et al: Interaction of lower esophageal sphincter pressure and length of sphincter in the abdomen as determinants of gastroesophageal competence. Am J Surg 143:40–47, 1982.
13. Pettersson GB, Bombeck CT, Nyhus LM: The lower esophageal sphincter: Mechanisms of opening and closure. Surgery 88:307–14, 1980.
14. Randolph J: Experience with the Nissen fundoplication for correction of gastroesophageal reflux in infants. Ann Surg 198:579–584, 1983.
15. Tunnel WP, Smith EI, Carson JA: Gastroesophageal reflux in childhood: The dilemma of surgical success. Ann Surg 197:560–565, 1983.

Keith W. Ashcraft

# 10

# Thal Fundoplication

> The real unsettled clinical controversy is not whether the full fundoplication is a tighter antireflux valve—which it is in both human and animal studies—but whether a less tight partial fundoplication coupled with placement of an intact esophageal wall in an intra-abdominal position, which is also known to control reflux, will do so with less gas bloat syndrome and inability to belch or vomit.[10]

The subject of gastroesophageal reflux and its surgical treatment is one that has received a great deal of attention in recent years. Malfunction of the gastroesophageal junction is poorly understood, although surgical procedures which restore the lower end of the esophagus to the abdominal cavity and hold it there by whatever means are a part of all successful antireflux operations. Nissen's fundoplication is probably the most likely to stop reflux,[5,9] although, when properly performed in childhood, some measurable reflux is not infrequently seen.[7,8,12] The Nissen procedure has been the one most frequently used and hence the one most frequently studied.

Alternatives to the 360 Nissen wrap are the partial wraps of Belsey, Hill, and Thal[11] or Dor,[6] and the gastropexy designed by Boerema. There is a large body of available information on the Belsey and Hill repairs in adults. Johnson has reported on the Boerema gastropexy in children (see Chapter 9). The Thal procedure (or Dor-Nissen) is presented here and experience in 675 pediatric patients over the course of 12 years is described.

The anterior fundoplication procedure which has been called the Thal fundoplication was described in 1968 to the American Surgical Association by Alan Thal. Thal's primary use of this procedure was as an onlay patch of gastric fundus for the treatment of distal esophageal stricture wherein the stricture was incised into the esophageal lumen, and the serosa of the stomach (or a skin graft applied to the serosa) was used as a basis for covering the defect.[11]

The same fundoplication has been in use since at least 1962, when Gavriliu began using it for the treatment of achalasia in adults.[6] He was enthusiastic about the operative results in a series of 180 patients reported in 1975. He attributed the origin

Pediatric Esophageal Surgery  
ISBN 0-8089-1776-5



209

of the operation to Professor J. Dor of Marseille. Dor, Gavriliu, and Thal have all agreed that a partial fundoplication is effective treatment for gastroesophageal reflux. Clinical experience with the Thal (or Dor-Nissen) partial fundoplication has demonstrated, in the author's opinion, a success rate and recurrence rate comparable to that of Nissen's fundoplication with probably fewer perioperative complications and certainly fewer long-term problems.[1,2]

The normal function of the gastroesophageal junction has been detailed in previous chapters, but it must be emphasized here that burping and vomiting are normal events, particularly in childhood. Use of the Thal fundoplication has stemmed from the fact that patients having undergone a fundoplication of this sort are usually able to burp and are always able to vomit if necessary. If, then, successful correction of the gastroesophageal reflux is accomplished at a rate comparable to that achieved by other operative procedures, it seems only logical that the partial wrap be considered superior to the Nissen, where gas bloats are common and vomiting is often impossible.[12] The experience of the author's group has been analyzed in the follow-up of these 675 patients with this sort of comparison in mind.

## THE OPERATIVE PROCEDURE[3]

Once the diagnosis has been established and nonoperative therapy either proven to be unsuccessful or contraindicated, the patient is admitted the morning of scheduled operation. After induction of anesthesia, a #14 or #18 sump-type nasogastric tube is inserted into the stomach for ease in palpating the esophagus at the hiatus and for overnight postoperative gastric drainage. A transverse upper abdominal incision is made from nipple line to nipple line inside the costal margins as high up on the abdomen as feasible. Even in the older child with a relatively narrow costal angle, transverse incisions are preferred because they allow adequate exposure of the upper abdominal contents while the transverse colon shields the small bowel from exposure. Additional procedures such as incidental appendectomy are avoided because, in the few patients who had had postoperative intestinal complications, all but one had undergone incidental procedures or incisions which required manipulation or exposure of the small intestine.

*Step 1.* Following entry into the abdominal cavity, the stomach is retracted downward, the left lobe of the liver is grasped with a sponge and lifted out of the wound while the left upper portion of the incision is retracted with a Richardson retractor. This counter-traction delineates the peritoneal attachment of the left lobe of liver to the diaphragm, which is then cut either with scissors or with electrocautery. One or two small blood vessels usually traverse this filmy attachment. The left lobe is taken down across the hiatus, but short of hepatic veins. The left lobe of the liver is then folded downward and retracted to the right by the second assistant, who stands above the surgeon on the right side. A Deaver retractor with a folded sponge is used on the liver for protection and traction.

*Step 2.* The peritoneum overlying the hiatus is then sharply incised transversely at the hiatus, which allows exposure of the anterior wall of the esophagus. This incision line is made clearer by lifting the hiatus with a forcep. The anterior (left) vagus nerve branch comes across the esophagus at this level and should be protected. Once the esophageal muscle is exposed, a spreading instrument is used to dissect on either side of the esophagus. A Waterston's Ductus Dissector is preferred, although a right-angled clamp may be used for this purpose. It is easier to pass the instrument behind the esophagus from right to left. This maneuver is used to pull back a dacron umbilical tape, which is then used for traction purposes. With downward traction on the esophagus, each limb of the crura is then grasped and pushed upward, away from the gastroesophageal junction, freeing the lower two–four cm of esophagus (Fig. 10-1).

*Step 3.* This same instrument is then passed once again behind the esophagus to clear the filmy attachments posteriorly, completing the exposure of the entire distal esophagus—front, sides, and back. Inspection then reveals whether or not the poste-

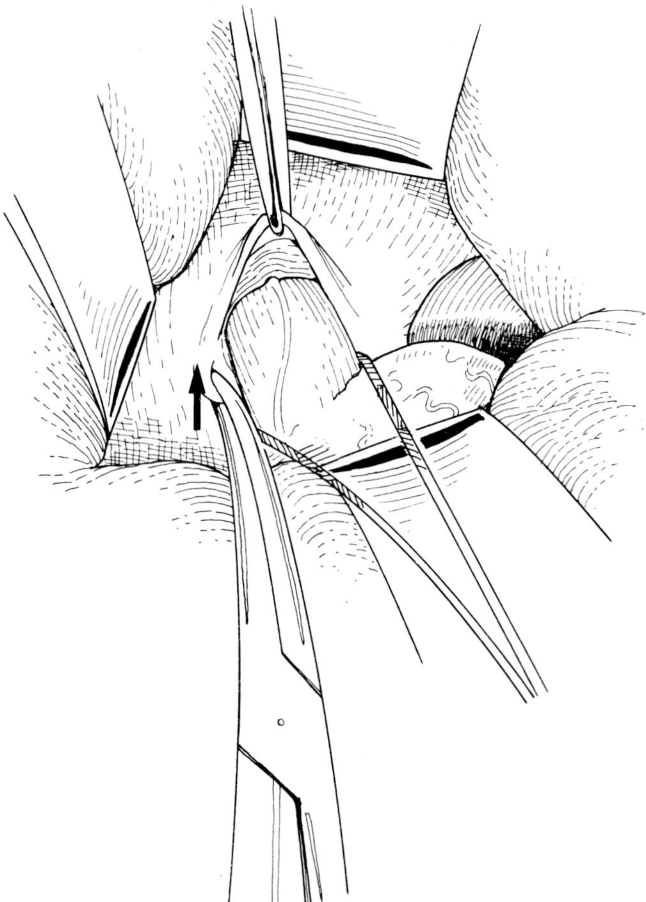

**Figure 10-1.** The lower esophagus has been exposed. The esophagus is surrounded by a dacron umbilical tape for traction purposes. Using counter-traction produced by this tape, the hiatus on both sides of the esophagus is pushed cephalad, exposing the lower two–four cm of esophagus.

rior branch of the vagus nerve has been included within the dacron tape. If it has not, the tape is replaced.

*Step 4.*  The distal esophagus is then lifted with a small retractor to allow exposure of the hiatus. A #2-0 silk cardiovascular suture is used to place a figure-of-eight suture in the hiatus, thus "repairing" the hiatus hernia (Fig. 10-2). Even in the absence of a hiatus hernia, this suture is placed because it thus limits the size of the hiatus postoperatively. This limiting stitch seems to have nearly eliminated the problem of postoperative herniation of the fundoplication through the hiatus into the mediastinum. This same suture is then used to affix the posterior wall of the esophagus to the closure of the hiatus, thus fixing the distal esophagus within the abdominal cavity posteriorly (Fig. 10-3).

*Step 5.*  The fundoplication is then carried out by suturing the anterior free wall of stomach up against the lower portion of the anterior half of the esophagus (Fig. 10-4). A running 2-0 or 3-0 prolene suture is used, beginning at the greater curve gastroesophageal (GE) junction and proceding cephalad. Once the desired apex of the fundoplication is achieved, the suture line is turned across the anterior half of the esophagus. (The surgeon must be careful to avoid the anterior branch of the vagus nerve.) Esopha-

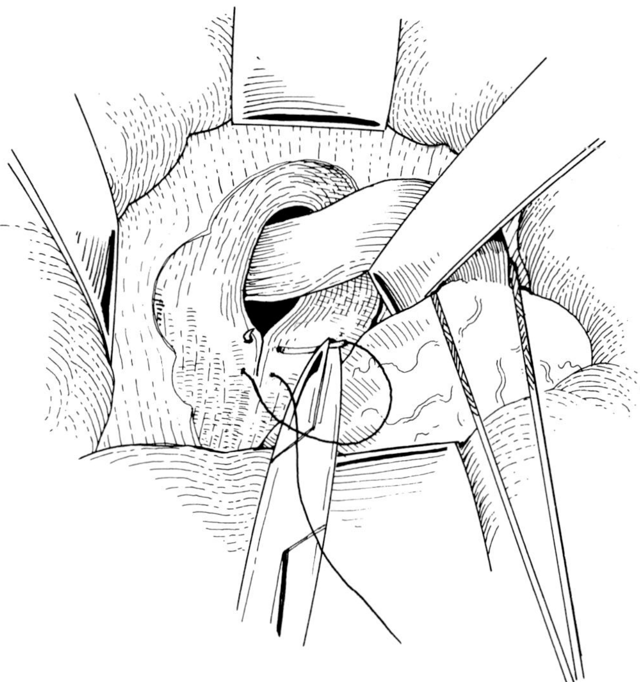

**Figure 10-2.**  The "limiting stitch" is placed to approximate the crura behind the esophagus. The older patients on solid-food diets require more room in this repaired hiatus than do the babies whose only intake is liquid. This suture must be tied carefully so as not to cut or necrose the crural muscle.

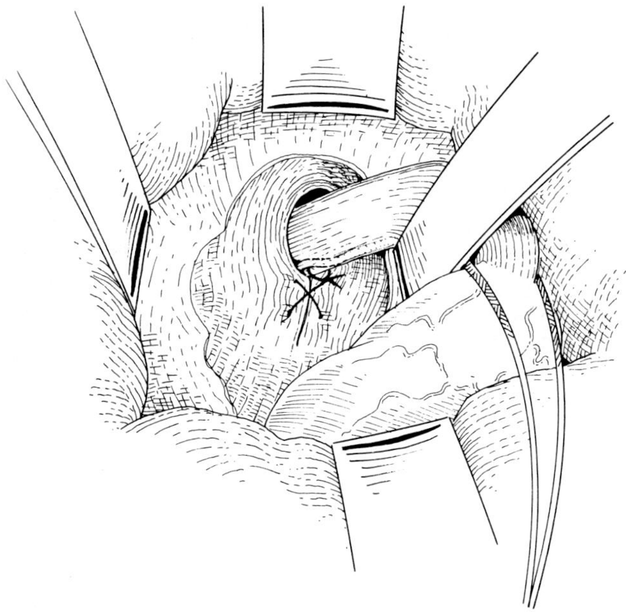

**Figure 10-3.** The "limiting stitch" is then used to affix the posterior wall of the esophagus. Great care is taken to avoid injury to the posterior (right) branch of the vagus nerve.

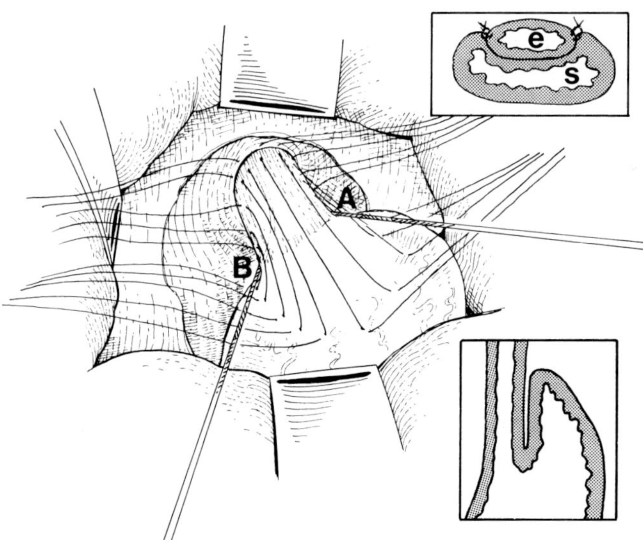



**Figure 10-4.** Although illustrated with interrupted sutures, the fundoplication is performed using a continuous Prolene suture (2-0 or 3-0) starting at the greater curve GE junction (A), proceding up the left side of the esophagus across the hiatus and down the right side of the esophagus to end at the lesser curve GE junction (B). The insets show the relationship of stomach and esophagus in cross-section and in sagittal section.

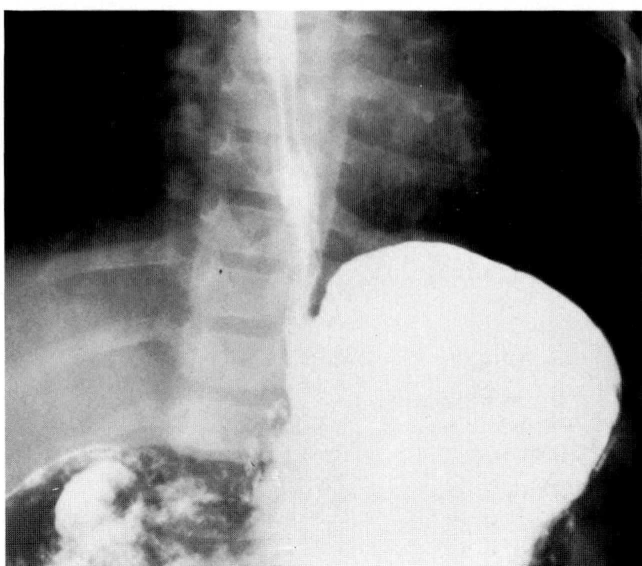

**Figure 10-5.**   The postoperative barium study should demonstrate the fundoplication within the abdominal cavity, without
obstruction or reflux.

gus, stomach, and the hiatus margin are included in the suture until the right lateral
aspect of the esophagus is reached. The suture line then turns caudad, sewing the
stomach to esophagus until the lesser curve GE junction is reached, where the suture is
tied to complete the fundoplication. The umbilical tape is removed, the liver replaced
in its normal position, and the wound closed with running dexon.

Postoperative management consists of overnight nasogastric suction with removal
of the tube the following morning and *immediate institution* of diet for age. Usually, by
72 hours postoperatively the patient has demonstrated adequate oral intake and is
ready for dismissal.

Follow-up consists of a visit to the office or clinic approximately a week after
dismissal from the hospital and again at four–six weeks to determine the result of the
operation. Four months postoperatively a barium esophagram is obtained to determine
if the GE junction is well below the diaphragm, to affirm that the fundoplication is
intact and that there is no esophageal narrowing and no reflux (Fig. 10-5). Because of
the necessity of hospitalization and the expense involved, the author's group does not
routinely repeat the diagnostic pH studies unless symptoms persist.


## RESULTS

In the series of 675 fundoplications done by the author's group over a span of 12
years, 625 procedures were initially successful in stopping the reflux (96.3 percent).
Twenty-five procedures (3.7 percent) have been done for *recurrent* reflux. Twelve of
these were done because the fundoplication came apart—eleven of these were among
the first 300 patients treated. Three were redone because a repaired hiatus hernia did
not hold; seven were redone because a hiatus hernia developed where none had been

present before (only one of which occurred after institution of the "limiting" stitch). One boy who had esophageal atresia and tracheoesophageal fistula as a neonate underwent three fundoplications but, because he had a micro stomach, none were successful. There was simply not enough stomach to provide an adequate fundoplication. This patient eventually came to esophagectomy with colon interposition. After the second of these fundoplication procedures, he developed the dumping syndrome, which has been a difficult management problem requiring gastric augmentation. Four patients have developed asymptomatic paraesophageal hiatus hernias following their original fundoplications but have not undergone reoperation.

There have been no instances of the gas bloat syndrome and no instances of inability to vomit. Three patients developed incisional hernias, two of them of whom were chronic ventilator patients. Six patients underwent operation for small intestinal obstruction. There have been no incisional hernias or bowel obstructions in the last 450 patients. Since the institution of the limiting stitch, which closes the hiatus and affixes the esophagus posteriorly, two paraesophageal hiatus hernias have developed. One was repaired although the patient was asymptomatic. At reoperation, it was discovered that the limiting suture had torn through the hiatus.

There have been no deaths attributable to the operation or complications of the operation.

Not all patients were relieved of their symptoms even after successful fundoplication. The explanation for this probably rests in the indirect association between gastroesophageal reflux (GER) and respiratory disease. When the manifestation of GER is esophagitis, intractable vomiting, or nutritional inadequacy due to regurgitation, fundoplication is virtually always curative. The author's group has found, in a group of 144 patients with chronic respiratory problems attributed to known GER, that 13 (9 percent) were not improved by successful fundoplication.[4] With apneic spells as the presumed result of known GER, ten of 95 patients (10.5 percent) continued to have apnea after successful fundoplication.

In the group of 144 patients undergoing the Thal fundoplication for chronic respiratory disease, however, there were six patients who required repeat fundoplication (four percent). Additionally, there were three patients (two percent) who had Grade 2 GER in the postoperative study, but who no longer had respiratory symptoms; these three patients were simply followed. These 144 patients were followed for an average of 32 months. These were our most extensively followed patients (4).

Errors of selection occur at about the same rate (4.5 percent) when fundoplication is done with the expectation of preventing apnea as when it is done to cure recurrent croup. These data compare favorably with those of other reported series.[8,12]

Lastly, but not of least importance, are factors of morbidity and economics. The procedure which carries a low morbidity and short hospitalization (at lower cost), all other things being equal, is the superior procedure.

## REFERENCES


1. Ashcraft KW, Goodwin CD, Amoury RA, et al: Thal fundoplication: A simple and safe operative treatment for gastroesophageal reflux. J Pediatr Surg 13:643–647, 1978.
2. Ashcraft KW, Holder TM, Amoury RA: Treatment of gastroesophageal reflux in children by Thal fundoplication. J Thorac Cardiovasc Surg 82:706–712, 1981.

3.  Ashcraft KW, Holder TM, Amoury RA, et al: The Thal fundoplication for gastroesopha-geal reflux. J Pediatr Surg 19:480–483, 1984.

4.  Ashcraft KW, Holder TM, Amoury RA, et al: Fundoplication as treatment for chronic respiratory distress in children, presented at the 7th Annual Gross Symposium. In Press.

5.  DeMeester TR, Johnson LF, Kent AH: Evaluation of current operations for the preven-tion of gastroesophageal reflux. Ann Surg 180:511–525, 1974.

6.  Gavriliu D: Aspects of esophageal surgery. Cur Probl Surg 12:32, 33, 1975.

7.  Harnsberger JK, Corey JJ, Johnson DG, et al: Long-term follow-up of surgery for gastro-esophageal reflux in infants and children. J Pediatr 102:505–508, 1983.

8.  Leape LL, Ramenofsky ML: Surgical treatment of gastroesophageal reflux in children. Am J Dis Child 134:935–938, 1980.

9.  Menguy R: A modified fundoplication which preserves the ability to belch. Surg 84:301–307, 1978.

10.  Skinner D, discussion in Leonardi HK, Lee El-Kurd MF, et al: An experimental study of the effectiveness of various antireflux operations. Ann Thorac Surg 24:215–222, 1977.

11.  Thal AP: A unified approach to surgical problems of the esophagogastric junction. Ann Surg 168:542–550, 1968.

12.  Tunell WP, Smith SI, Carson JA: Gastroesophageal reflux in childhood. Ann Surg 197:560–565, 1983.

Eric W. Fonkalsrud

# 11

# The Role of Surgery in the Treatment of Gastroesophageal Reflux and Gastric Dysmotility Disorders in Childhood

During the past decade, gastroesophageal reflux (GER) has been recognized with increasing frequency in infancy and childhood. Although chalasia is a benign and self-limited cause of repeated emesis in small infants,[3] chronic reflux of gastric contents into the esophagus may be a pernicious cause of malnutrition, growth retardation, recurrent aspiration, pneumonia, asthma, esophagitis, esophageal stricture, and a variety of other symptoms.[9,19] As more sophisticated techniques have been developed to identify children with GER, the condition has been recognized with increasing frequency, particularly in young infants. Although most previous reports on the subject have referred to "hiatus hernia" as the clinical condition requiring operative correction, more recent experience indicates that less than 10 percent of children with symptomatic reflux have radiographically demonstrable hiatus hernia.

The lower esophageal sphincter pressure (LESP) has been considered to be abnormally low in most children with reflux, although the etiology of this is unclear. The normal LESP in infants and children ranges from 15 to 30 mmHg. Periodic increases in intra-abdominal pressure in infants appear to accentuate the symptoms of reflux. Transient elevation of the LESP has been achieved therapeutically by administering cholinergic drugs such as bethanecol and metoclopramide. Histamine antagonists such as cimetidine have a similar effect, although these drugs are not administered safely for long periods of time in infants and children with reflux. With increased recognition in infants and young children of symptomatic reflux which is refractory to medical therapy, a large number of children have been relieved of their symptoms by an antireflux operation, most commonly the gastroesophageal fundoplication (GEF).

During the past few years, delayed gastric emptying has been observed with increasing frequency in children who experience symptoms of GER.[13,15] Using the most sophisticated techniques currently available, including the incorporation of isotopes into solid or semi-solid foods, it is estimated that approximately 50 percent of children with symptomatic reflux may have abnormal gastric emptying. Radionuclide studies with Tc 99m sulfur colloid in feedings of normal consistency for age have made it feasible to determine the magnitude of retention after varying time intervals.[14] Patients with abnormally long gastric retention may benefit from pyloroplasty in combination with or without fundoplication.

It has been noted during the past few years that more than one-third of the children who experience symptomatic GER also have esophageal motility disorders. Children with central nervous system disorders, esophageal atresia, and certain other conditions have been identified as frequently having absent or markedly abnormal propulsive waves in the esophagus. In this circumstance, GER may produce particularly severe symptoms because of the delayed clearance of gastric contents from the esophagus.

The realization that symptomatic GER is frequently accompanied by delayed gastric emptying and/or esophageal dysmotility has led to a careful and comprehensive evaluation of the symptomatic child with the "GER syndrome" in order to select the appropriate medical or surgical treatment.

The present report is based upon the clinical experience at the University of California at Los Angeles (UCLA) Medical Center with 304 infants and children suffering from symptomatic GER, 290 of whom underwent GEF during the years between 1969 and 1985. It has become apparent that predominantly severe gastric dysmotility disorders are best treated by pyloroplasty alone, as in the 14 additional children in this report, whereas those with symptomatic GER and normal gastric emptying should be treated by fundoplication alone. A small group of children with GER has experienced a combination of low LESP and delayed gastric emptying, and thus requires both fundoplication and pyloroplasty.


## CLINICAL EXPERIENCE

During the 16-year period of study, more than 425 children underwent evaluation for GER at the UCLA Medical Center. From this group, 290 children were selected to undergo GER for symptomatic reflux; 14 additional children underwent pyloroplasty alone. Among the 183 male and 121 female patients, 170 (56 percent) were younger than one year of age at the time of operation. The age at operation varied from 12 days to 18 years (median: 10.5 months). A summary of the major symptoms in this group of pediatric patients who underwent GEF is shown in Table 11-1. Repeated emesis was present in almost all patients; 45 percent experienced repeated respiratory infections or pneumonia; and 34 percent had poor growth and were considered as failure to thrive.

Associated medical conditions were present in 157 (54 percent) of the 290 children selected to undergo fundoplication (Table 11-2); six children had two other disorders. Reflux was found in 97 children with neurologic disorders, including 72 with central nervous system damage and/or retardation. An additional 14 children had cerebral palsy. Thus, one-third of the patients who underwent fundoplication had neurologic disorders, five of whom were microcephalic. The majority of these patients

**Table 11-1**

*Major Clinical Symptoms of 290 Children*
*Who Underwent Fundoplication*

| Symptom | Percentage |
|---|---|
| Repeated emesis | 94 |
| Pneumonia or repeated respiratory infections | 46 |
| Failure to thrive | 34 |
| Asthma | 16 |
| Dysphagia caused by stricture | 6 |
| Apnea or near-miss SIDS* | 5 |
| Anemia | 4 |
| Epigastric pain | 2 |

* Sudden infant death syndrome

required assistance with feedings, which was most effectively provided with a feeding gastrostomy. Since children with central nervous system disorders of severe magnitude often have a decreased LESP, it is very common for such patients to aspirate frequently after a feeding gastrostomy is performed. It is therefore the recommended policy in patients at UCLA, as well as in many other hospitals,[6] to perform a GEF at the time of feeding gastrostomy for such patients.

Twenty-two infants and children with previously repaired esophageal atresia and tracheoesophageal fistula experienced repeated reflux and aspiration with pneumonia. One of these children suffered 17 episodes of pneumonia during the seven years after repair of the esophageal atresia before GER was identified. Of these patients, 18 underwent fundoplication during the first three months of life when esophagrams and/or gastrograms (via gastrostomy tubes) showed frequent reflux up to or above the

**Table 11-2**

*Associated Medical Conditions of 290 Children*
*Who Underwent Fundoplication*

| Condition | No. of Cases | |
|---|---|---|
| Central nervous system damage and/or retardation | 72 | |
| Cerebral palsy | 14 | 97 pts. |
| Down's syndrome | 9 | (33% of total) |
| Systemic dysmyotonia | 2 | |
| Esophageal atresia | 22 | |
| Congenital heart disease | 14 | |
| Immunodeficiency | 6 | |
| Achalasia | 5 | |
| Gastroschisis or omphalocele | 4 | |
| Familial dysautonomia | 3 | |
| Other | 12 | |
| Total | 163 | |

esophageal anastomosis. Each of these children also experienced moderate to severe dysmotility in the esophagus between the anastomosis and the lower esophageal sphincter (LES).

A group of 32 children had symptomatic esophagitis, 19 of whom had strictures that produced dysphagia and required dilatation. Among these children, seven had esophageal atresia with severe reflux; seven children with strictures had neurologic disease or brain damage.

Fourteen children had congenital heart anomalies which were not believed to affect the development of reflux; however, the repeated pulmonary aspiration mandated fundoplication to treat the heart defect most safely. Immunodeficiency syndromes with repeated pulmonary infections and reflux were present in six children, and five other children underwent fundoplication concomitant with esophageal myotomy for achalasia. Three children had familial dysautonomia with recurrent pulmonary aspiration. Repeated reflux was experienced in four patients with gastroschisis or omphalocele during the first two years of life, requiring fundoplication.

## DIAGNOSTIC STUDIES

Although various tests have been used to document GER in children with symptoms, 24-hour esophageal pH monitoring has consistently been the most efficient study (Table 11-3). This study was 100-percent accurate in diagnosing GER when the pH in the esophagus was four or below for more than five percent of the total time monitored.[7] In patients with severe symptomatic reflux, an esophageal pH study of eight– 12 hours was adequate to confirm the diagnosis. In patients who have recurrent pulmonary infections, asthma, or a variety of other conditions in which frequent severe emesis is a less prominent symptom, the 24-hour esophageal pH record has been invaluable. This procedure is performed without sedation and usually includes overnight hospitalization when a 24-hour analysis is desired. The esophageal pH study should be performed with the patient awake, asleep, upright, and reclining. Measurement of the total number of reflux episodes, the number of episodes of low pH exceeding five minutes, and the duration of the longest single episode, combined with the total percentage of time that the esophageal pH is low, will determine if the study is diagnostic of reflux.

GER was demonstrated by a thin barium esophagram with slight pressure applied to the abdomen in 85 percent of the children who underwent operation. Only 12 children had roentgenographic evidence of a hiatus hernia.

**Table 11-3**
*Procedures Diagnostic of Pathologic Reflux*
*(evaluation of 425 children)*

| Test | Positive Results |
| --- | --- |
| 24-hour esophageal pH monitoring | 98% |
| Thin barium esophagram | 85% |
| Esophageal manometry (LESP) | 61% |
| Technetium scintigraphy | 60% |
| Esophagoscopy (esophagitis) | 32% |

Esophageal manometric studies were considered abnormal in 61 percent of the children undergoing fundoplication in whom the study was performed, as evidenced by an LESP of less than 14 mmHg. Gross esophagitis was demonstrated by esophagoscopy in 19 percent of children who were studied. Esophageal biopsy specimens showed microscopic evidence of esophagitis in the presence of grossly normal-appearing mucosa in 13 percent of children who underwent endoscopy.

The demonstration of the radioactive marker technetium in the lung by scintigraphic studies following ingestion of milk containing the isotope led to the positive diagnosis of reflux in 60 percent of the children on whom the study was performed. This study was most frequently positive in children who had central nervous system disorders.

## GASTRIC EMPTYING DISORDERS

Gastric emptying as measured by the radionuclide marker Tc 99m sulfur colloid incorporated into liquid, solid, or mixed solid and liquid meals was abnormal in 48 percent of the children examined. The marker is nontoxic and nonabsorbable from the stomach and does not alter the osmolality of the gastric contents. The marker is homogeneously distributed in the meal, in particle form, comparable with that of normal food for the appropriate age patient (in formula for infants; cereals for toddlers;

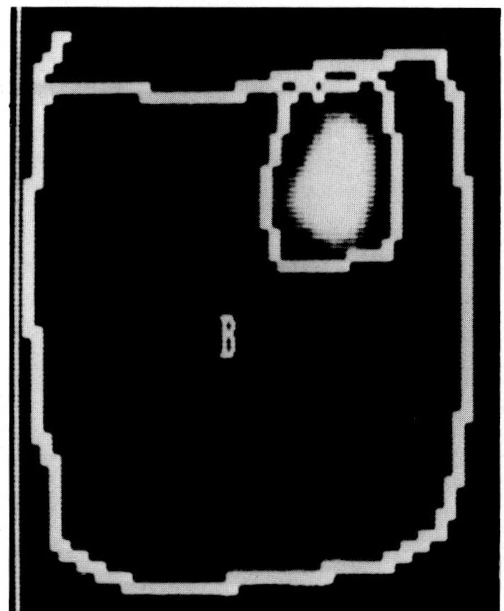
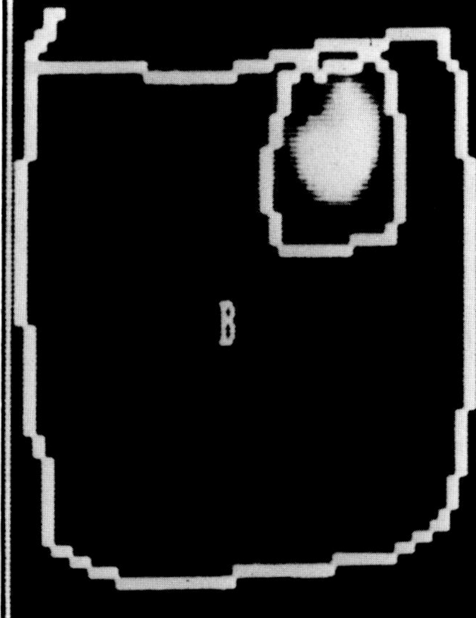

**Figure 11-1.**   Radionuclide gastric emptying study in an infant with antral dysmotility syndrome showing 96 percent retention of a labeled milk meal at 60 minutes. More than 50-percent retention is considered abnormal. From: Mulvihill S, Fonkalsrud EW: Pyloroplasty in infancy and childhood. J Pediatr Surg 18:930–936, 1983. With permission.

sandwiches for older patients). If more than 50 percent of the marker is retained in the stomach at 60 minutes, the study is considered abnormal. In 14 patients younger than three years, gastric retention of the isotope marker and meal exceeded 80 percent in 90 minutes and was considered sufficiently abnormal to warrant pyloroplasty alone (Fig. 11-1). In each of these patients, the LESP was normal or elevated, none being lower than 28 mmHg. The 24-hour esophageal pH record was also only mildly abnormal in these 14 young children. The pylorus was not obstructed or considered abnormal in any of these patients. Pyloroplasty alone was performed in each of these children, nine of whom are believed to have the antral dysmotility syndrome.[7]

In 18 children, the gastric emptying study and the 24-hour lower esophageal pH monitoring were both abnormal. The LESP was also low in each of these patients. Each of these 18 children (median age: 16 months) underwent GEF and pyloroplasty. In eight of these patients, the pyloroplasty was performed at a second operation when the patient continued to experience delayed gastric emptying after fundoplication which was verified by delayed clearance of isotope from the stomach.

An upper gastrointestinal series identified congenital anomalies of the duodenum in four patients, including congenital web or diaphragm and malrotation during the evaluation for reflux; each patient was treated by repair of the anomaly rather than by fundoplication or pyloroplasty.


## ESOPHAGEAL DYSMOTILITY

Esophageal dysmotility was identified in 36 percent of the children studied and was characterized by abnormal peristalsis as measured by a 5-lumen tube that records pressures at five-mm intervals in the lower esophagus. Eight children had abnormal motor transit of a liquid bolus on esophageal scintiscan. Dysmotility was present in each of the 22 children who had esophageal atresia and reflux, as well as in most patients with neurologic disorders. The presence of esophageal dysmotility did not appear to correlate with abnormal gastric emptying in the children studied.


## MANAGEMENT

After the diagnosis of GER without gastric outlet obstruction, each child underwent a trial of medical therapy before the decision for operation was made. For infants, this included upright positioning at approximately a 60° angle in an infant seat designed for this purpose. Frequent, low-volume feedings were given to those who were vomiting and failing to thrive. For older children, the head of the bed was elevated at least eight inches. Patients were instructed not to eat for at least two hours prior to bedtime. When esophagitis was documented, cimetidine or antacids were given as necessary. Bethanecol and/or metaclopramide or other medications that increase the LESP were tried in more than 45 percent of patients who eventually were selected for operation. These drugs were rarely effective in permanent relief of severe reflux. Children with recurrent pneumonia and/or aspiration were selected for early operation; those with asthma were selected for operation only after carefully documenting the presence of reflux by 24-hour esophageal pH testing and by evidence of reflux on esophagram. Prolonged medical therapy was not employed for any child who had symptomatic esophageal stricture.

## OPERATIVE TECHNIQUE

Each of the 290 children with GER underwent a transabdominal Nissen fundoplication under general anesthesia.[9,18] A rubber nasogastric catheter was passed in order to decompress the stomach and facilitate mobilization of the esophagus. Bougies were not placed in the esophagus. An upper midline abdominal surgical incision provided excellent exposure in infants and children, even for patients who had undergone previous transthoracic repair. After mobilization of the left lobe of the liver from the diaphragm, the gastrocolic ligament along the upper third of the greater curvature of the stomach was divided, as were the short gastric vessels. The peritoneum was incised on each side of the esophagus and a plane was developed around the esophagus by blunt dissection; the vagus nerves and major branches were preserved. In no case was it necessary to remove the spleen. The dissection did not extend below the cardioesophageal junction on the lesser curvature in order to avoid injuring the hepatic branches of the vagus nerve. The esophagus was mobilized over a distance of 2.5–4.0 cm. In no instance was a short esophagus identified in which an adequate length could not be obtained for repair below the diaphragm. The crura of the diaphragm were approximated posterior to the esophagus with one–two nonabsorbable sutures with one stitch attached to the esophagus. A "wraparound" was made from two to three cm in length, depending on the size of the patient. Initially, small bites of esophageal muscularis were included in the repair to prevent slippage of the wraparound; however, with the last 210 patients, this step was omitted in favor of placing two–four sutures between the upper edge of the wraparound and the diaphragm near the hiatus. A large clamp was placed between the wraparound and the esophagus during the repair to assure that the fundoplication was loose. Although the fundoplication was placed around the intra-abdominal esophagus, it was not specifically intended to increase the LESP. The mean increase in LESP after surgery was only 5.5 mmHg in those patients in whom the study was performed.

All patients younger than three years underwent a tube gastrostomy, as did many of the older children, in order to facilitate postoperative feeding, reduce the incidence of gas bloat, and to serve as a modified gastropexy. The gastrostomy was removed in the majority of patients within three weeks. In 69 patients who had feeding disorders, central nervous system damage, and/or esophageal dysmotility, however, the tubes were left in for longer periods in order to facilitate feedings. Moreover, in nine of the patients with stricture, the tubes were retained in order to permit postoperative dilatation. Except for occasional mild skin irritation around the tube, no complications developed from the gastrostomy tube in any patient, and only four have required surgical closure of the gastrostomy wound (all after six months).

None of the patients with esophageal strictures caused by reflux have experienced complications caused by postoperative dilatations, and none have required subsequent esophageal resection. Moreover, only seven of the 22 children with esophageal atresia required dilatation of anastomotic strictures subsequent to fundoplication.

## RESULTS OF OPERATION

Two of the 290 children who underwent fundoplication died during the first three weeks after operation (Table 11-4), one of whom had familial dysautonomia and suffered a severe dysautonomic crisis ending in death four days later. The other patient had undergone repair of gastroschisis at another hospital after birth and had experienced necrosis of a large segment of small intestine after complete repair of the defect. She subsequently required total parenteral nutrition and developed superior vena caval obstruction as well as bilateral pleural effusions. Gastrostomy feedings were followed by massive GER. A fundoplication was performed to permit enteric feedings, since the intravenous routes for alimentation were not available. This patient died three weeks after operation. Seven additional patients have died of the underlying disease at times ranging from one month to three years after fundoplication.

Seven children developed posterior paraesophageal hernias extending into the mediastinum that caused dysphagia and recurrent symptoms of emesis and aspiration. In six of the patients, the crura had not been approximated posterior to the esophagus. Each of these patients required reoperation, with repair of the crura and tightening of the fundoplication.

Frequent use of the gastrostomy tube in infants and young children who were often aerophagic after operation provided easy egress for swallowed air. Nonetheless, six patients who had gastric dysmotility experienced transient gas bloat syndrome after the gastrostomy was removed, two of whom eventually underwent secondary pyloroplasty. Two patients may have experienced mild injury to the vagus nerves during operation. The majority of patients were able to eructate within four weeks after operation; however, none has evidenced clinical recurrence of reflux except for those with paraesophageal hernia. In addition to those with severe neurologic disorders, seven children experienced transient dysphagia from five days to two weeks after surgery during the early phase of the study when the fundoplication was made somewhat tighter than it was later. Persistent delay in gastric emptying was believed to be due to a primary gastric dysmotility disorder in six patients after fundoplication, each of whom required subsequent pyloroplasty.

Table 11-4

*Complications Following Fundoplication*
*(290 children)*

| Complication | Number |
| --- | --- |
| Deaths (within 3 weeks) | 2 |
| Deaths (late due to underlying disease) | 7 |
| Postoperative paraesophageal hernia | 7 |
| Gas bloat syndrome | 6 |
| Transient dysphagia | 7 |
| Delayed gastric emptying | 14 |
| X-ray recurrenct of reflux | 10 |
| Wound infection | 6 |
| Pulmonary infection or atelectasis | 24 |
| Intestinal adhesions | 6 |

Of the 290 children treated, 24 developed pulmonary infection and/or atelectasis during the early postoperative period, requiring extra measures for clearing pulmonary secretions and requiring prolonged use of antibiotics. Each of these patients had experienced repeated pulmonary infections and/or asthma before operation.

Wound infection developed in six patients. Six children developed intestinal adhesions requiring laparotomy, one of whom required resection of a segment of small intestine. Small intestinal herniation behind the gastrostomy had caused obstruction in two of these patients; care is taken at the time of operation to interpose the transverse colon between the small intestine and gastrostomy.

Repeated vomiting was relieved in each of the 273 patients in whom this was a major preoperative symptom (Table 11-5). Of the 133 infants and children with recurrent pulmonary disease, 125 were either markedly improved or were cured of the pulmonary symptoms. All but five of the 46 children with asthma experienced considerable relief of symptoms and six others who had been receiving high-dose asthmatic medications are no longer receiving continuous therapy. Of the 99 infants with failure to thrive, each demonstrated catch-up growth (in some cases spectacular) during the first six months subsequent to operation. One infant gained 10.5 pounds in three months after operation, although he had gained only 3.5 pounds during the first nine months of life.

Each of the 19 patients with esophageal strictures due to esophagitis or after anastomosis was relieved or required only occasional dilatations after fundoplication.

Dysphagia was relieved in three of five patients who underwent esophageal myotomy in combination with fundoplication for achalasia.

The majority of children with neurologic disorders required feeding gastrostomies and concomitant fundoplication. Sixty-nine of the children were considered long-term gastrostomy feeders.

Follow-up esophagrams were obtained in 162 of the 290 patients from two months to 12 years postoperatively. In ten patients, esophagram showed a trace of reflux into the lower third of the esophagus within one year after operation, although each of the patients was asymptomatic. No reoperations were required for recurrent reflux in the absence of a paraesophageal hernia.

Similarly, postoperative lower esophageal pH monitoring performed on patients from six weeks to six years postoperatively has shown reflux in only eight patients, six of whom had paraesophageal hernia requiring reoperation. In the other two patients,

**Table 11-5**

*Results Following Fundoplication (290 children)*

| Result | No. Relieved/No. with Symptoms |
|---|---|
| Relief of reflux symptoms | 273/273 |
| Relieved or cured of pulmonary symptoms | 125/133 |
| Weight gain in "failure to thrive" patients | 99/99 |
| Improvement in asthmatic symptoms | 41/46 |
| Relief of strictures | 19/19 |
| Relief of dysphagia in achalasia patients | 3/5 |
| Long-term gastrostomy feeders | 6/9 |

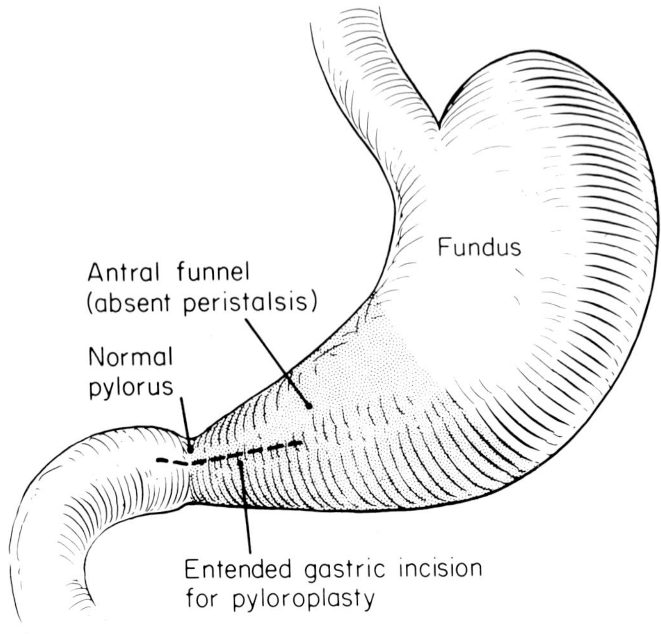


**Figure 11-2.** In infants and children with severe delay in gastric emptying who do not respond to medical management, a two-layer Heineke-Mikulicz pyloroplasty is constructed with approximately 75 percent of the vertical incision made through the antrum. From: Mulvihill S, Fonkalsrud EW: Pyloroplasty in infancy and childhood. J Pediatr Surg 18:930–936, 1983. With permission.

the reflux was much milder than that noted before operation, and the clinical symptoms were sufficiently mild to indicate that reoperation was unnecessary. In each of the 31 patients who underwent pyloroplasty with or without fundoplication, the symptoms of reflux and gastric stasis were relieved. Four of the patients developed transient diarrhea believed to stem from dumping; however, in no patient did these symptoms persist beyond three weeks after surgery. A Heineke-Mikulicz pyloroplasty was performed in each of the patients, with the incision extending over two-thirds of its distance onto the antrum and less than one-third of its distance onto the duodenum (Fig. 11-2). A two-layer suture repair was used in each case. None of the patients experienced pyloric leak or obstruction after operation.

## DISCUSSION

Infants with symptomatic GER may benefit transiently, and in many cases permanently, from medical therapy consisting of the use of thickened feedings, keeping the infant in a semi-upright position, and the use of bethanecol or metoclopramide to increase the LESP, in addition to other measures. It is evident, however, that prolonged medical therapy for the majority of infants with symptomatic reflux may be more time-consuming and expensive, as well as less likely to produce relief of symptoms, than is an antireflux operation. There has been an increasing trend, as evidenced by UCLA clinical experience and that of Ashcraft et al.,[1,2] Johnson and Jolley,[11] Tunnell et al.,[21] and others, to recognize symptomatic GER that is unresponsive to medical therapy in infants. More than 50 percent of antireflux operations performed in the pediatric age group are carried out in those younger than one year. The antireflux operation provides prompt relief of the severe and disabling symptoms of growth failure, repeated pulmonary infections, esophagitis, etc., in more than 95 percent of cases, and is associated with an operative mortality rate of less than 0.4 percent and a morbidity rate of less than seven percent.

Although various techniques have been used to identify symptomatic reflux, it was not until continuous 24-hour lower esophageal pH monitoring became widely used that a standard and easily reproducible technique was available.[8] For patients with severe symptomatic reflux, only six–eight hours of esophageal pH monitoring may be necessary to establish the diagnosis; however, in infants with more insidious symptoms, measurement of esophageal pH during sleep, in the upright and supine positions, and after feedings over a 24-hour period is most helpful. When the lower esophageal pH decreases to four or lower for more than five percent of the time the patient is monitored, the patient with symptomatic reflux is considered to have symptoms severe enough to warrant a fundoplication. The esophageal pH monitor has also served as the most reliable technique for determining the success of the antireflux operation months or years later.[4]

Although the LESP is helpful in identifying severe symptomatic reflux when the pressure is lower than 15 mmHg, more than 60 percent of patients undergoing fundoplication in the present series had an LESP in the normal range. Similarly, esophagoscopy is much less likely in children to show esophagitis either grossly or microscopically than it is in adults with reflux, and esophagoscopy is therefore usually only confirmatory in infants and young children with severe symptoms who have abnormal esophageal pH.

The transabdominal Nissen fundoplication is technically easier and less traumatic to the child than is transthoracic repair.[9,19] The tightness of the fundoplication is determined most safely and easily by inserting a clamp beneath the wraparound and opening gently rather than by inserting a bougie down the esophagus. Since in the UCLA experience the incidence of esophageal dysmotility in children undergoing fundoplication approximates 40 percent, it is imperative that the operation avoid constricting the gastroesophageal junction and/or increasing the LESP. The average increase in LESP in more than 50 patients measured both before and after operation has not exceeded 5.5 mmHg. The loose wraparound has permitted more than 60 percent of patients to burp within a few weeks after surgery. The fundoplication appears to prevent reflux by placing a nipple valve between the stomach and esophagus. Similar success in relieving reflux symptoms in children has been reported by Ashcraft et al.,[1,2] using the Thal fundoplication.

Inasmuch as one of the most serious and common complications subsequent to fundoplication is development of a paraesophageal hernia, it is essential to approximate the crura posterior to the esophagus and, if possible, to position the entire repair within the abdomen. Nonetheless, in the two patients in whom a portion of the fundoplication extended above the diaphragm, the symptoms of reflux were relieved. In the group of 290 operations for reflux, no patient was found to have an esophagus so short that transabdominal repair was not feasible. Paraesophageal hernia was recognized in 12 of 191 patients undergoing Nissen fundoplication by Bettex and Kuffer[5] and in ten of 117 patients reported by Tunnell et al.[21] In patients with asthma, cystic fibrosis, or chronic pulmonary disease, particular attention should be directed toward constructing a strong repair of the crura. In three of the patients with paraesophageal hernia, the sutures in the fundic wrap separated with partial dissolution of the fundoplication, most likely due to tension on the sutures associated with frequent coughing, when the stomach and wraparound slipped into the mediastinum, as observed by Randolph.[19] When a paraesophageal hernia develops, it is likely to increase in severity and to exert pressure against the lower esophagus, causing both dysphagia and recurrece of reflux. Transabdominal repair shortly after establishing the diagnosis is recommended, approximating the crura with several nonabsorbable sutures, and, when necessary, attaching the repair to the median arcuate ligament.

The relationship of gastric dysmotility to GER has been clarified only recently as a result of the radionuclide techniques introduced in 1966 by Griffith et al.,[10] who used $CR^{51}$ mixed with porridge. Since most clinically significant gastric motility disorders alter the emptying of solids more than that of liquids, combining Tc 99m sulfur colloid into hepatic Kupffer cells has provided a technique for evaluating emptying of solids, and is now considered the most accurate test for diagnosing gastric motility disorders.[13,17] Children who retain more than 50 percent of the isotope feedings in the stomach after 90 minutes are considered to have gastric dysmotility. These children do not have pyloric stenosis. Currently available information is insufficient to indicate how long gastric dysmotility will persist in the infant or young child; however, if the patient is symptomatic and does not improve with medical therapy, it is the opinion of the UCLA group that pyloroplasty alone should be performed, as in 14 of the UCLA patients. It is estimated that at least ten percent of children with symptomatic reflux sufficiently severe to warrant operation will require pyloroplasty (10.5 percent in the present series). If the 24-hour esophageal pH monitor shows reflux and if the LESP is low, it is advisable to perform a concomitant fundoplication (as was done in 18 of the 304 children). If the patient has moderate to severe gastric dysmotility and moderate reflux on esophageal pH monitoring but normal LESP, it is difficult to determine whether a concomitant fundoplication is necessary. Similarly, if the child has severe reflux with borderline gastric dysmotility, it is difficult to determine whether a concomitant pyloroplasty should be performed with fundoplication. Further refinements of the diagnostic studies may be helpful in answering these questions in the future. In six patients from the present clinical experience, it was necessary to perform a pyloroplasty at a second operation after fundoplication. The antral dysmotility syndrome as described by Byrne et al.[7] appears to be an extreme variant of gastric dysmotility disorders seen in patients younger than one year of age. Although many such patients may be treated successfully with metoclopramide and continuous feedings, approximately half will eventually require pyloroplasty. It is likely that many children who have undergone fundoplication performed for reflux, but who have experienced symptoms of gas bloat and poor feeding postoperatively, may have gastric dysmotility disorders, and have a type of closed-loop obstruction. An algorithm has been developed to assist in defining which patients with symptomatic reflux will benefit from which type of operation (Fig. 11-3).

As noted previously,[9] esophageal stricture due to esophagitis or after repair of esophageal atresia dilates far more easily after successful fundoplication than before. Only eight of the 19 children in the present clinical experience required one or more

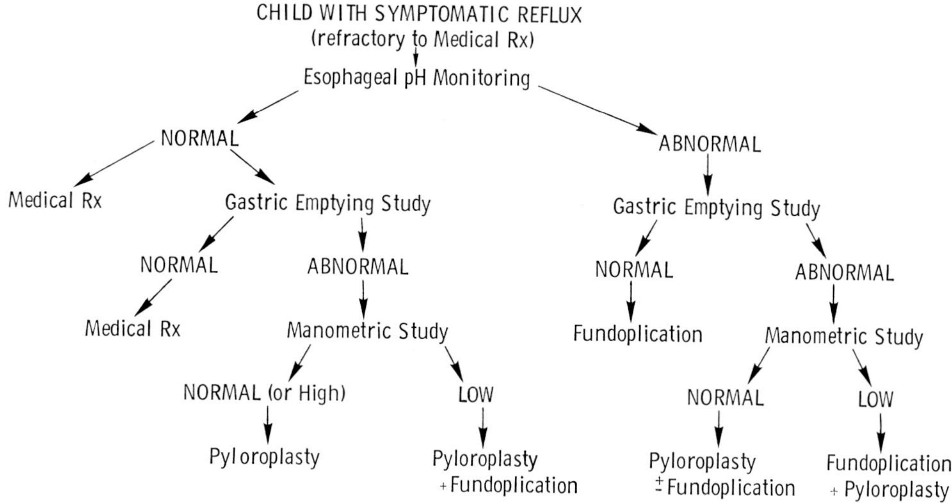


**Figure 11-3.**    Algorithm indicating the diagnostic studies which are most helpful in determining which children with symptomatic reflux may benefit from GEF alone, pyloroplasty alone, or both procedures.

dilatations of strictures subsequent to fundoplication. The incidence of significant reflux after repair of esophageal atresia is higher than 60 percent in patients from the UCLA Medical Center, and is similar to that reported by others.[16] Jolley et al.[12] have observed that tension on the esophageal anastomosis may correlate with the high incidence of reflux after repair of esophageal atresia; delayed gastric emptying is also common in these patients. The close correlation between delayed gastric emptying and abnormal esophageal motor function in patients with reflux has been observed by Velasco et al.[23] and others. Russell et al[20] have shown that radionuclide screening serves as a sensitive test for esophageal motor dysfunction, and corroborates the results obtained by serial esophageal pressure studies.

As noted by Byrne et al.,[6] retarded infants and children are likely to experience recurrent GER and aspiration with growth failure. Vane et al.[22] have demonstrated that the LESP is lowered after acute and chronic brain injury. Many of these patients have abnormal esophageal motility patterns. The large number of patients in the present review (33 percent) with chronic central nervous system disorders and severe reflux who were treated by fundoplication and gastrostomy corroborates the view that these procedures will greatly benefit these patients with respect to chronic care. If a feeding gastrostomy is necessary in a brain-damaged child, a concomitant fundoplication is advisable to avoid subsequent reflux when feedings are administered.

## REFERENCES


1.    Ashcraft KW, Holder TM, Amoury RA, et al: The Thal fundoplication for gastroesophageal reflux. J Pediatr Surg 19:480–483, 1984.
2.    Ashcraft KW, Holder TM, Amoury RA: Treatment of gastroesophageal fistula in children by Thal fundoplication. J Thorac Cardiovasc Surg 82:706–712, 1981.

3. Berenberg W, Neuhauser EBD: Cardioesophageal relaxation (chalasia) as a cause of vomiting in infants. Pediatrics 5:414–418, 1950.

4. Berquist WM, Fonkalsrud EW, Ament ME: Effectiveness of Nissen fundoplication for gastroesophageal reflux in children as measured by 24-hour intraesophageal pH monitoring. J Pediatr Surg 16:872–875, 1981.

5. Bettex M, Kuffer F: Long-term results of fundoplication in hiatus hernia and cardioesophageal chalasia in infants and children. Report of 112 consecutive cases. J Pediatr Surg 4:526–530, 1969.

6. Byrne WJ, Euler AR, Ashcraft E, et al: Gastroesophageal reflux in the severely retarded who vomit: Criteria for and results of surgical intervention in 22 patients. Surgery 91:95–98, 1982.

7. Byrne WJ, Kangarloo H, Ament ME, et al: Antral dysmotility: An unrecognized cause of chronic vomiting during infancy. Ann Surg 193:521–524, 1981.

8. DeMeester TR, Johnson LF: Evaluation of Nissen anti-reflux procedure by esophageal manometry and 24-hour pH monitoring. Am J Surg 129:94–98, 1975.

9. Fonkalsrud EW, Ament ME, Byrne WJ, et al; Gastroesophageal fundoplication for the management of reflux in infants and children. J Thorac Cardiovasc Surg 76:655–660, 1978.

10. Griffith GH, Owen GM, Kirkman S, et al: Measurement of rate of gastric emptying using chromium-51. Lancet 1:1244–1245, 1966.

11. Johnson DG, Jolley SG: Gastroesophageal reflux in infants and children: Recognition and treatment. Surg Clin N Am 61:1101–1115, 1981.

12. Jolley SG, Johnson DG, Roberts CC, et al: Patterns of gastroesophageal reflux in children following repair of esophageal atresia and distal tracheoesophageal fistula. J Pediatr Surg 15:857–862, 1980.

13. McCallum RW, Berkowitz DM, Lerner E: Gastric emptying in patients with gastroesophageal reflux. Gastroenterology 80:285–291, 1981.

14. Meyer JH, MacGregor IL, Gueller R, et al: 99mTC-tagged chicken liver as a marker of solid food in the human stomach. Am J Dis Child 21:296–304, 1976.

15. Mulvihill S, Fonkalsrud EW: Pyloroplasty in infancy and childhood. J Pediatr Surg 18:930–936, 1983.

16. Parker AF, Christie DL, Cahill JL: Incidence and significance of gastroesophageal reflux following repair of esophageal atresia and tracheoesophageal fistula and the need for antireflux procedures. J Pediatr Surg 14:5–8, 1979.

17. Pellegrini CA, Broderick WC, VanDyke D, et al: Diagnosis and treatment of gastric emptying. Am J Surg 145:143–151, 1983.

18. Randolph JG: Experience with the Nissen fundoplication for correction of gastroesophageal reflux in infants. Ann Surg 198:579–584, 1983.

19. Randolph JG, Lilly JR, Anderson KD: Surgical treatment of gastroesophageal reflux in infants. Ann Surg 180:479–483, 1974.

20. Russell COH, Hill LD, Holmes ER, et al: Radionuclide transit: A sensitive screening test for esophageal dysfunction. Gastroenterology 80:887–892, 1981.

21. Tunnell WP, Smith ER, Carson JA: Gastroesophageal reflux in childhood: The dilemma of surgical success. Ann Surg 197:560–565, 1983.

22. Vane DW, Shiffler M, Grosfeld JL, et al: Reduced lower esophageal sphincter (LES) pressure after acute and chronic brain injury. J Pediatr Surg 17:960–963, 1982.

23. Velasco N, Hill LD, Gannan RM, et al: Gastric emptying and gastroesophageal reflux: Effects of surgery and correlation with esophageal motor function. Am J Surg 144:58–62, 1982.

Keith W. Ashcraft

# 12

# Vascular Ring

Anomalies of the aorta and the great vessels which arise from it may be the cause of dysphagia by compression or constriction of the esophagus. These lesions had been described at autopsy more than 200 years prior to Gross' first successful division of a vascular ring in 1945.[8] These anomalies are estimated to affect nearly three percent of the population,[16] although only a few of them are symptomatic; because they some-times present as esophageal obstruction, they are included in this text.

The most constricting of the lesions are the complete vascular rings formed by a double aortic arch. There are various forms of open or incomplete rings formed by an aberrant vessel in combination with a patent ductus or ligamentum arteriosus. The open rings may also produce symptoms by compression of the trachea or esophagus but are not as likely to be symptomatic as are the complete rings.

## SYMPTOMS

The symptoms of vascular ring may be respiratory or esophageal. Stridor, retrac-tion, and repeated infections are the usual respiratory symptoms. An affected child may develop severe respiratory distress at times of stress or crying. The opistho-tonic position is sometimes assumed by the child because this seems to provide some relief from the respiratory obstruction. Dysphagia, coughing, or choking with ingestion of foods are the usual esophageal signs and symptoms of vascular ring abnormalities.

Each of the five vascular ring abnormalities shall be described in turn.

Pediatric Esophageal Surgery
ISBN 0-8089-1776-5



231

## EMBRYOLOGY

The aortic arch and great vessels develop from the gill arch arteries, of which there are six pair. Normal formation of the aortic arch requires resorption of the right portion of the paired dorsal aortas with remolding of the right subclavian and common carotid from the right fourth arch, and the ventral and dorsal aortas which adjoin it. The right innominate is the first great vessel off the arch. The left common carotid is the second branch off the arch of the aorta and the left subclavian the final vessel off the arch. These latter two vessels result from the anterior portion of the left ventral aortic root and the left third arch. A double aortic arch results when the resorption of the right dorsal aorta fails to occur.[7] If both arches persist, the right is generally the larger of the two. Usually, the posterior portion of the left arch behind the takeoff of the left subclavian and in front of the ligamentum or ductus arteriosus is the narrowest portion. Division of this left arch should be done at its narrowest position.

## DOUBLE AORTIC ARCH (Fig. 12-1)

Seventy-five percent of double aortic arch malformations are symptomatic.[11,12] Stridor and opisthotonos are common airway manifestations of double aortic arch. Dysphagia is always present if sought. It is because a "complete" work-up for stridor in any child includes a barium esophagram that the double aortic arch is often discovered as a result of evaluation for respiratory symptoms.

Radiographically, the double aortic arch vascular ring should be suspected when

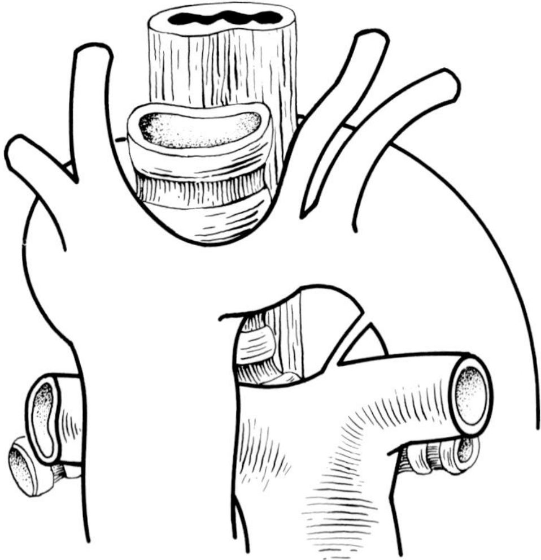

**Figure 12-1.** The most symptomatic of the vascular rings involving the aorta is the double aortic arch. In addition to a patent ductus or ligamentum arteriosus, the left arch forms a constricting ring around the trachea and esophagus. Almost always the right arch is the larger of the two and division of the ring therefore should be done at the narrowest point in the left arch. This lesion is best approached via a left thoracotomy.

a right aortic arch is present on the plain chest roentgenogram.[5,17] The barium study, however, is the definitive diagnostic test and reveals a posterior indentation of the esophagus above the level of the carina with offset of the longitudinal axis of the esophagus in the frontal projection (Fig. 12-2).[12] This posterior indentation is also seen with an aberrant subclavian artery crossing behind the esophagus. Angiography is really not very helpful either in making the diagnosis or planning the operative approach, except when the predominant arch is on the left.[5] Endoscopy, if performed, will reveal a pulsatile narrowing in the trachea with indentation, usually anteriorly and laterally and in the esophagus posteriorly. Pulsation may be felt when the esophagoscope passes over the posterior arch.

## SURGICAL TREATMENT

Surgical division of the double aortic arch is indicated whenever the diagnosis is established, even though symptoms may be minimal.[1] Prolonged compression of the trachea by a vascular ring will produce tracheomalacia, which often will complicate the postoperative course.[5] It is sometimes necessary to dissect the trachea and esophagus from the inside of the vascular ring in order to allow expansion of the ring. Occasionally, it is necessary to suture the anterior component of the divided ring to the underside of the sternum in order to relieve pressure upon the softened tracheal cartilages. Experience with 13 patients having a double aortic arch revealed that five had a patent ductus arteriosus, while the remaining eight had a ligamentum arteriosus. Patent or not, this structure requires division in most patients. Only one of these 13 patients had a right-sided descending aorta. All were operatively approached via a left thoracotomy. The site of division of the vascular ring was proximal to the left common carotid in one patient, while in 12 the site of division was posterior to the origin of the left subclavian. There were no deaths from the operative procedure or in the postoper-

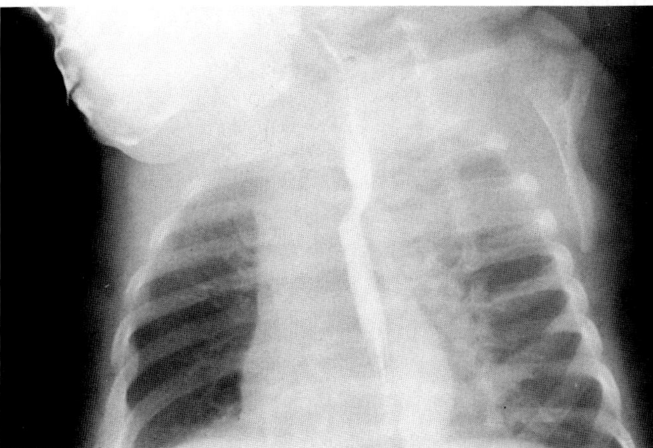

**Figure 12-2.** The barium esophagram in a child with a double aortic arch is shown. The longitudinal axis of the esophagus is offset, which distinguishes the double aortic arch from other aberrant vessels which impinge upon the esophagus.

ative period. The median age at division was three months (range: one–108 months). Late sequellae from division of a vascular ring are rare.[15]

## INCOMPLETE RINGS

An incomplete vascular ring is formed by: (1) a right-sided aortic arch with left-sided ductus arteriosus with left-sided descending aorta; (2) a left aortic arch with an aberrant right subclavian artery; (3) a right aortic arch with an aberrant left subclavian artery and ligamentum or ductus arteriosus; or, (4) the so-called pulmonary vascular sling or aberrant left pulmonary artery.

The incidence of a right-sided aortic arch with left-sided ductus arteriosus and left descending aorta is impossible to determine (Fig. 12-3). In the majority of these patients, the aorta crosses behind the esophagus, but the ligamentum forming the left lateral portion of the ring is not short enough to constrict the airway or the esophagus. The predominant symptom in this group of patients is dysphagia from the posteriorly compressing aortic arch. The presentation of this form of vascular ring is often subtle because it is an open ring. The author's group has treated three patients suffering from this malformation over the last 13 years, two of whom also had ventricular septal defects which required open patch repairs at another operation. All were approached operatively through a left thoracotomy with division of the ligamentum arteriosus in two patients and the ductus arteriosus in the other patient. One patient died from an exsanguinating hemorrhage; she had previously undergone patch closure of her ventricular septal defect. When the vascular ring was approached through a left thoraco-

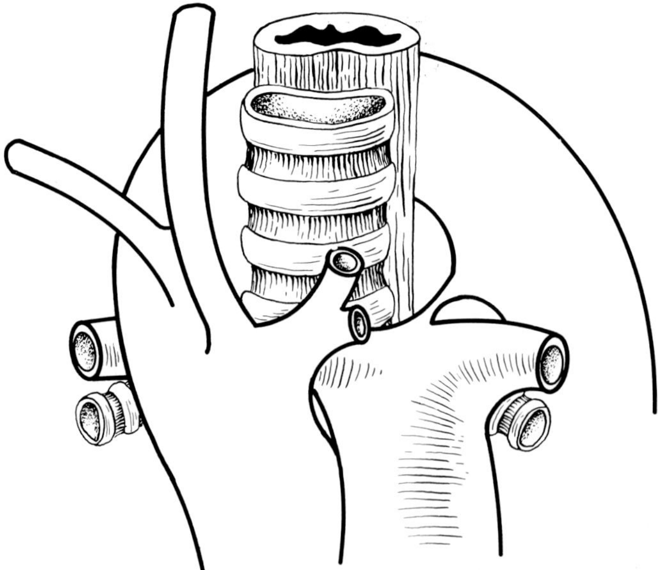

**Figure 12-3.**   The right-sided aortic arch and left descending aorta with ductus or ligamentum is sketched. This lesion is often not very symptomatic. Its treatment consists of division of the ligamentum arteriosus or patent ductus arteriosus.

tomy, the ligamentum was divided. Edema in the anterior mediastinum prompted dissection in this area, which resulted in uncontrollable hemorrhage from a pseudoaneurysm at the aortic cannulation site used for cardiopulmonary bypass.

An aberrant right subclavian artery coming behind the esophagus from a left-sided aorta is the most common form of vascular ring abnormality (Fig. 12-4). It is estimated to occur in more than one percent of the United States population. Instead of arising from the innominate artery, the right subclavian arises as the most distal vessel from the arch. It crosses the mediastinum behind the esophagus, producing its symptoms by posterior compression. Since there is no ligamentum on the right side except in the exceedingly rare instance,[10] most of these patients are asymptomatic.[4] The term dysphagia lusoria was established to characterize this specific group of patients.

The diagnosis is established by barium esophagram, which shows an oblique indentation of the esophagus from below upward toward the right axilla. The long axis of the esophagus above and below the indentation, however, is continuous—as opposed to the double aortic arch, where an offset is almost always the case. It is sometimes difficult to postulate that the slight amount of indentation on the back wall of the esophagus can be the cause of significant dysphagia. Many surgeons do not expect a great symptomatic improvement from the division of an aberrant right subclavian artery.[4]

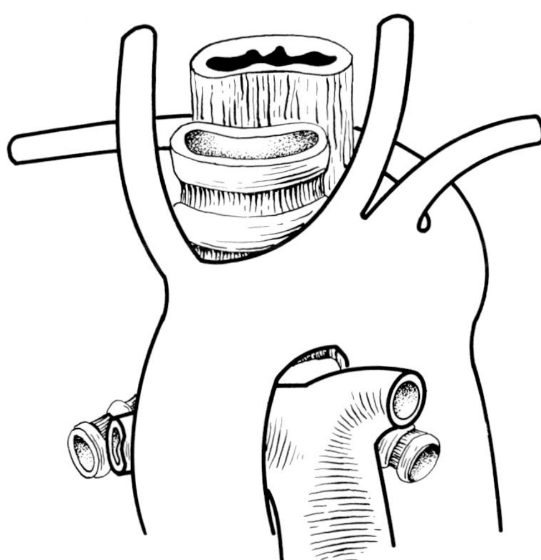

**Figure 12-4.** The right common carotid comes off of the left side of the aortic arch with the left common carotid and left subclavian being the next two vessels. The final vessel to come off the descending aorta is the right subclavian, which crosses behind the esophagus. This is the most common and the most open of the vascular rings; it is therefore least likely to produce symptoms. The operative approach is division of the subclavian artery behind the esophagus done through a right thoracotomy. Both ends of the subclavian artery are oversewn. Blood supply to the right arm thereafter is by way of collateral vessels.

Surgical treatment consists of a right thoracotomy with division and suture of the aberrant subclavian artery as far behind the esophagus as possible. It is not necessary in the pediatric patient to re-establish flow through this vessel by anastomosis to the innominate artery or to the ascending aorta, because collateral circulation will certainly keep the arm well vascularized. In the adult patient, particularly the older adult patient in whom atherosclerosis may be prevalent, re-establishment of vascular continuity by anastomosis is recommended. One patient has been reported to have developed subclavian steal syndrome long after division of the subclavian artery.[14]

The author's group has divided this aberrant vessel in two patients in 13 years. There was marked relief of the dysphagia following operation.

It is unusual to see a right aortic arch, right descending aorta, anomalous left subclavian with left ductus (Fig. 12-5). This anomaly produces more obstruction than does the left arch, aberrant right subclavian because the ring is tighter.

The diagnosis is established with the barium esophagram showing a posterior esophageal indentation directed from below upward to the left shoulder.

The author's group has had two patients with this lesion in its series. Division

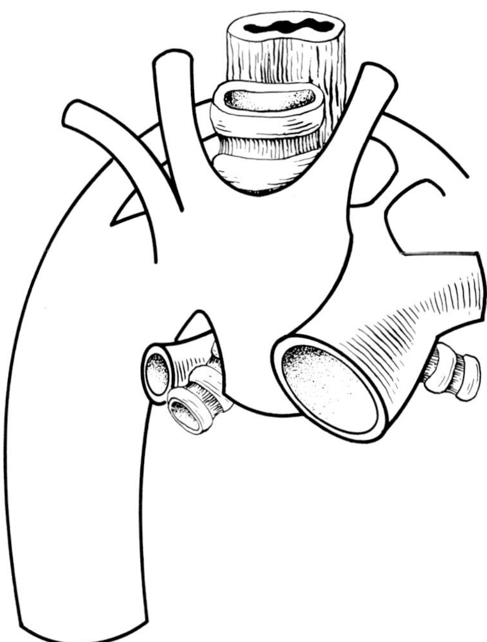

**Figure 12-5.** The right-sided arch with right descending aorta and aberrant left subclavian artery is sketched. This ring is another which is formed by the presence of the ligamentum or ductus arteriosus on the left side (see Fig. 12-3). Unless the indentation of the esophagus is severe, probably the only therapy for this lesion is division and suture of the patent ductus arteriosus or ligation of the ligamentum arteriosus. It may be, however, that division of the aberrant left subclavian artery will be necessary, as it is in the case of the aberrant right subclavian artery. The operative approach is through the left chest.

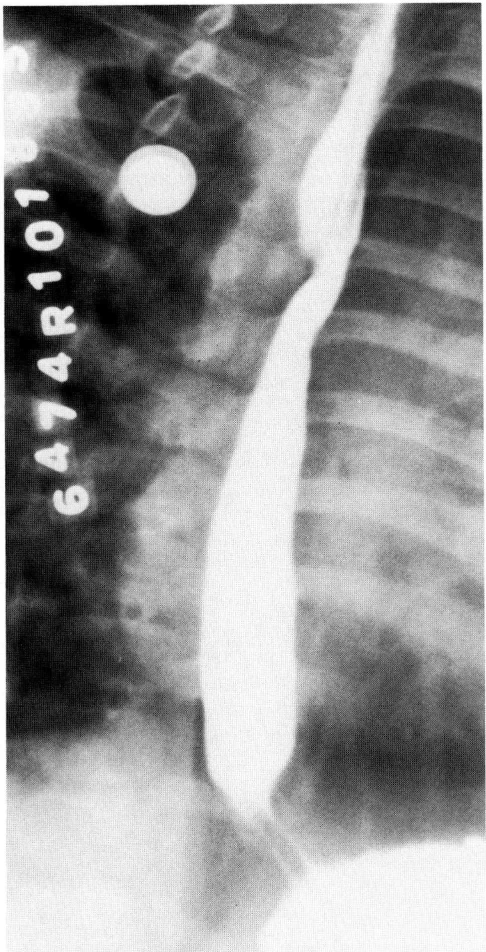

**Figure 12-6.**   This young patient has a vascular ring composed of a right-sided aortic arch and right descending aorta, left aberrant subclavian artery with ligamentum arteriosus. The patient was six months old at the time of this diagnosis. He had previously undergone colostomy as a newborn for imperforate anus with rectourethral fistula. Following the abdomino-sacroperineal pull-through at five months, he underwent colostomy closure. While en route to his home about 150 miles distant, he experienced a cardiorespiratory arrest. He was resuscitated by his parents and taken to a nearby hospital emergency room, where he was found to be alert and well. He was immediately returned to our hospital. Evaluation for a known ventricular septal defect was then carried out, which revealed the above vascular ring malformation. This lesion was corrected by division of the ligamentum arteriosus via a left thoracotomy. Three weeks later, the ventricular septal defect was patched using extracorporeal circulation, deep hypothermia, and circulatory arrest. 12 years now follow his most recent operation and he is doing well.

and suture of the ductus in one patient and of the ligamentum arteriosus in the other was all that was required to open the ring. Both patients had associated ventricular septal defect and one had an imperforate anus as well (Fig. 12-6).

The vascular sling, or aberrant left pulmonary artery, is the most difficult of the vascular ring malformations (Fig. 12-7). This is generally a very serious lesion and is associated with cartilaginous malformation of the airway which will preclude survival

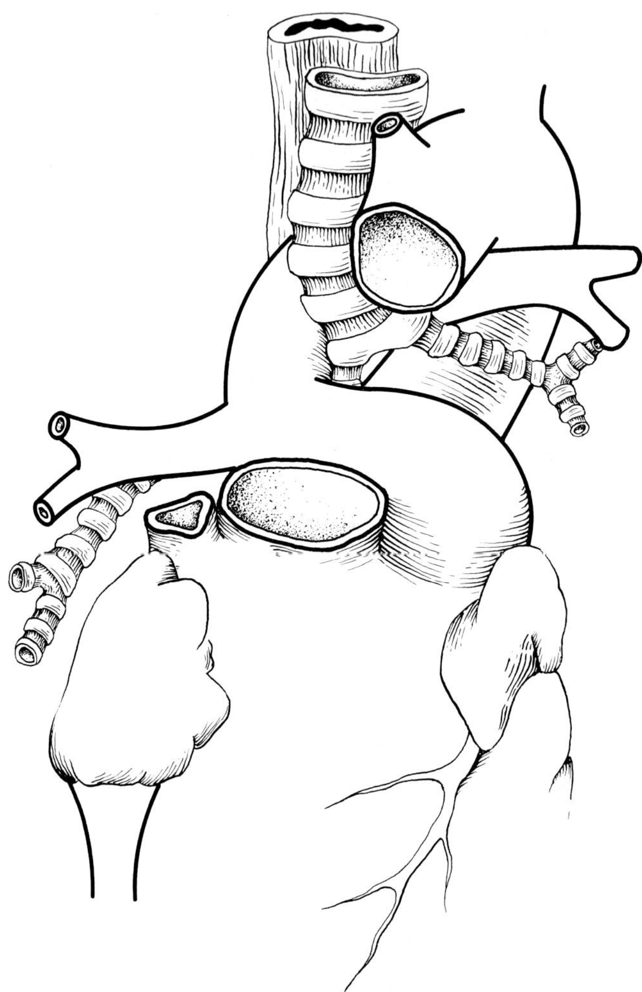

**Figure 12-7.** The pulmonary vascular sling shows an aberrant left pulmonary artery coming off the right pulmonary artery rather than the main pulmonary artery. It wraps around the right main bronchus, crosses between the trachea and esophagus and reaches the left lung by that route. The most significant symptom produced by this lesion is airway obstruction. Not illustrated in this drawing are the frequently very stenosed complete cartilaginous rings in the trachea and the proximal bronchi which attend this congenital defect in about 50 percent of patients.

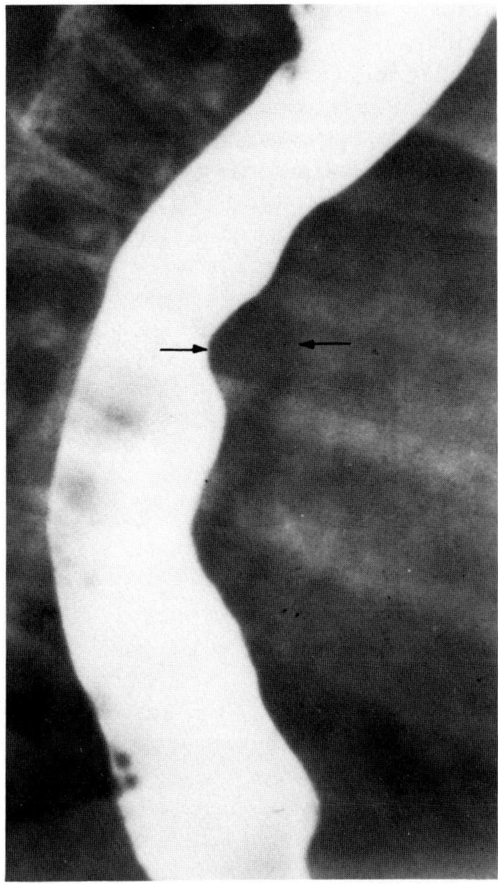

**Figure 12-8.** The patient with a pulmonary vascular sling showing the anterior indentation of the esophagus with displacement of the tracheal air column forward is pictured (arrows). The trachea is considerably narrowed in this patient. Her operative procedure at two months of age consisted of an anterior median sternotomy and the use of extracorporeal circulation, deep hypothermia, and circulatory arrest. At this time, the left pulmonary artery was taken off of the right pulmonary artery and re-attached to the main pulmonary artery to eliminate tracheal and esophageal compression. Because of complete cartilaginous rings which were exceedingly narrow, the lower nine rings of trachea were excised, with the carina being anastomosed to the upper trachea. At about ten days postoperatively, the patient disrupted this anastomosis. She was dilated a number of times but continued to have recurrent respiratory infections and sepsis. She suffered major central nervous system damage following one cardiac arrest and finally expired two-and-a-half months following operative procedure for another cardiorespiratory arrest.

in nearly half of patients.[6,14] If the cartilage rings are normal, the lesion will produce airway obstruction by pressure upon the backside of the distal trachea and esophageal symptoms by indentation of the anterior wall of the esophagus where the aberrant left pulmonary artery goes between these two structures.

The diagnosis of vascular sling is usually made in the very young child because of serious airway obstruction. The plain roentgenogram of the chest may show a somewhat serpentine course for the narrowed lower trachea. The barium esophagram is diagnostic, showing an anterior indentation in the esophagus just below the level of the aortic arch where the aberrant left pulmonary artery courses between trachea and esophagus (Fig. 12-8). Bronchoscopy and bronchography are necessary in order to assess the extent of the airway malformation which is so often seen with the vascular sling.[3] Since the incidence of associated cardiac malformations is about 50 percent, cardiac catheterization should be part of the preoperative evaluation.[9,11] Angiography is probably not absolutely necessary, but should be done in conjunction with of cardiac catheterization.[6]

## Surgical Treatment

Division of the aberrant left pulmonary artery with re-anastomosis anterior to the trachea is the treatment of choice for a pulmonary vascular sling. Although this is possible through a left thoracotomy, a more reasonable approach is a median sternotomy using cardiopulmonary bypass with deep hypothermia and circulatory arrest. Replacement of this pulmonary artery should be successful unless there are complicating factors, although in many reported follow-up studies, little or no blood flow has been detected.[14]

Unfortunately, nearly 50 percent of the children with this anomaly succumb to the associated major airway anomalies.[3,14] Rather than having C-shaped rings of the normal airway, these infants have complete rings with tracheal stenosis which may extend from the cricoid cartilage to the carina and beyond. The author's group has had two patients with vascular sling, both of whom had severe airway malformations which proved fatal. One survived several months following resection of the nine lowest tracheal rings. Her death occurred as a result of disruption of the anastomosis of the carina to the upper trachea, probably because of tension created with the resection of such a large portion of her trachea.

Most of the reported cases of vascular sling have been corrected by the left thoracotomy approach. If tracheal resection is necessary, the anterior approach using cardiopulmonary bypass to simplify anesthetic management for the tracheal resection is recommended.

## ASSOCIATED ANOMALIES

Other congenital defects involving the heart are commonly associated with vascular ring.[2,12,13] The experience of the author's group reveals three ventricular septal defects in 22 patients. Surgical treatment for these defects must be individualized and the most significant lesion treated first. Other than for vascular sling, either a right or left thoracotomy is used for the division of a vascular ring, and, although it is theoretically possible to divide these from a sternotomy approach, it is quite difficult in fact.

**REFERENCES**


1. Arciniegas E, Hakimi M, Hertzler JH, et al: Surgical management of congenital vascular rings. J Thorac Cardiovasc Surg 77:721–727, 1979.
2. Binet JP, Langlois J: Aortic arch anomalies in children and infants. J Thorac Cardiovasc Surg 73:248–252, 1977.
3. Castadena AR: Pulmonary artery sling. Ann Thorac Surg 28:210–211, 1979.
4. Comer TP, Weinberger M, Sirak HD: Aberrant right subclavian artery. Ann Thorac Surg 13:559–563, 1972.
5. deLaval M: Vascular rings. In Stark J, deLaval M (Eds.): Surgery For Congenital Heart Defects. London: Grune & Stratton, 1983.
6. Dunn JM, Gordon I, Chrispin AR, et al: Early and late results of surgical correction of pulmonary artery sling. Ann Thorac Surg 28:230–238, 1979.
7. Gray SW, Skandalakis JE: The thoracic aorta. In Gray SW, Skandalakis JE (Eds.): Embryology for Surgeons. Philadelphia: W.B.Saunders Company, pp. 809–857, 1972.
8. Gross RE: Surgical relief for tracheal obstruction from a vascular ring. N Engl J Med 233:586–590, 1945.
9. Koopot R, Nikaidoh H, Idrill FS: Surgical management of anomalous left pulmonary artery causing tracheobronchial obstruction. J Thorac Cardiovasc Surg 69:239–246, 1975.
10. Murthy K, Mattioli L, Diehl AM, et al: Vascular ring due to left aortic arch, right descending aorta, and right patent ductus arteriosus. J Pediatr Surg 5:550–554, 1970.
11. Rheuban KS, Ayers N, Still JG, et al: Pulmonary artery sling: A new diagnostic tool and clinical review. Pediatrics 69:472–475, 1982.
12. Richardson JV, Doty DB, Rossi NP, et al: Operation for aortic arch anomalies. Ann Thorac Surg 31:426–432, 1981.
13. Roesler M, deLeval M, Chrispin A, et al: Surgical management of vascular ring. Ann Surg 197:139–146, 1983.
14. Sade RM, Rosenthal A, Fellows K, et al: Pulmonary artery sling. J Thorac Cardiovasc Surg 69:333–346, 1975.
15. Shumacker HB, Burford TH: Unusual sequel to operative intervention for vascular ring. J Thorac Cardiovasc Surg 65:124–126, 1973.
16. Sissaman NJ: Anomalies of the aortic arch complex. In Moss AJ, Adams FH (Eds.): Heart Disease in Infants, Children and Adolescents. Baltimore: Williams and Wilkins, 1968.
17. Swischuk LE: Plain Film Interpretation in Congenital Heart Disease. Philadelphia: Lea & Febiger, pp. 176–191, 1970.

# Index